A SHORT TEXTBOOK OF
MEDICAL MICROBIOLOGY

UNIVERSITY MEDICAL TEXTS

General Editors

SELWYN TAYLOR D.M., MCh. (Oxon), F.R.C.S., Hon. F.R.C.S. (Ed),
Hon. F.C.S. (SA).
H. J. ROGERS M.A., M.B., B.Chir, Ph.D., M.R.C.P.

A complete list of titles in the series is available from the publishers.

A Short Textbook of Surgery
SELWYN TAYLOR D.M., M.Ch. (Oxon), F.R.C.S.
L. T. COTTON M.Ch. (Oxon), F.R.C.S.

A Short Textbook of Medicine
J. C. HOUSTON M.D., F.R.C.P.
C. L. JOINER M.D., F.R.C.P.
J. R. TROUNCE M.D., F.R.C.P.

A Short Textbook of Chemical Pathology
D. N. BARON M.D., D.Sc., M.R.C.P., F.R.C. Path.

A Short Textbook of Clinical Oncology
R. D. RUBENS M.D., B.Sc., M.R.C.P.
R.K. KNIGHT M.B., F.R.C.P.

A Short Textbook of Psychiatry
W. LINFORD REES B.Sc., M.D., F.R.C.P., D.P.M.

**A Short Textbook of Preventive Medicine
for the Tropics**
A. O. LUCAS M.D., D.P.H., D.T.M.&H., F.R.C.P., S.M.Hyg., F.M.C.P.H.
H. M. GILLES M.D., F.R.C.P., F.F.C.M., F.M.C.P.H., D.T.M.&H.

A SHORT TEXTBOOK OF
MEDICAL MICROBIOLOGY

Fifth Edition

D. C. TURK
DM, MRCP, FRCPath.

*Consultant Microbiologist,
Regional Public Health Laboratory, Sheffield
Hon. Clinical Lecturer in Medical Microbiology,
University of Sheffield*

I. A. PORTER
MD, FRCPath.

*Consultant Bacteriologist, City Hospital, Aberdeen
Hon. Clinical Senior Lecturer in Bacteriology, University of Aberdeen*

B. I. DUERDEN
BSc(Med. Sci.), MD, MRCPath.

*Senior Lecturer in Medical Microbiology, University of Sheffield
Hon. Consultant in Bacteriology, Sheffield Health Authority*

T. M. S. REID
BMed Biol, MB, ChB, MRCPath

*Consultant Bacteriologist, City Hospital, Aberdeen
Hon. Clinical Senior Lecturer in Bacteriology, University of Aberdeen*

HODDER AND STOUGHTON
LONDON   SYDNEY   AUCKLAND   TORONTO

Cover illustration: showing an electronmicrograph of a longitudinal section through three vertebrate cardiac muscle cells. Courtesy of Y. Uehara, G. R. Campbell and G. Burnstock, Department of Anatomy, University College, London.

British Library Cataloguing in Publication Data

A Short textbook of medical microbiology.—5th ed.
—(University medical texts)
1. Medical microbiology
I. Turk, D. C.
616′.01   QR46

ISBN 0 340 32388 4

First published 1965
Second edition 1969   Reprinted 1971, 1972
Third edition 1974   Reprinted 1975, 1976, 1977
Fourth edition 1978   Reprinted 1979, 1980 (with amendments), 1982
Fifth edition 1983   Reprinted 1984

Typeset by Macmillan India Ltd., Bangalore

Printed and bound in Great Britain
for Hodder and Stoughton Educational,
a division of Hodder and Stoughton Ltd,
Mill Road, Dunton Green, Sevenoaks, Kent,
by Richard Clay (The Chaucer Press) Ltd, Bungay, Suffolk

EDITOR'S FOREWORD

With this the fifth edition, Turk and Porter's *Short Textbook of Medical Microbiology*, which first appeared in 1965, takes on an entirely new lease of life since the senior authors are now joined by Brian Duerden and Tom Reid. The book is no larger than it was before, but the accent has changed as well as the contents being thoroughly updated.

Change is most noticeable in the space now devoted to immunology, a sound knowledge of which is so essential today throughout the whole of medicine. In addition, the importance of anaerobic infections has latterly taken on a new significance and these now receive the attention they merit.

The antimicrobial drugs are constantly being added to and the chapter devoted to them has been thoroughly revised and notes about many new substances have been included, not least the third generation of cephalosporins.

This book has always been a good source of information about infections rarely seen in the United Kingdom. This naturally makes it popular with readers overseas, and in these days of ever increasing air travel it behoves all of us to know something about them. There are a number of additions to this group including Legionnaire's disease, viral haemorrhagic fevers and Campylobacter infections.

Students will continue to find this compact work the ideal introduction to the subject, but it is a real compliment and a measure of its excellence, that many more senior 'students' turn to it for revision when preparing for higher and specialist examinations.

Selwyn Taylor

AUTHORS' PREFACE

Our aim as we have prepared each edition of this book has been to provide medical students with a concise, readable, up-to-date account of Medical Microbiology, which will help them to understand man's relationships with his microbial parasites and will prepare them for further reading in the subject and for an informed approach to the investigation of patients and to the prevention and treatment of microbial disease. We have repeatedly asked ourselves two questions: 'What is essential for this purpose?' and 'What can we safely leave out?'; and of course our answers to these have changed with the passage of time, and each new edition has involved substantial alterations. We are happy that this book, as well as being popular with medical students in our own and various other countries, has been found helpful by many others – notably by para-medical workers and also by qualified doctors, even including trainee bacteriologists; but we continue to regard it as primarily a book for medical students.

The two of us who have been responsible for the book through its first 17 years of life are delighted that, for the preparation of this Fifth Edition and with an eye to the future, we have been able to recruit two highly suitable younger colleagues. They both have wide experience in clinical microbiology and have made their impacts on all parts of the book; but they have also brought valuable special interests and knowledge, particularly about anaerobic bacteria (Dr. Duerden) and medical immunology (Dr. Reid).

As before, we have avoided details of laboratory methods, as we have assumed that our readers have opportunities to learn all that they need to know about these in practical classrooms or from other sources. Nor have we catered for readers who want practical instructions about the use of sterilizers, antiseptics, immunizing agents or antimicrobial drugs, though we trust that what they read here will enable them to understand the principles of the use of all these.

Suggestions for further reading are given at the ends of most chapters, but two major textbooks are relevant to so many chapters that they are mentioned here instead. The first volume of *Medical Microbiology*, 13th. edition, edited by J. P. Duguid and others (Churchill Livingstone, Edinburgh and London, 1978) is entitled 'Microbial Infections' and contains a great deal that is of interest to medical students and clinical doctors. (Its second volume, 12th. edition 1975, 'The Practice of Medical Microbiology', contains more technical laboratory information.) The clinical pictures, epidemiology and management of diseases due to micro-organisms are clearly and authoritatively described in *Infectious Diseases* by A. B. Christie (Churchill Livingstone, 3rd. edition 1980).

Margaret A. J. Moffatt, B.Sc., Ph.D., Senior Lecturer in the Department of Bacteriology, University of Aberdeen, has once again given valuable advice on the revision of the chapter on viruses. We are also grateful to Ian Geary, F.I.M.L.S. for redrawing our diagram of bacterial morphology (Figure 5, page 81), and to our publishers for their sustained interest and unfailing helpfulness.

D.C.T.
I.A.P.
B.I.D.
T.M.S.R.

CONTENTS

PART I

INTRODUCTION

CHAPTER 1

'MEDICAL MICROBIOLOGY'

Microbiology, largely a paramedical subject during its childhood and adolescence, has matured into a wide-ranging science with medical microbiology as just one of its many subdivisions. In this book we shall confine ourselves almost exclusively to that subdivision, and indeed to those parts of it which are most important to medical students; but first, to get our subject in perspective, we will contrast some of the widely different ways of approaching the study of micro-organisms.

Naturally enough, the medical microbiologist has always been interested chiefly in micro-organisms that are parasites of man, especially those that are able to cause disease. He has tended to regard other organisms as unimportant, or as nuisances that contaminate his cultures or confuse him in other ways; but in general he has managed to keep clear of them by using cultural conditions more favourable to the growth of parasites. His culture media have mostly been made from meat broth, blood and other complex animal materials; their exact composition has not greatly concerned him provided that they have suited the requirements of the species which he has wanted to grow. In his attempts at classification he has been preoccupied with the problem of recognizing pathogens; and as ability to produce disease is not consistently linked with other microbial properties, he has used a different set of criteria for the subdivision of each group of organisms. Many of his tests have been, and still are, empirical and scientifically crude—for example he talks of bacteria producing 'acid' and 'gas' from a sugar or an alcohol without reference to the nature of the acid or gas or the mechanism of their production. Yet by such means he has gone a long way towards unravelling the problems of human microbial diseases and has provided clinicians with much valuable information. Similar empirical techniques have been successfully applied in other fields, such as veterinary medicine, agriculture and industry.

In sharp contrast to the view-point of the medical microbiologist is that of the academic microbiologist who is interested in micro-organisms for their own sake, and to whom the question whether they can cause disease is merely one aspect of their biology. He wants to know the minutiae of microbial structure, and his knowledge of these has increased greatly following the development of electron microscopy. He wants to know the details of microbial metabolism, and for this purpose he has to use media of defined chemical composition and apparatus that maintains continuous control of that compostition even while metabolism is going on. He investigates mechanisms of microbial reproduction and genetics, and attempts to evolve classifications based upon the properties of the organisms themselves rather than upon what they do to other creatures. In all of these respects his discipline differs widely from the traditional approach of the medical microbiologist.

Paradoxical though it sounds, there are other students of microorganisms who are not primarily interested in the organisms themselves or in the effects that they produce on other creatures. Many biologists, physiologists and biochemists use bacteria or fungi as relatively simple and manageable models in which to study processes that also occur in the cells of more complex organisms. Such workers have incidentally added much to our knowledge of micro-organisms. So have those biochemists who use them either as sources of interesting compounds or as tools with which to carry out chemical manipulations, and the genetic engineers who have programmed them to synthesize useful materials, including therapeutic agents such as insulin and interferon.

Although we have described them separately, these various disciplines overlap and learn from each other. Medical microbiology today owes an increasing amount to workers in other parts of the microbiological field. Medical microbiologists should keep abreast of the conceptual and technical advances made by such colleagues, in order to apply them in their own territory; but medical students and clinicians are not under any such obligation, and they need to know only a little of the technology of medical microbiology. What matters to them is the help that medical microbiology can give in the understanding, investigation, treatment and (best of all) prevention of microbial diseases of man. That is what this book is about.

New Methods

The traditional task of the routine medical microbiology department is to look for and to identify actual or potential disease-producing microorganisms in material from patients, and then to determine, so far as laboratory tests permit, which antimicrobial drugs—if any—are likely to be effective against them when given to the patients. The usual approach to these problems is to examine some of the material, suitably stained, under the microscope for preliminary clues to the presence and nature of any infection; to grow the organisms in culture; and to make such subcultures as are necessary to purify and identify them and to test their sensitivities to various drugs. Such procedures may take several days to produce results that are useful in the management of patients, and they have all been carried out by hand because of the technical problems of designing machines that can handle large numbers of specimens without cross-contamination.

Recent years have seen exciting advances in the development of rapid methods and of automation in medical microbiology. There are new ways of detecting and precisely identifying organisms in specimens shortly after their arrival in the laboratory—for example, by staining them with fluorescein-labelled specific antibodies (*immunofluorescence micro-scopy*— p. 16); or by using *countercurrent immuno-electrophoresis* (CIE—p. 241) to detect specific microbial antigens; or by using *gas–liquid chromatography* to detect specific microbial products. At a later stage, when they have been grown in sufficient quantity, it may be possible to identify bacteria by *pyrolysis gas–liquid chromatography* far more rapidly and precisely than by older methods. A *sensitive turbimetric system* can provide early evidence of bacterial multiplication in a suitable liquid, as can measurement of *release of radio-active CO_2* from a culture medium containing ^{14}C-labelled glucose; and since such procedures can also give indications, within the first few hours, of failure of bacterial multipli-cation in the presence of certain drugs, it may well be possible to recommend the appropriate treatment for an infection well before the offending organism is identified. *Electrical impedance monitoring* is a highly sensitive means of early detection of bacterial growth in fluids—e.g. in urine or blood or broth cultures. The number of bacteria in a liquid (e.g. a urine specimen) can be rapidly determined by *microcalorimetry* (a very sensitive means of detecting their heat output), or by *luminescence biometry*, in which the amount of bacterial adenosine triphosphate—and thus the number of bacteria—in a given amount of the liquid can be assessed by measuring the brightness of the flash of light emitted when that amount is mixed with a standard preparation of luciferin-luciferase (the 'lighting system' of fireflies); such methods make it possible to recognize many specimens as not requiring further bacteriological investigation because they do not contain bacteria in the numbers found when there is a true infection. Problems of automated processing of microbiological specimens are being overcome, and the consequent increase in the capacity of laboratories to process large numbers of specimens will doubtless lead to the development of more screening tests. These will make possible the rapid exclusion of some of the possible diagnoses in appropriate cases—a contribution which is often at least as useful to the clinician as the belated production of a positive report.

The developments outlined in the previous paragraph are likely to bring about major changes in the practices of routine diagnostic laboratories, and ultimately to be of benefit to clinicians and patients; but as yet, for economic and other reasons, such methods are not in general use.

CHAPTER 2

HISTORICAL PERSPECTIVE

Man has always lived in an environment that abounds with minute living organisms, and he has always carried them in countless billions around and within his person; but because of their tiny size they escaped his direct observation until recent times. However, from the beginning of history some of their effects—especially those that he did not like—have commanded his attention and interest. The science of microbiology can be said to be little more than a century old, having its origins in the work of Louis Pasteur in the 1850s, but that great breakthrough was preceded by many centuries of speculation and investigation.

The Concept of Contagion

From the most ancient writings we learn that plagues and pestilences were already well-recognized features of human existence. Not being able to see their immediate causes, man attributed them to all sorts of real and hypothetical factors in his environment, such as divine anger, cosmic influences, witchcraft, the seasons of the year or bad air. It was appreciated at an early date that the introduction of a sick person into a community could result in spread of the disease to the local population. The book of Leviticus indicates that the methods of spread of certain skin and venereal diseases were known, and that their victims were accordingly excluded from contact with their fellow men. In his *De Contagione* published in 1546, Fracastorius struck a remarkably modern note with the statement that diseases could be spread by direct contact between individuals, by the agency of inanimate objects such as clothing and personal possessions (which he called *fomites*—a three-syllable Latin word originally meaning 'kindling wood') or through the air. He suggested that this spread involved the passage of small infective particles, 'seminaria', from an affected person to others, but since he could not demonstrate the existence of these particles, his theory received little attention.

In the late eighteenth and early nineteenth centuries the theory of contagion was again propounded vigorously by certain medical men. In 1795 Gordon of Aberdeen showed that an epidemic of puerperal fever 'seized such women only as were visited or delivered by a practitioner or taken care of by nurses who had previously attended patients affected with the disease'. He recommended washing and the changing of clothes to prevent carriage of contagion from one puerperal woman to another. Almost 50 years later Semmelweiss showed that the spread of puerperal infection by students and practitioners who commonly went straight from the post-mortem room to the maternity wards could be reduced by cleanliness and the washing of their hands in a solution of chloride of lime. Both these men believed that the carriage of 'something' from one patient to another was responsible for the development of puerperal fever.

Early Observers of Micro-organisms
In 1671 Kircher reported the presence of little worms in the blood of patients with plague, and claimed that they were responsible for the disease. However, it is likely that what he saw were aggregations of red blood cells, and that the honour of being the first observer of micro-organisms belongs to Antony Leeuwenhoek, the linen-draper of Delft in Holland. His hobby was the making of simple but ingenious microscopes, and with these he was able, in 1674, to observe minute living creatures in rain, sea and pond water, and in various other fluids. He communicated his findings in a series of letters to the Royal Society in London, but neither he nor his contemporaries appear to have realized the significance of his observations. During the eighteenth century several workers suggested that small creatures such as he had described might be responsible for various diseases, but their ideas were not accepted for lack of any factual support.

By the early nineteenth century improvements in microscope design had made possible the beginning of systematic description of micro-organisms. In 1838 Ehrenberg, in his work on 'Infusoria' (the small creatures found in infusions), introduced such terms as *bacterium, vibrio, spirillum* and *spirochaete*. Meanwhile, in 1835, Agostino Bassi had described the fungus (later named *Botrytis bassiana*) which caused muscardine, a disease of silkworms, and he had suggested that this disease was transmitted by contact or by infection of food. This, the first reliable report of a disease caused by a transmissible parasitic micro-organism, was followed in 1839 by Schoenlein's description of the fungus that causes the human disease favus. In 1850 Rayer and Davaine reported the presence of rod-shaped organisms in the blood of animals that had died of anthrax, and Davaine later showed that this disease could be transmitted by inoculation of blood containing such rods but not of blood from which they were absent. During this era other claims to have found microbial causes of disease were put forward with inadequate experimental backing, and in 1840 Henle pointed out that a micro-organism causing a disease should be present in every case and should produce a similar disease in animals into which it was inoculated—criteria which were later expanded into 'Koch's postulates' (see p. 41).

The Theory of Spontaneous Generation

Up to the seventeenth century philosophers and scientists had generally accepted that at least some animals could develop entirely from non-living materials. Thus putrefying meat was believed to give rise to maggots and the mud of the Nile to snakes, whereas corn and a linen cloth stored in a jar were considered suitable ingredients for the production of mice! However, in 1688 Redi showed that putrefying meat did not produce maggots if flies were kept away from it, and thereby convinced many that the theory of spontaneous generation was inaccurate, at least in relation to flies and larger creatures. It survived in relation to microscopic creatures for another 200 years, and in the latter half of the eighteenth century it was the subject of a fierce controversy, with the Italian abbot Spallanzani and the Irish priest Needham as the central figures. Needham's claim that micro-organisms reappeared in infusions which had previously been heated to kill all living creatures was countered by Spallanzani's demonstration that this did not occur if the heating was vigorous enough and if air was subsequently excluded from the container. According to Needham, this was because excessive heat destroyed a 'vegetative force' that was necessary for the generation of organisms. In 1854 Schroeder and Dusch showed that the growth of micro-organisms which took place in a previously heated infusion if air was allowed to enter the container could be prevented by first passing the air through a cotton-wool filter—in other words, that the important component of the air was particulate. However, their later findings were erratic and confusing because the amount of heat that they used was inadequate to sterilize all of the fluids tested.

Pasteur, Lister and Koch

To the French chemist Louis Pasteur belongs the credit both for terminating the dispute about spontaneous generation and for establishing beyond doubt the role of micro-organisms in transmissible diseases. He entered the field of microbiology at a point far removed from medicine—the study of fermentation. This phenomenon had been known to man from very early times but was without an explanation until 1837, when Schwann and Cagniard-Latour discovered independently that the yeasts always associated with alcoholic fermentation of sugar solutions were living organisms. Their belief that these organisms actually caused the fermentations was disputed by Liebig and others who upheld purely chemical explanations. In a series of brilliant experiments and papers between 1855 and 1860 Pasteur showed conclusively that lactic and butyric acid fermentations were the work of bacteria, and that the fermentations involved in the production of beer and wines were the work of yeasts. He also showed that there was a relationship between the type of micro-organism involved and the type of fermentation produced. He then proceeded to destroy the theory of spontaneous generation (though its supporters were slow to admit defeat) by showing that living micro-organisms were invariably derived from exactly similar living organisms. In the course of this work he learnt a great deal about the scrupulous care needed in dealing with bacteria and fungi, and about their differing nutritional requirements, and so he laid the foundations of modern microbiological technique. But he was far more than a careful technician. His brilliance lay in his ability to see the far-reaching significance of his discoveries. From problems of preparation and preservation of wine, beer and vinegar he went on to rescue the silkworm industry from the scourge of an infectious disease called pebrine, to show farmers how the spread of anthrax among their animals could be prevented, and then to discover how to immunize these animals against anthrax, fowls against chicken cholera and finally man against rabies.

Meanwhile, news of Pasteur's work on fermentation reached Joseph Lister, the Professor of Surgery in Glasgow. At that time virtually all wounds suppurated and the mortality following surgery was fearful. Failure of wounds to produce 'laudable pus' was in fact considered a bad sign—quite rightly, as we can see today, for all wounds were infected and lack of suppuration frequently meant absence of resistance to infection on the part of the patient. Lister concluded that if micro-organisms caused fermentation they might also cause suppuration of wounds, and that in their absence wounds might heal cleanly and without risk to the patients' lives. So he introduced his *antiseptic technique*, which he first described in 1867. By washing wounds with carbolic acid, spraying this substance into the air of the operating theatre and applying protective dressings to keep fresh organisms from entering the wounds, he achieved a striking reduction of post-operative sepsis and mortality. Because carbolic acid was toxic to patients and to their attendants, it was far from being the perfect answer to the surgeon's problems, and today more emphasis is placed upon preventing the introduction of organisms into wounds (*asepsis*) than upon their destruction, but Lister's procedure proved their importance and prepared the way for modern surgery.

In 1870 a young German general practitioner, Robert Koch, began to follow up the work of Davaine on anthrax. He was able to grow in artificial culture the rod-shaped organisms seen in the blood of animals suffering from this disease, and to reproduce the disease by injecting his cultures into animals. He also showed that the rods could turn into resistant spore forms and then back into rods. During the last quarter of the nineteenth century, Koch and his bacteriological pupils identified the causative organisms of tuberculosis, cholera, typhoid, diphtheria and many other major diseases of man and animals, and began to establish a systematic classification of bacteria. This work was made possible by technical advances for which Koch himself was largely responsible, including the use of aniline dyes for staining micro-organisms, of oil-immersed microscope objectives for examining them and of media solidified with agar for growing them.

Immunology

Sometimes slowly and sometimes more rapidly, immunology has grown during the past century from being a branch of medicine, primarily concerned with immunity to infectious diseases, to being a wide-ranging science that has made valuable contributions to the development of biology and of medicine. Some of these contributions have been in the field of prevention or treatment of infectious diseases by artificial induction of immunity—i.e. immunization. Such work began long ago. Immunization against smallpox, by inoculation with material from a lesion of a patient (*variolation*), had been practised for centuries in the East before its introduction into Britain in 1721. It was a hazardous procedure, but smallpox was a widespread and terrible disease. In 1796 Jenner discovered that protection against smallpox could be achieved much more safely by inoculation with material from a lesion of cowpox, a natural disease of cattle. This process became known as *vaccination*, from the Latin *vacca*, a cow. We now know that its success was due to the close relationships between the viruses of cowpox and smallpox (variola). The final stages of this story are outlined on p. 256.

Almost a century after Jenner's discovery Pasteur found that fowls inoculated with an old laboratory culture of the organism of chicken cholera developed only a mild illness and were subsequently resistant to infection with fresh cultures of the organism. Then he discovered that sheep could be protected against anthrax by inoculation with cultures of anthrax bacilli attenuated (i.e. rendered harmless) by growing them at 42 °C. This work provided a basis for a rational approach to the prevention of microbial diseases, and it was found possible to attenuate many other pathogenic organisms. Then in 1890, following the discovery by Roux and Yersin that the symptoms of diphtheria were mainly due to the release of a soluble poison (toxin) from the bacteria, Behring showed that guinea-pigs could be protected against this disease by injections of diphtheria toxoid (toxin treated to make it harmless). With Kitasato he similarly immunized animals against tetanus. The sera of such immunized animals were shown to neutralize the appropriate toxins specifically, and also to give protection against the appropriate diseases to other animals into which they were injected. Within a few years the treatment of human diphtheria was greatly advanced by the introduction of effective antitoxic sera (animal sera that neutralized diphtheria toxin) which could be injected into human beings with reasonable safety.

Meanwhile, in 1884 Metchnikoff had shown that cells called phagocytes are important in the development of immunity to infection. This set the scene for a fierce battle of words between those who believed that immunity is essentially 'humoral' and the 'cellular' school of thought. As we shall see in Chapters 7 and 8, there was no need for a battle; both types of mechanism are important, and they are closely interrelated.

The branch of immunology known as diagnostic serology can be said to have started in 1896, when Gruber and Durham demonstrated the clumping of cholera organisms by specific antiserum—a means of definitive identification of these organisms. Later in the same year Widal described his diagnostic test for typhoid, which consisted of showing that the patient's serum would clump (agglutinate) typhoid bacilli. Some of the innumerable later developments of diagnostic serology are discussed in later chapters, notably in Chapter 15.

Thus the second half of the nineteenth century saw not only the establishment of the microbial origins of many diseases and the identification of many of the responsible organisms, but also the introduction of the first specific weapons for dealing with them. The pace of development in the present century precludes a brief historical summary, but two major advances in clinical microbiology deserve mention before we end this preliminary survey.

Antimicrobial Drugs

Naturally occurring compounds have been used with success in the treatment of infections for several centuries—at least since the first recorded use of an extract of cinchona bark (quinine) for malaria in 1619; but it was in the opening years of the present century that Paul Ehrlich began the search for synthetic substances specifically designed to attack harmful microbes (his 'magic bullets'). His arsenical compounds were effective against a limited number of such organisms, notably those causing syphilis and trypanosomiasis; but it was from 1935 onwards, with the introduction first of the sulphonamides and then of the antibiotics and sundry other antimicrobial drugs, that major advances were made, so that by now virtually all bacterial, fungal and protozoal infections and even a few due to viruses have come within the reach of effective drug treatment. Many diseases that were virtually untreatable and commonly fatal a mere 40 years ago can today be treated with almost invariable success. Medical bacteriology has been transformed by these developments, since its contributions have become far more relevant to patient care and are more urgently needed; but the transformation has included the whole of medical practice and indeed the way of life and life-expectation of us all. In almost any branch of medicine a doctor frequently has to decide whether to use an antimicrobial drug, and, if so, which to choose from the increasingly and confusingly wide selection available to him. A firm grasp of basic microbiological facts and principles provides the best foundation for his decisions.

Virology

In the very early days of bacteriology it became apparent that some undoubtedly infectious diseases had no detectable bacterial causes. Pasteur, for example, demonstrated the infectivity of rabies and the possibility of preventing it by immunization, but he could not find its aetiological agent. He suggested that this might be because it was very small. In 1892 the Russian botanist Ivanovsky transmitted tobacco mosaic disease to healthy plants by means of a bacterium-free filtrate of sap from affected plants—work which was corroborated by the Dutch bacteriologist Beijerink. Six years later Loeffler and Frosch showed that foot-and-mouth disease of cattle was also transmissible by means of a bacterium-free filtrate. From that time onwards it was generally accepted that some diseases are due to living agents even smaller than bacteria. For many years their further study was hampered by lack of suitable techniques. By light microscopy it was possible to detect single particles of some of the larger viruses ('elementary bodies') and others could be seen as cytoplasmic or intra-nuclear aggregates of particles ('inclusion bodies') inside infected cells. A certain amount could be learned by transmission experiments in living animal hosts. But whereas from the time of Koch almost any hospital laboratory could provide a diagnostic bacteriological service, medical virology remained a subject for research workers because it lacked any equivalent to bacteriology's routine 'microscopy and culture' approach. The overcoming of these problems in the 1950s opened the way to the provision of a routine diagnostic virological service. Today this is generally available and is being steadily developed. As more effective antiviral drugs become available, rapid diagnosis of virus infections becomes increasingly important and useful.

Suggestions for Further Reading

The Life of Pasteur by R. Vallery-Radot (Constable, London, 1923).

Microbe Hunters by P. de Kruif (first published 1926, currently available as paperback, Pocket Books Inc., New York).

Milestones in Microbiology trans. and ed. by T. D. Brock (Prentice-Hall, London, 1961).

A History of Bacteriology by W. D. Foster (Heinemann, London, 1970)—for the period 1840–1940.

Changing Patterns: An Atypical Autobiography by Sir Macfarlane Burnet (Heinemann, Melbourne and London, 1968)—for developments in bacteriology, virology and immunology as seen and influenced by an eminent worker in these fields.

Microbes and Men by R. Reid (British Broadcasting Corporation, 1974).

PART II

PART II

BIOLOGICAL BACKGROUND

CHAPTER 3

'CONCERNING LITTLE ANIMALS'
(Leeuwenhoek, 1676)

Micro-organisms can be defined as living creatures so small that individuals cannot be seen without the aid of a microscope; and microbiology is the study of such organisms. The 'little animals' which Leeuwenhoek saw and described in various natural fluids (see p. 6) doubtless included micro-organisms that we should today classify as bacteria, fungi, protozoa and algae, but we now know of other groups far too small to have been seen with his instruments.

Micro-organisms of medical importance can be classified in five large groups: (1) Bacteria; (2) Rickettsiae and Chlamydiae; (3) Viruses; (4) Fungi; (5) Protozoa. The cells of fungi and protozoa are essentially similar in structure to those of higher plants and animals, and these organisms are therefore known as *eukaryotic*, whereas bacteria, rickettsiae and chlamydiae are known as *prokaryotic* because their cells have a much simpler nuclear structure, do not have nuclear or other internal dividing membranes and have in their walls a mucopeptide substance not found in eukaryotic cells (see below). Viruses are even simpler in structure and cannot be described as living cells.

Bacteria
These are cellular (usually unicellular) organisms. A typical bacterial cell is able to carry out many different metabolic activities and to increase its size and reproduce itself by fission. Individual cells are of the order of 0.5–1 μm broad by 0.5–8 μm long (1 μm = a micrometre, a thousandth of a millimetre). The shape of a bacterial cell is determined by its rigid but permeable *cell wall*, which also prevents it from swelling up and bursting as the result of osmosis. The main structural component of this wall is

mucopeptide (or *peptidoglycan*), which consists of chains of alternating molecules of *N*-acetylglucosamine and *N*-acetylmuramic acid cross-linked by peptide chains. Within the cell wall is the *protoplast*, which is mainly semi-solid *cytoplasm* surrounded by a thin elastic semi-permeable *cytoplasmic membrane*—a complex structure which is of great importance in determining what substances can enter or leave the cell and is the site of most of its enzymic activities. In some bacteria the cytoplasmic membrane forms highly convoluted, invaginated membranous organelles called *mesosomes*, which appear to be the sites of specialized metabolic activity and are prominent during cell-wall synthesis and during sporulation. Among the structures to be found within the cytoplasm are many granular *ribosomes*, which contain much of the cell's ribonucleic acid (RNA) and a *chromosome* or *nuclear body* (sometimes more than one), consisting of a long double-stranded deoxyribonucleic acid (DNA) molecule in the form of a much twisted and contorted ring; other DNA may be present in the form of small extra-chromosomal portions called *plasmids*. Both chromosomes and plasmids are anchored to membrane attachment sites that control their replication. Some bacteria form *capsules*, usually composed of polysaccharide, outside their cell walls. Some have fine whip-like organs of locomotion called *flagella* (singular *flagellum*) protruding from their surfaces. Some have numerous shorter hair-like protrusions called *fimbriae* or *pili*; most of these are apparently organs of adhesion, enabling the bacteria to attach themselves to surfaces such as those of host cells, and may be important in the production of disease, but some have a special role in bacterial conjugation (*sex-fimbriae*, p. 28). A few bacterial species form non-reproductive *spores*, which develop intracellularly and have thick walls, greatly reduced metabolic activity and greatly increased resistance to adverse conditions. (For more detail about these and other morphological features of bacteria see pp. 73–4).

Bacteria reproduce by *binary fission*, one cell enlarging and then dividing into two approximately equal parts. This division is preceded by simple replication of the nuclear ring, without the polarized mitosis that is part of the reproductive process of most other types of nucleated cell, and therefore without the possibility of segregation and re-assortment of chromosomal genes.

Bacteria are divisible into large groups that differ in the shapes of their bacterial cells. Cells that are spherical, or nearly so, are called *cocci*. These are commonly grouped together. If in pairs, they are often referred to as diplococci. Repeated division in the same plane produces chains; division in two or three planes at right angles produces regular packets of four, eight or more; and division without any definite orientation produces irregular clusters. The *bacilli* or rods are elongated cylindrical forms, straight or slightly curved, with ends that are rounded, square, pointed or sometimes swollen to form clubs. Certain bacteria which resemble bacilli but are more definitely curved are known as *vibrios* or comma bacilli. The *spirochaetes* are corkscrew-like spirals. Some of these (e.g. the lepto-spirae) are tightly coiled, whereas others (e.g. the borreliae) have large open coils. Actinomycetes and other *higher bacteria* (so called because they are thought to represent a more advanced state of evolution although they are still prokaryotes) resemble the fungi (eukaryotes) in forming branched filaments. The mycoplasmas are an exception to the rule that bacterial cells are encased in rigid cell walls. Their cells are esentially protoplasts, and are smaller in size than those of other bacteria (c. 0.25μm diameter). They can grow and reproduce like other bacteria, but their lack of cell wall means that they are of variable shape and can survive only in roughly isotonic conditions. They have much in common with the mutant forms of normal bacteria known as *L-forms* (p. 74).

Rickettsiae, Coxiella burneti and Chlamydiae
These organisms resemble bacteria in that they contain both RNA and DNA, have muramic acid in their outer coats, reproduce by binary fission and are susceptible to the action of antibacterial drugs that have no effect on viruses. On the other hand, with diameters of only 0.25–0.5 μm they are nearer in size to viruses than to bacteria, and they are also (with only one known exception) virus-like in being unable to reproduce except inside the cells of the host organisms.

Viruses
Though some viruses are similar in size to the organisms just described, most of them are smaller—some very much smaller—than any other known living organisms, and are too small to be seen with an ordinary light microscope ('ultra-microscopic') unless they form inclusion bodies (p. 162). The virus particle is called a *virion*, not a cell. At its simplest, as in the viruses of poliomyelitis, this is a mere 25–30 nm in diameter (1 nm = a nanometre, a thousandth of a micrometre) and consists only of a nucleic acid core, the *genome*, packed within a protein coat, the *capsid*, which protects the genome during transmission between host cells. At the other end of the range, the virions of pox viruses measure about 200×300 nm and are chemically and structurally a good deal more complex, though they are still developments of the same basic plan. The nucleic acid found in a virus of any given type is either RNA or DNA, but not both as in bacteria and other cellular organisms. Viruses increase in number not by fission but by *replication* inside bacterial, plant or animal host cells which they have converted into virus-production units (p. 157). A virion has no metabolic activity of its own, but those of some viruses contain enzymes that initiate host cell activities.

Fungi
These are generally larger than bacteria, and are commonly multicellular. Their relatively thick cell walls owe their rigidity not to mucopeptide, as do those of bacteria, but to chitin or other components. The *moulds* grow as tubular branching filaments (hyphae) which become interwoven to

form a network (mycelium). In some families the hyphae are divided into short lengths by cross-walls (septa). Such fungi reproduce by forming asexual or sexual spores of various kinds. The *yeasts* are oval or spherical cells which commonly reproduce by budding, but may also form sexual spores. (These reproductive spores differ in nature and function from bacterial spores.)

Protozoa

These unicellular organisms, mostly much larger than bacteria, show clear differentiation of their protoplasm into nucleus and cytoplasm (i.e. they are eukaryotes). Their reproductive mechanisms vary from simple binary fission, with nuclear replication by mitosis, to complex life-cycles involving sexual and asexual phases and the formation of cysts.

THE MICROSCOPE—THE MICROBIOLOGIST'S BASIC TOOL

Leeuwenhoek's simple optical instruments opened the door to the microbial world. Our subsequent exploration of it has been largely dependent upon improvements in microscope design and in methods of preparing organisms for microscopic examination. The ordinary light microscope has been joined by other instruments which have given important additional information. Detailed theoretical descriptions of these different microscopes are to be found in larger textbooks, and the practical knowledge which is essential for their efficient use should be learned in the laboratory. Here we deal only with the general principles of microbial microscopy.

Ordinary Light Microscopy

Organisms to be examined with the light microscope may be:

1 *Unstained* ('*wet preparation*'). A drop of fluid culture or any other suspension of organisms is placed on a glass slide, covered with a coverslip and examined with the high-power dry objective of the microscope, using a restricted amount of light. Objects such as bacteria that diffract light appear dark against a bright background. In this way it is possible to determine the size and shape of the organisms and whether they are motile. True spontaneous motility must be carefully distinguished from the Brownian movement to which all small particles in a fluid medium are subject, and from drifting due to currents in the fluid. Differentiation between organisms in such preparations cannot be carried very far, and some bacterial groups, notably the spirochaetes, are so feebly refractile that they cannot be seen at all in this way. When wet preparations are examined by *phase-contrast* microscopy, the diffracted light is also retarded by a quarter of a wavelength; consequently, details of the structure of organisms stand out sharply against a grey background.

2 *Stained.* Bacteria are commonly examined by fixing them to a glass slide (usually by heating) and applying stains. They can then be examined with the oil-immersion objective of the microscope, using a bright light source. Even with only a simple stain such as methylene blue or carbol fuchsin, this procedure usually enables us to see more of the shape, arrangement and structure of the organisms than is visible in unstained preparations, though allowance has to be made for artefactual changes due to drying and staining. Additional valuable information can be obtained by using differential staining techniques. Gram's method (p. 77), the most widely used of these, divides bacteria into Gram-positive (retaining the blue stain) and Gram-negative (decolorized, but taking up the red counterstain), a distinction which is of true biological significance and also of considerable practical value. The Ziehl–Neelsen staining procedure (p. 132) makes it possible to recognize a relatively small but important group of bacteria which are 'acid-fast'—i.e. cannot be readily decolorized with acid after being stained with hot carbol fuchsin.

Dark-Ground Microscopy
Some bacteria too feebly refractile to be seen by ordinary light microscopy—e.g. the spirochaetes of syphilis and leptospirosis—can be seen by dark ground illumination, which also shows up fine details of their shape.

Dark ground illumination is obtained by focusing a hollow cone of light from below on to the top surface of the microscope slide in such a way that, unless deviated from its path, the light will diverge again and miss the front lens of the objective. Thus the only light to enter the objective and reach the eye of the observer is that which has been deflected by striking bacteria or other objects on the slide. These objects shine brightly against a dark background. The process is essentially the same as that by which one sees fine dust particles when looking from the side at a shaft of bright sunlight. Dark-ground microscopy is usually applied to unstained wet preparations, with water or oil between the condenser and the slide to prevent total internal reflection of light within the condenser, and between the cover-slip and the objective to prevent scattering of light.

Fluorescence Microscopy
Certain dyes fluoresce when exposed to light of appropriate wave-length (usually ultra-violet). Tubercle bacilli can be selectively stained with one such dye, auramine, by a Ziehl–Neelsen-like procedure in which the auramine replaces the carbol fuchsin. They can therefore be recognized in smears of sputum or other material stained in this way and examined microscopically by ultraviolet light.

In the fluorescent-antibody technique (immunofluorescence) fluorescent dyes are coupled with the serum proteins known as antibodies (p. 55). When such an antibody combines with its appropriate antigen, the antigen-antibody complex is fluorescent. Micro-organisms and other antigens can be located and identified in sections and smears by 'staining' these preparations with dye-conjugated specific antibodies. Two fluorescent dyes commonly used, fluorescein isothiocyanate and lissamine-rhodamine, give green and orange fluorescence respectively. This technique is discussed further on pp. 244–5.

Electron Microscopy
This procedure has much greater resolving power than light microscopy, and permits much greater magnification (× 300 000 or more, as against × 1500). It has made possible the determination of the size, shape and structure of viruses, and has added greatly to our knowledge of the finer structure of bacteria and larger micro-organisms. A beam of electrons, derived from an 'electron gun', is passed through a series of electromagnetic fields which correspond to the lenses in an optical microscope in that they bring about convergence of the beam. The material to be examined is mounted on a thin membrane of collodion, polyvinyl formal or carbon, which is supported on a metal grid, and the examination is carried out in a high vacuum which inevitably produces some distortion. Ultra-thin sections of tissue or of suitably embedded microbial or other cells can be examined, and so can films made from suspensions of very small particles, such as the smaller viruses. To be clearly visible these objects must differ from their surroundings in their opacity to the electron beam. This can be achieved by supplying a background of more electron-opaque material, such as sodium phosphotungstate ('negative staining'); or by 'positive staining' with some electron-opaque material that will selectively adhere to the particles (e.g. various heavy-metal compounds, or ferritin-labelled antibodies); or by 'shadow casting'—i.e. projecting a shower of metal atoms over the film obliquely, so that a thin layer of metal is formed all over it except in the 'shadows' of particles. After the electron beam has passed through the material to be examined it is made to produce a visible image on a fluorescent screen or to produce photographs that can usually be much enlarged. Whereas ordinary electron microscopy can show outlines and structural details in a flat plane, the more sophisticated technique of scanning electron microscopy can produce clear 'aerial views' of particles such as microbial and other cells, showing the contours, irregularities and texture of their surfaces.

CHAPTER 4

ECOLOGY

Micro-organisms are virtually ubiquitous. The distribution of any particular species is limited by its growth requirements and by its compatibility with other species, but micro-organisms of some sort are to be found in almost any environment. They are present in soil, water and air and in most kinds of inorganic or organic non-living matter, as well as within and on the surfaces of living creatures.

An important part in the balance of nature is played by the many bacterial and fungal species which live by breaking down and recycling the bodies of dead animals and plants. Micro-organisms are at both the beginning and the end of some food chains, which thus become cycles. 'If microscopic beings were to disappear from our globe, the surface of the earth would be encumbered with dead organic matter and corpses of all kinds, animal and vegetable. . . . Without them, life would become impossible because death would be incomplete' (Louis Pasteur, 1861). Such organisms that live on dead organic matter are described as *saprophytic*. Some normally saprophytic species can occasionally invade the tissues of living animals and humans, but this is rare. Some writers also use the term saprophytic for organisms that are superficial and harmless parasites, but these are better described as commensals (see below).

A small minority of micro-organisms, including nearly all those of medical importance, are commonly or necessarily *parasitic*—i.e. they live inside or on the surfaces of other living organisms. Bacteria themselves harbour parasitic viruses called bacteriophages, and plants and animals act as hosts to large and varied microbial populations. Parasites may be *commensal, symbiotic* or *pathogenic*. A *commensal* (literally, one that shares the table) derives nourishment from its host but does nothing in return—a non-paying guest. Many examples are found in the secretions of human skin and mucous membranes. A *symbiont* lives in partnership with its host, receiving nourishment but rendering service in return—a paying guest. Such are the nitrogen-fixing bacteria of the root nodules of leguminous plants, the cellulolytic bacteria that digest plant food in the intestine of herbivores (but not of man), and the vitamin-synthesizing bacteria of the human intestine. Some bacteria commonly regarded as commensals are in fact beneficial to their hosts because they make it difficult for potential pathogens to colonize his surfaces (see also Chapter 7, Non-specific Host Defences). A *pathogen* does harm to its host. These terms refer to relationships between parasites and hosts, not simply to properties of micro-organisms; the same micro-organism may exhibit different forms of parasitism in different hosts, or even in the same host at different times or in different sites. Pathogenicity is as much an expression of the host's susceptibility as it is of the organism's intrinsic power to cause disease. To use a well-worn analogy, the soil is as important as the seed in determining the outcome of infection.

MAN'S NORMAL MICROBIAL POPULATION

There is evidence that in at least some species an apparently healthy young animal may harbour in its tissues viruses which it derived from its mother *in utero* and which may cause it to develop leukaemia later in life. We do not know whether such transmission involves only leukaemia viruses, or whether anything of the sort occurs in man. With this reservation we can say that the healthy human foetus has no resident microbial population up to the time of its birth. It acquires on its surface or swallows or inhales an assortment of micro-organisms from the mother's birth canal, and these are soon reinforced by contributions from various human and inanimate (and possibly also animal) sources in the newborn infant's immediate environment. Those organisms which find themselves in suitable environments, whether on the outer or inner body surfaces, begin to multiply and to enter into complex competitive relationships with other potential colonizers. Within hours of birth the infant has begun to acquire a resident microbial population—or rather, a number of different populations, since some organisms thrive on the skin, others do better in the mouth or throat or nose, others in the intestine and so on. By degrees—and at speeds that depend on many factors, such as frequency and method of washing, diet and living conditions—the combinations of organisms that have taken up residence in different areas of the growing child's external and internal surfaces form fairly stable, balanced, interdependent populations and come to resemble those commonly found in such sites in adults (often described as the *normal flora*). Some idea of the nature of these combinations is given in Chapter 14 (pp. 224–36). The bacterial population of a single human body is of the order of 10^{14}; a skin scale may carry many bacterial micro-colonies, each consisting of many thousands of cells; and there are around 10^{12} bacteria in a gram (wet weight) of colonic contents or faeces. Two points need to be remembered: that the range of organisms detectable in any situation depends on the methods used in looking for them as well as on the actual population, and that throughout life there are fluctuations and marked personal differences in the 'normal' microbial populations of the body, dependent on general health, diet, hormonal activity, age, race and many other factors.

It is important to appreciate that the very large microbial populations that we have been discussing consist of micro-organisms that are in commensal or symbiotic relationships with man. The pathogenic relationship is of course highly important in medicine and will be dealt with at length in the chapters that follow, but it is the exception—indeed, the rare exception. Normal microbial populations should be treated with due respect. In many different spheres man has discovered by costly trial and error that problems and dangers as well as advantages may result when he applies his advancing knowledge to the alteration of complex established ecological system—in popular language, to upsetting the balance of nature. When our modern anti-microbial weapons are used against pathogens, their powerful effect on normal microbial populations is too often forgotten, sometimes with disastrous results. Pathogens have had most of the limelight, and we know all too little about the ways in which man benefits from the activities of his normal microbial flora (though a few ways are mentioned in later chapters, notably on p. 46); but it is increasingly clear that the doctor must not take as his motto words that we once saw in an insecticide advertisement: 'The only good bug is a dead bug'!

'Germ-free' Animals
An animal born by Caesarian section to avoid microbial contamination, and then maintained in a germ-free environment and fed sterilized food, develops no microbial population. Because of the uncertainty about intra-uterine transmission of viruses (see above) the term 'germ-free' may not be an accurate description of such animals, and the alternative term *gnotobiotic* has been coined. They can be exposed to specified bacteria with the knowledge that their responses will not be complicated by previous unknown contacts with these or similar organisms, or by the presence of other bacteria. Study of such highly unnatural situations is helping to elucidate the roles of normal flora, and the mechanism of pathogenicity and host resistance.

Suggestion for Further Reading
Invisible Allies: Microbes and Man's Future, by Bernard Dixon (Temple Smith, London, 1976).

CHAPTER 5

PHYSIOLOGY

Micro-organisms are of diverse sizes, shapes and structures, and live in widely varied environments. It is not surprising that they also differ widely in the details of their physiology, even though their biochemical mechanisms in general are similar to those of all living creatures, including man. This chapter deals mainly with bacteria. The physiology of rickettsiae, viruses and most medically important protozoa is less easily studied because it is inextricably intertwined with that of their host cells. Points of special importance in relation to individual groups of micro-organisms will be discussed in the appropriate places in Part IV.

METABOLIC NEEDS

The bacterial cell is a complex structure. Within its minute confines are included a wide variety of proteins, nucleic acids, polysaccharides, lipids and their derivatives. Some bacteria are motile, some generate light, but the main activity of bacteria as a whole is reproduction—that is, the making of new bacteria. This process may go on at an amazing speed. Under optimal conditions some species divide as often as three or four times per hour, which means that a single bacterium, visible only by microscopy, may grow overnight into a colony several millimetres in diameter made up of billions of its progeny. (The word 'grow' in relation to micro-organisms is generally used to mean 'increase in numbers'.)

Such a formidable synthetic operation requires an adequate supply of energy and raw materials and appropriate environmental conditions. The precise needs of a particular organism depend largely upon the equipment with which it is provided for carrying on its work—in other words, upon the range of *enzymes* that it possesses, in consequence of its genetic make-up or *genotype*. Some enzymes are *constitutive*, produced by the organisms in almost all circumstances, and others are *inducible*, produced (after some initial delay) in response to special circumstances, usually the presence of their specific substrates.

Sources of Energy

Some micro-organisms are *phototrophs*, able to derive their energy from sunlight. The majority, however, are *chemotrophs*, getting their energy from the oxidation of chemical compounds. Those that are parasites of man or animals are called *chemo-organotrophs* because they utilize organic compounds.

Oxygen

Organisms that grow readily in the presence of air are described as *aerobes*. (The word 'grow' in relation to micro-organisms is generally used to mean 'increase in numbers'.) Some species are *obligate* (or *strict*) *aerobes*, unable to grow in the absence of free oxygen, but others are *facultative* organisms able to grow in the presence or absence of oxygen, though they often grow more vigorously under aerobic conditions. *Obligate anaerobes* require a highly reduced environment and cannot grow if more than a trace of free oxygen is present. The energy-producing pathways (see below) in anaerobes can operate only at a very low redox potential that cannot be sustained in the presence of free oxygen. Moreover they poison themselves in the presence of oxygen by making peroxides and superoxides, which they cannot destroy since they do not possess effective catalase and superoxide dismutase enzymes. Anaerobes are thought to be the most primitive micro-organisms in the evolutionary scale. *Micro-aerophiles* are organisms that grow best in the presence of a little oxygen, though the term is often applied loosely and incorrectly to CO_2-dependent bacteria (see below).

The oxidations on which chemotrophs depend for their energy can be carried out in three different ways: *aerobic respiration*, with free oxygen as the final hydrogen-acceptor in a chain of oxidation-reduction reactions; *anaerobic respiration*, with inorganic compounds (nitrates, sulphates and carbonates) as final hydrogen-acceptors; and *anaerobic fermentation* of a carbohydrate or other organic substance, the hydrogen-acceptor being another molecule of the energy source or some other organic molecule. Various organic acids and the gases CO_2 and H_2 may be formed as end-products of fermentation. (In medical microbiological writings the word fermentation is commonly used in a less precise sense—see p. 77). Some bacterial species use only one of these three ways; others are more versatile.

Carbon Dioxide

This is probably necessary in small amounts, such as are present in the atmosphere, for the growth of most micro-organisms. A higher concentration, $5-10\%$, improves the growth of many parasitic species, notably of *Neisseria gonorrhoeae* and many anaerobes, and is usually necessary for the primary isolation of *Brucella abortus* from pathological materials. Some bacteria, such as *Streptococcus milleri*, have an absolute requirement for a higher concentration of CO_2 and are called CO_2-*dependent* or *carboxyphilic*. Free CO_2 can be the sole carbon source for autotrophs.

Raw Materials

Some chemotrophic bacteria (called *autotrophs*) can grow in simple inorganic salt solutions. At the other end of the scale are the leprosy bacillus and the spirochaete of syphilis, which cannot be grown in non-living media, and rickettsiae and viruses, which depend upon their host cells for essential enzymes as well as for raw materials. Between these extremes are innumerable gradations. Among common parasites of man, *Escherichia coli* can grow in a solution containing glucose, ammonium sulphate and a few other inorganic salts. In contrast, *Haemophilus influenzae* has very exacting requirements; as well as a suitable carbohydrate, various minerals and an assortment of amino-acids, purines and vitamins, this species must be supplied with nicotinamide-adenine dinucleotide or its phosphate as a codehydrogenase, and with haemin or some closely related substance for the synthesis of respiratory enzymes (p. 123). Such differences in the nutritional requirements of organisms are of great importance to the medical microbiologist in his choice of culture media.

Temperature

Psychrophiles grow best at low temperatures, some below $0°C$. They are important in connection with cold storage of food and blood, but otherwise are not relevant to medical microbiology. *Thermophiles*, found in such situations as hot springs and rotting vegetable matter, are of no medical importance except as sensitizing agents in 'farmer's lung', etc. (p. 64); but the term 'thermophilic' is applied to some medically important species that differ from related species in being more tolerant of temperatures over $40°C$ (e.g. certain *Campylobacter* species—p. 122). Most bacteria, including all parasites of man, are *mesophiles*, with optimal growth temperatures somewhere between 20 and $40°C$; they vary considerably in the ranges of temperature over which they will grow. As might be expected, nearly all of man's parasites are best suited by temperatures around $37°C$. Many of them will multiply at lower temperatures, down to $20°C$ or less, but few at more than $45°C$. Some will grow only within a narrow temperature range—e.g. *Neisseria gonorrhoeae*, $30-39°C$. Unusual among human pathogens is *Yersinia pestis*, the causative organism of bubonic plague. Its optimal growth temperature of about $27°C$ is probably related to the fact that multiplication in the proventriculus of the rat-flea is an important stage in its transmission (pp. 117–8).

Hydrogen Ion Concentration

Micro-organisms differ widely in their preferences and tolerances concerning the pH of their environment. Most of those of medical importance grow best in slightly alkaline conditions. Artificial culture media must be carefully buffered to prevent the rapid lowering of the pH value by acid metabolic products to a level at which organisms can no longer multiply. Lactobacilli are unusual among the bacterial flora of the human body in preferring an acid medium (pH 4.0). Indeed, they help to protect the adult vagina because they form lactic acid from the glycogen of the mucosa and thereby keep the vaginal secretion too acid for the growth of most other organisms. The medium devised by Sabouraud for the isolation of relatively slow-growing fungi uses their ability to grow at pH 5.4; this is inhibitory to bacteria which would otherwise overgrow them. At the other end of the scale, *Vibrio cholerae* grows best around pH 8.5.

METABOLIC PRODUCTS

Obviously the most important product of bacterial metabolism is more bacteria. This section deals with some others, which for convenience of discussion are somewhat arbitrarily classified under four headings— toxins, extracellular enzymes, pigments and other products. Antibiotics are considered later, on pp. 33–6.

Toxins

The potent toxins that some living bacteria liberate into their environment are called *exotoxins*; they are proteins with enzymic activity, and are heat-labile. One of the most powerful poisons known is the toxin produced by *Clostridium botulinum*, a soil bacterium that sometimes grows in human or animal foods and renders them highly lethal (pp. 103 and 287). Similar exotoxins are released by the causative organisms of tetanus, diphtheria and scarlet fever while they are growing in host tissues, and travel to other parts of the body where they produce the characteristic clinical features of these diseases. The bacteria which cause cholera and some types of dysentery multiply in the lumen of the host's intestine and produce exotoxins that damage the intestinal mucosa and are consequently known as enterotoxins. Other exotoxins named according to their effects include the haemolysins (red-cell-destroying toxins) and leucocidins (leucocyte-destroying toxins) of streptococci and staphylococci, and the phospholipase C (lecithinase) of *Clostridium perfringens* (one of the gas-gangrene bacilli) which hydrolyses the phospholipid lecithin, a constituent of cell membranes. The important exotoxins are discussed more fully in later chapters.

Gram-negative bacteria have, outside the mucopeptide structural layer of their cell walls (p. 13), a thicker phospholipid–polysaccharide–protein layer. The name *endotoxin* is given to complex lipopolysaccharide-containing material derived from this layer. It is more heat-stable than exotoxins and, unlike them, is mostly liberated on the death and disintegration of the bacteria, though some organisms shed it from their surfaces during life. The endotoxins of different species differ somewhat in composition and effect, but all are weight-for-weight less potent than most exotoxins and much less specific in their effects. When in the human or animal blood-stream, endotoxin can cause fever, intravascular coagulation and the clinical state known as shock—or, in such circumstances, more specifically called bacteraemic shock or even 'Gram-negative shock'. These changes are mainly consequences of macrophage activation by endotoxin (p. 61). A sensitive test for the presence of endotoxin in body or other fluids is provided by its ability to cause a lysate of amoebocytes from the horseshoe crab *Limulus polyphemus* to form a gel (the Limulus lysate test).

Extracellular Enzymes

Some of these enzymes have already been mentioned in their capacity as exotoxins. Others, although not so directly harmful to the host, still contribute to the pathogenicity of the organisms, and may be called *aggressins*. The coagulase produced by most pathogenic staphylococci may give some protection against host defences by coating the cocci with fibrin formed from plasma fibrinogen. The pathogenicity of these organisms may also be enhanced by the fact that clumps of cocci in fibrin clots become trapped in capillary blood vessels and multiply there, whereas isolated cocci are removed from circulation by phagocytosis as described on pp. 47–8. Conversely, the streptokinase of haemolytic streptococci probably facilitates their passage through clots by activating plasminogen to the fibrinolytic enzyme plasmin. The hyaluronidases formed by various species are spreading factors that open up connective tissues to bacterial invasion by destroying hyaluronic acid in the cement substance.

Many micro-organisms depend for their survival on enzymes that destroy toxic substances. We have already mentioned catalase, which destroys peroxides (p. 22), and we shall refer repeatedly to another group of enzymes which have acquired great medical importance—β-lactamases, by means of which many bacteria can destroy penicillins and cephalosporins.

Other extracellular enzymes are concerned with the nutrition of their producers. Before an organism can use nutrients of high molecular weights, they must be broken down into molecules small enough to pass through its cytoplasmic membrane. Extracellular digestion by excreted enzymes is of particular importance to saprophytic organisms (p. 18).

Pigments

Phototrophic micro-organisms trap the energy of sunlight by means of their pigments, in much the same way as do the blue-green algae and higher plants. All chemotrophs also contain pigments—flavoproteins and cytochromes—which participate as electron donors and acceptors in their respiratory pathways. The pyocyanin of *Pseudomonas aeruginosa* (formerly *pyocyanea*), which gives a characteristic green colour to its cultures and also to pus from infected wounds, may have a respiratory function; whereas the black or brown pigment of *Bacteroides melaninogenicus* is merely a by-product of its metabolism of the haemoglobin in the culture medium. Red, yellow, violet and other pigments are produced by some bacteria, mostly saprophytes of no medical importance, and also by many moulds. Growths of such organisms have been responsible for a number of curious episodes, such as 'bleeding' of statues and strange discolourations of foods. Pigment production may help in the identification of organisms. For example, some of the ringworm fungi can be differentiated by the characteristic colours that they release into media on which they are growing.

Other Products
Some of man's essential vitamins are synthesized for him by his intestinal flora—a point which it is sometimes dangerous to forget. We have seen signs of severe deficiencies of vitamins B and K appear with startling speed in a patient with ulcerative colitis whose intestinal tract has been virtually sterilized by antibiotic treatment. In nature the end-products of the metabolism of one species are often the food supplies of another—an important factor in maintaining stable populations. For example, dextran produced by oral streptococci may be broken down for their own use by *Bacteroides* species in dental plaque. A well-known laboratory illustration of the same principle is the satellite growth of *Haemophilus influenzae* around colonies of other bacteria which supply it with V factor (p. 123).

However, many products of microbial metabolism are probably of no use to any organisms, and indeed accumulated waste products are often fatal to their producers and to others. The precise nature of the end-products of the metabolism of any particular organism depends in part upon the organism itself and in part upon the substrates available and the conditions of growth. If the substrates and conditions are standardized, analysis of the end-products may help to identify the organism. This principle underlies many of the tests used in medical microbiology. We have mentioned the crude but informative procedure of testing an organism's ability to produce acid and gas from various sugars and alcohols (p. 1). Such investigations provide a basis for the classification of Gram-negative bacilli and of several other groups of bacteria and fungi. Some other tests commonly used for similar purposes are mentioned on p. 110. Gas-liquid chromatography (p. 3) can be used to identify products of bacterial metabolism, principally short-chain fatty acids and alcohols produced by anaerobes. These can be detected in cultures, and also in some clinical specimens—a rapid means of detecting the presence of the relevant organisms in the specimens.

REPRODUCTION

Genetics
In general, micro-organisms reproduce themselves either by simple fission of one cell into two or by some form of sexual process in which genetic material from two or more cells is pooled and subsequently redistributed. Virus reproduction (or replication) does not conform to either of these patterns; it is discussed in Chapter 11. Some of the pathogenic protozoa,

notably the malarial parasites, have complex life cycles with sexual and asexual phases (see Chapter 13). Many fungi also show both types of reproduction, but most of those of medical importance have no known sexual phase; they form reproductive spores, but these are asexual.

A bacterium that reproduces by simple binary fission, as described on p. 13, gives rise to two identical organisms, and consistent repetition of this process would produce a population of identical organisms. However, changes in the genetic composition (*genotypic variation*) of bacteria can happen in several ways. These include:

1 *Mutation.* The bacterial chromosome consists of double-stranded DNA, which in many bacteria at least is in the form of a loop. Each intertwined spiral strand is a long sequence of nucleotide units; and each unit consists of a deoxyribose component which is part of the backbone of the strand and a projecting nitrogenous base component which is linked with that of a unit on the other strand. The base is any one of four substances—the purines adenine and guanine and the pyrimidines cytosine and thymine. The sequence in which these four bases occur down the length of the strand constitutes a code or formula which determines the structure of the cell's enzymes and structural proteins and therefore the properties of the organism. The two strands are not identical but are complementary. The deoxyribose units are orientated in opposite directions, and the adenine on one strand is always matched by and linked with thymine on the other, whereas guanine is paired with cytosine. When the cell is about to divide, the two strands separate and each acts as a template or guide for the construction of its new partner, so that if all goes well two new double-stranded molecules are formed, each identical with and containing one strand of the original molecule. On the great majority of occasions all does go well; but this complex and delicate process is occasionally disturbed by factors that break the strands or cause errors of copying and consequent changes in the code. The altered pattern is then faithfully handed on to later generations, provided that it is compatible with survival.

Spontaneous mutations that cause recognizable changes in properties are relatively rare. Any given 'mistake' will arise in ordinary circumstances only once in several millions of divisions, though its likelihood can be considerably increased by exposing the dividing organisms to ultraviolet or X-irradiation or to one of various 'mutagenic' chemicals. However, bacteria reproduce so fast that mutants are continually appearing, and reliable occurrence rates can be calculated for many specific mutations. The significance of mutation is greatly enhanced by circumstances that favour the mutants. For example, if 100 million bacteria, including one streptomycin-resistant mutant, are added to a suitable streptomycin-containing broth, the broth will soon be populated entirely by streptomycin-resistant descendants of the one mutant. (Environmental selective mechanisms are similarly important in determining the significance of any other form of genotypic variation.)

Note that mutation occurs within a single cell. Each of the other three processes described below involves movement of genetic material from one cell to another.

2 *Transformation.*   Certain bacteria can acquire genetic characteristics by soluble-DNA-mediated transformation. The first clear evidence of the central role of DNA in inheritance was provided in 1944 by Avery, McLeod and McCarty's report of their studies of pneumococcal type-transformation. If pneumococci of one capsular type (p. 90) are grown under defined conditions in the presence of soluble DNA from pneumococci of another type, a minute proportion of the dividing cells take up the 'foreign' DNA, incorporate it into their genetic make-up, and produce progeny that make capsular material appropriate to the type which provided the DNA. Transformation can occur in many bacterial species other than pneumococci, but only when donor and recipient strains are of the same or closely related species.

3 *Transduction.*   Sometimes when a bacterial culture is infected by a virus (called a bacteriophage—p. 193) from another strain, a small minority of the recipient organisms acquire some property of the donor strain and transmit it as a stable genetic character to their descendants. This happens because the bacteriophage brings with it some of its previous host's DNA—usually in place of some of its own DNA, and transducing phages are therefore often defective. Since as a rule any bacteriophage has only a narrow host range, transduction is usually between closely related strains. *Lysogenic conversion*, a different form of genotypic variation due to bacteriophage, is described on p. 194.

4 *Conjugation.*   The genetic material of bacteria is not all located in the nuclear chromosome. In some bacteria at least, part of it is in the form of extra-chromosomal DNA units known as *plasmids*, some of which alternate between being free and being integrated into the chromosome. Free plasmids replicate independently of the chromosomes. They determine possession of properties that are not essential for the survival of the bacterium in a favourable environment, but provide a pool of 'optional' characters that may confer advantages in other circumstances. Individual bacterial cells of many different species contain special plasmids, *transfer factors*, which confer on them the ability to form *sex fimbriae* (p. 13) by which they attach themselves to and conjugate with other bacterial cells that do not already have transfer factor plasmids. In conjugation genetic material—the transfer factor with or without one or more other plasmids or part of the chromosome—is transferred from the initiating cell to its partner, which can then pass on some or all of the newly acquired genetic material (and therefore the associated properties) to its progeny, and to other transfer-factor-negative cells by conjugation. This form of genetic transfer is a great deal more complex than our brief outline suggests, and there are a number of variants of it. Although transfer occurs most readily between related strains, it is not restricted to donor and recipient strains with close taxonomic relationships. This has important medical implications; for example, antibiotic-resistant but harmless organisms in the human or animal intestine can confer antibiotic resistance, by plasmid transfer, on potentially pathogenic but previously antibiotic-sensitive bacteria of other genera which the host happens to ingest. The practical significance of such *transferable* or *infective drug resistance* is discussed in Chapter 21.

Phenotypic variations are changes of appearance or behaviour which depend on environmental factors and involve no alteration of genetic structure. The microscopic and colonial appearance of bacteria, their possession of flagella or of capsules, and many of their metabolic activities vary according to their circumstances. Particularly clear examples of phenotypic variation are provided by bacteria that show enzymic induction; these inherit a potential ability to make certain enzymes but only 'learn' to do so after being exposed for a while to appropriate substrates (p. 21).

Phases of Growth

Many laboratory investigations of bacteria depend upon introducing them into or on to sterile culture media where they can multiply; and many experiments have been worthless because the experimenter failed to appreciate some of the factors determining their subsequent rate of multiplication. Each bacterial strain has its own maximal rate which it can achieve under optimal conditions; but it does not necessarily begin to reproduce at this rate straight away.

Figure 1 shows a typical growth curve of a bacterial culture in broth. The logarithm of the count of living bacteria is plotted against the time after the inoculation of the broth. The exact shape of the curve depends on many factors, including the nature of the organism, the size of the inoculum, the age of the culture from which it was taken, the composition of the medium and the conditions of incubation; but four stages of activity can usually be discerned. In the first stage, called the *lag phase*, the inoculated bacterial cells adapt themselves to their new environment and prepare for division. They increase in size, but there is little increase in numbers. In due course division speeds up and is soon occurring at the maximal rate for the system. The increase in numbers is now exponential, the population doubling at regular intervals. Since such an increase takes the form of a straight line when plotted against a logarithmic scale, this stage is called the *logarithmic phase* of growth. The maximal rate of division continues until it is slowed by one or both of two factors— exhaustion of nutrients or accumulation of toxic metabolites. The population increase gradually comes to a standstill, the *stationary phase*, in which the rate of production of new cells by division equals the rate of loss by death. This is succeeded by the *phase of decline*, in which the

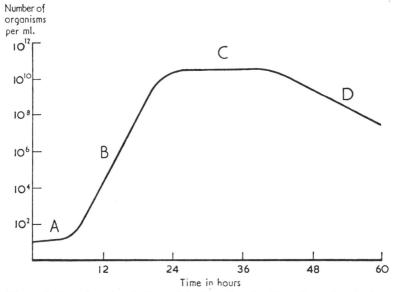

Figure 1 Growth curve of a bacterial culture in a liquid medium, showing lag phase (A), logarithmic phase (B), stationary phase (C) and phase of decline (D).

number of living bacteria slowly decreases. The speed and shape of this decline depends upon the susceptibility of the organisms to their own waste products; some delicate species are extinct within a few days, whereas cultures of others may continue to yield survivors for years. The total number of bacteria, living and dead, in a broth culture remains constant for a long period after the stationary phase, unless the organism is autolytic, producing enzymes that destroy its own cells.

One reason why it is important to know about these phases of growth is that the rapidly multiplying bacteria of the logarithmic phase are particularly susceptible to damage by antiseptics and antibiotics. They are also able to multiply at maximal speed immediately, without a lag phase, if transferred to suitable fresh medium. Therefore many *in vitro* comparisons between organisms are meaningless because the inocula are taken from cultures in different phases of growth.

A logarithmic rate of multiplication can be maintained indefinitely if the culture medium is repeatedly or continuously renewed. Such *continuous culture* has important industrial applications—e.g. in the manufacture of antibiotics—and also makes possible the study of bacterial metabolism under constant and controllable conditions.

SURVIVAL AND DEATH

Micro-organisms vary greatly in their resistance to adverse physical and chemical conditions. Some fail to survive minor environmental changes, whereas others are difficult to kill. Spore-forming species are the most durable. Spores have the physical protection of their thick coats, their water content is low, their metabolic activity is minimal and since they do not divide they avoid the increased susceptibility of dividing cells to various noxious agents. The tubercle bacillus and related organisms do not form spores, but having waxy hydrophobic surfaces and low rates of metabolism they are more resistant than most bacteria to drying and to chemical agents. They do not share the heat-resistance of the spore-formers.

In the sections and chapters that follow we use a number of technical terms relating to antimicrobial processes or substances. *Sterilization* means the killing or removal of *all* micro-organisms, including bacterial spores. *Disinfection* has a less precise meaning. The word suggests freeing an object from *potentially harmful* micro-organisms, but there is no process for doing so which differentiates between these and non-pathogens. In practice, disinfection means use of chemicals (*disinfectants*—p. 32) to eliminate nearly all micro-organisms—*nearly* all because chemicals cannot be relied on to destroy bacterial spores, and some widely used disinfectants are ineffective against viruses. The meanings of the terms *chemotherapeutic agent* and *antibiotic* are given on pp. 34–5. We have abandoned the terms *antisepsis* and *antiseptic*, which were formerly used in much the same senses as disinfection and disinfectant. Applications of the processes of sterilization and disinfection are discussed in Chapter 17.

Effects of Physical Agents on Micro-organisms

DRYING   Drying, as by exposure to ordinary atmospheric conditions, rapidly kills many bacteria and viruses, but some important non-sporing pathogens, such as *Mycobacterium tuberculosis, Staphylococcus aureus* and the smallpox virus, can survive in dust for long periods and sporing organisms can do so almost indefinitely.

FREEZING   Freezing kills some organisms, especially if they are in a liquid medium that is frozen slowly, but in other circumstances it can be a valuable means of preserving microbial viability. Even delicate organisms such as viruses and *Haemophilus influenzae* survive for many months at temperatures between -20 and $-70\,^{\circ}$C if they are frozen rapidly.

A combination of drying and freezing known as *freeze-drying* or *lyophilization* is the most satisfactory method for long-term storage of bacteria. Broth cultures or bacterial suspensions are rapidly frozen and then evaporated to dryness in high vacuum. Alternatively, small volumes can be rapidly evaporated in the vacuum without preliminary freezing; they freeze in the early stages of this process as a result of loss of latent heat. Ampoules containing the lyophilized organisms are sealed while still attached to the vacuum pump, and can then be stored at room temperature.

HEAT   *Heat is the most effective agent for killing micro-organisms*, and is extensively used in sterilization. Most vegetative bacteria are killed in a few minutes at 60 °C, but killing of spores by dry heat may take as much as an hour at 160 °C. Moisture increases their susceptibility, but even so they may survive prolonged boiling. With steam under pressure sterilization can be achieved in 15 minutes at a pressure of 15 lb/sq. in. (i.e. at a temperature of 121 °C) or in 3 minutes at 30 lbs/sq. in. (134 °C).

RADIATION   Sunlight has an antimicrobial effect by virtue of its content of *ultraviolet light*, and artificial UV light is used in sterilization of air, of some forms of apparatus, and of materials such as plasma which would be rendered useless by heating or by chemical treatment. Although UV light has the merit of doing very little harm to the material treated, it has little power of penetration and can therefore sterilize only surfaces or thin layers of material. The efficacy of this non-ionizing radiation is greatly impaired by even a small amount of dust between the light source and the target. *X-rays, gamma-rays* and other penetrating ionizing radiations are much more efficient sterilizing agents, and under controlled conditions can be relied upon to kill all micro-organisms. In consequence they are used commercially for sterilizing disposable instruments and equipment.

Disinfectants
By this term we mean substances with useful antimicrobial activity which do not have serious general destructive effects such as are possessed by strong acids and alkalies, but which are too toxic for systemic use in the treatment of microbial infections. They are referred to as *bactericidal* when they kill bacteria (cf. fungicidal, germicidal) and as *bacteriostatic*** when they only prevent multiplication. It means nothing, however, to describe a substance as bactericidal or bacteriostatic without defining the concentration in which it is used, the identity and state of the organism and the conditions under which the two come into contact.

Some examples of well-known disinfectants are given in Table I. The useful applications of these varied compounds are determined by such properties as toxicity to human tissues, range of antimicrobial activity and degree of inactivation by organic matter. To give a few illustrations, cresols are too toxic to be applied to the skin, crystal violet is relatively ineffective against most Gram-negative organisms, and oxidizing agents are useless for the sterilization of faeces because they are reduced and inactivated by the large amounts of organic material present. But crystal violet is useful in the treatment of staphylococcal skin lesions, oxidizing agents can be used for the destruction of Gram-negative organisms so as to make water safe to drink, and cresols are suitable for sterilizing faeces. Other examples of the appropriate use of various disinfectants are given in later chapters, notably on pp. 266–9.

---

* The alternative spelling *bacteristatic* seems to be gaining support and is more consistent with *bactericidal*, but it is not yet generally accepted.

Table 1   Some properties of some commonly used disinfectants
Since the actions of disinfectants depend very largely on the conditions under which they are tested, entries in this table should be regarded as wide generalizations.

Class of compound	Examples and trade names	Vegetative bacteria killed[1]	Inactivation by organic matter	Toxicity to human tissues
Alcohols	Ethyl alcohol[2]	All	Moderate	Moderate
Aldehydes	Formaldehyde[3]	All	Moderate	Marked
	Glutaraldehyde ('Cidex')	All	Moderate	Moderate
Organic dyes	Crystal violet	Some	Moderate	Slight
	Proflavine	Some	Slight	Slight
Cationic detergents	Cetrimide[4] ('Cetavlon')	Most	Marked	Slight
	Chlorhexidine ('Hibitane')	Most	Marked	Slight
Soaps, anionic detergents		Some	Slight	Slight
Phenols	Carbolic acid	All	Slight	Marked
Clear phenolics	'Hycolin', 'Stericol' 'Clearsol'	All	Slight	Moderate
Cresols	'Lysol'	All	Slight	Marked
Chloroxylenols	'Dettol'	Some	Moderate	Moderate
Hexachlorophane	'Phisohex'	Most	Slight	Slight
Oxidizing agents	Iodine, chlorine, iodoform, chloroform, sodium hypochlorite, potassium permanganate, hydrogen peroxide	All	Marked	Slight to moderate
Salts of heavy metals	Mercuric chloride	All	Marked	Marked

[1]No available disinfectant is reliably effective against bacterial *spores*. The susceptibilities of rickettsiae, chlamydiae and viruses to disinfectants are considered on pp. 147 and 165.
[2]Absolute alcohol is a relatively ineffective disinfectant; its activity is increased by dilution to 70% v/v in water.
[3]Formaldehyde can be used either as a gas or in aqueous solution; formalin is a 40% aqueous solution of formaldehyde.
[4]An important feature of cetrimide is its inefficacy against *Ps. aeruginosa*. It is used in selective media for culture of this species.

Standardization of disinfectants presents serious problems. The Rideal–Walker coefficient was at one time widely used as a measure of the potency of a disinfectant. In fact it is only a measure of its superiority or inferiority to phenol for the single purpose of killing typhoid bacilli in the absence of organic matter. Even the Chick–Martin test, in which organic material is present in the form of sterilized faeces, tells us only what a disinfectant can do in those particular circumstances. Results obtained in a test-tube culture in a fluid medium may well be irrelevant to the choice of a disinfectant for the treatment of floors, furniture, or wounds. So far as practicable, such a choice should be based on 'in-use' tests specially designed to determine whether the disinfectant can do the job for which it is being used.

Chemotherapeutic Agents

These are synthetic chemicals active against micro-organisms *in vitro* and of sufficiently low toxicity to be administered systemically. Scientific chemotherapy began in the first decade of this century (p. 10), when Ehrlich introduced the therapeutic use of the organic arsenical compounds, starting with atoxyl for trypanosomiasis and arsphenamine for syphilis. Then in 1935 Domagk showed that the newly-discovered prontosil (sulphonamidochrysoidin) could cure streptococcal infections in mice or human beings. Other therapeutically useful sulphonamides followed, differing from one another in solubility, toxicity and degree of absorption from the intestine but all acting in the same way upon bacteria. Being derivatives of *p*-aminobenzene sulphonamide, they all closely resemble *p*-aminobenzoic acid (PABA). Many bacteria need PABA as a metabolite for synthesis of tetrahydrofolic acid—itself an essential co-enzyme for purine and pyrimidine synthesis.. If these organisms take up sulphonamide instead of PABA, their metabolism is arrested. Bacteriostasis depends upon there being a considerable excess of sulphonamide over PABA in the environment, and is reversible by the addition of more PABA. Sulphonamides are not bactericidal. Their discovery was one of the great events of medical history because they are effective against a wide range of bacteria of medical importance—e.g. haemolytic streptococci, pneumococci, meningococci, gonococci, dysentery bacilli and many of the Gram-negative bacilli causing urinary tract infections.

Many other chemotherapeutic agents are currently in clinical use, notably those mentioned on pp. 324–6 and those used for leprosy (p. 136), tuberculosis (pp. 338–9), virus infections (pp. 164–5) and protozoal infections (pp. 206–14).

Antibiotics

This term, coined in 1942 by Waksman to describe a newly-discovered class of antimicrobial agents, is now a household word. According to Waksman's definition, an antibiotic is a substance, produced by micro-organisms, which can inhibit the growth of or even destroy other micro-organisms (the reverse of symbiotic activity). He also specified that dilute solutions of the substance must have these properties, thus excluding, for example, the lactic acid produced by lactobacilli (p. 24). The limits of

Waksman's definition have been stretched by man's activities in synthesizing compounds similar to or identical with those made by microorganisms. It is hard to deny the name antibiotic to a substance such as chloramphenicol, which is now man-made but is chemically identical with an antibiotic produced by a bacterium. The semisynthetic penicillins and other antimicrobial substances produced by chemical alteration of microbial products are less easy to classify, and the dividing line between antibiotics and chemotherapeutic agents is now indefinite.

Very large numbers of antibiotics have been isolated from cultures of fungi or bacteria, notably from branching bacteria of the genus *Streptomyces*. Those with low toxicity to man coupled with high activity against his pathogens have been studied and exploited most fully. The first of these, *penicillin* (more strictly, benzyl penicillin), was isolated from the mould *Penicillium notatum* by Fleming in 1928 and made available for medical use by the work of Florey and Chain a decade later. It is remarkably non-toxic when pure; in concentrations which can be easily and safely achieved in the body it is bactericidal to many important pathogens; and in the form of its sodium salt it is reasonably stable, except in acid conditions. It continues to be one of the most valuable antibiotics for clinical use, but falls short of the ideal in several important respects. It is ineffective against many pathogenic bacteria, including the tubercle bacillus and most Gram-negative bacilli, and against all non-bacterial pathogens; its use has resulted in the emergence of resistant (usually penicillinase-producing) strains of many species, notably *Staph. aureus*; and its effectiveness when given by mouth is limited by its acid-lability. Subsequent research has therefore been directed to finding other antibiotics that do not have these defects. Very large numbers of streptomycetes and other organisms have been screened for signs of antibacterial activity, and a number of useful compounds have been found by this empirical approach. They have considerably expanded the range of pathogens susceptible to antibiotic treatment, which now includes the great majority of bacteria, the rickettsiae and the chlamydiae and some of the fungi. However, all of these compounds have at least some toxicity for man, and in concentrations that can be achieved in the body many are only bacteriostatic. Some of them can be given by mouth. Meanwhile it has been possible to produce variants of the penicillin molecule which do not share the defects of benzyl penicillin (pp. 327–8).

To be of clinical value an antibiotic must have *selective toxicity*—i.e. it must produce serious structural or metabolic lesions in the cells of microorganisms without doing significant damage to the cells of the human host. Hence the success of the β-lactams (pencillins and cephalosporins), which interfere with synthesis of cell-wall mucopeptide, a vital bacterial component not shared by human or other eukaryotic cells (p. 12); the consequences of such interference are, in some circumstances and with some organisms, the inability of bacteria to form cross-walls and so replicate themselves, and in other circumstances the formation of a faulty cell wall which, like a damaged cycle-tyre outer tube, allows rupture of the unsupported cytoplasmic membrane (the 'inner tube') by osmotic pressure. Other antibiotics—the aminoglycosides, chloramphenicol, the tetracyclines, erythromycin and clindamycin—interfere at various points in the protein-synthesizing activities of bacterial ribosomes, and their clinical usefulness depends on structural differences between bacterial and mammalian ribosomes. Both of these forms of interference with the processes of growth are effective only against multiplying bacteria, as is the inhibition of bacterial RNA synthesis by the rifamycins; but the damage that the polymyxins inflict on bacterial cytoplasmic membranes, leading to leakage of cell contents, is lethal even to resting cells.

Differences in drug sensitivities between bacterial species, or between strains within a species, are of great importance in medical microbiology and in the clinical management of bacterial infections. The mechanisms that underlie such differences are discussed on pp. 316–9.

Further information about chemotherapeutic and antibiotic agents in common use in clinical medicine is to be found in Chapter 21.

Suggestions for Further Reading
Biochemistry of Bacterial Growth by J. Mandelstam, K. McQuillen and I. W. Dawes, 3rd edn. (Blackwell, Oxford, 1980).

PART III

PART III

PATHOGENESIS OF MICROBIAL DISEASES

CHAPTER 6

TRANSMISSION OF PATHOGENS

The term *infection* and related words occur frequently in most discussions of microbial diseases, but there is no general agreement as to their precise meaning—in particular, as to whether they imply actual invasion of host tissues or merely the presence of potential invaders. We think that infection is best defined as the arrival or presence of potentially pathogenic organisms on the surface or in the tissues of an appropriate host. We can then refer to an infected person, to an infected wound or part of the body, or to an infected animal or plant—even to a bacterium being infected with bacteriophage—but not to infected inanimate objects. For the latter, when they are carrying potential pathogens, and also when they should be sterile but have ceased to be so, we prefer the term *contaminated*. An infectious disease is one that is transmissible from patient to patient by transfer of the causative organism, and an infectious patient is one from whom such a disease can be acquired. Infection is called *clinical* when it is causing overt disease, or *subclinical* when there is little or no impairment of the patient's health. Persistent subclinical infection that may be converted into clinical infection by changing circumstances (such as a reduction in the patient's general immunity) is described as *latent*.

Even these definitions do not eliminate all terminological difficulties, since an aura of uncertainty surrounds the words 'potentially pathogenic'. For example, all human beings carry in their intestinal tracts *Escherichia coli* and related Gram-negative bacilli capable of producing disease in the urinary tract, in wounds and elsewhere. If we are to retain any useful meaning for the words that we are attempting to define, carriage of normal commensal or symbiotic organisms in normal sites must be excluded from their scope, even if those organisms are sometimes pathogenic elsewhere, or when the host's defences are impaired (*opportunist* pathogens).

There is no ambiguity about the following terms commonly used in discussing microbial diseases; *epidemic*, a noun or an adjective, describing a temporary marked increase in frequency of a particular disease in a community; *pandemic*, referring to a world-wide epidemic; and *endemic*, used only as an adjective, describing a disease which is persistently present in a community. An endemic disease may from time to time flare up into an epidemic.

SOURCES OF PATHOGENS

Except when lowered local or general resistance makes a patient susceptible to the attacks of his resident parasites, pathogenic organisms are *exogenous*—that is, they come from outside the patient. With few exceptions (such as some fungi and possibly some clostridia), they come, directly or indirectly, from other human beings or from animals. These may themselves be clinically infected, or may be *carriers*, transmitting pathogens without showing any evidence of related disease. Carriers are important in the spread of epidemics, since they are hard to detect, mix freely with other people, and may disseminate large numbers of organisms over long periods; whereas victims of clinical disease are less 'successful' as distributors of the organisms because they are liable to be segregated, to some extent at least, and may even be permanently removed from circulation by death. Carriers may be *incubational* (or *precocious*) carriers, who will shortly develop the disease, or *convalescent* carriers, who have already had it. Often, however, they are *symptomless* carriers, whose infection is entirely sub-clinical. Duration of the carrier state, and of excretion, is widely variable. Typhoid is the classic example of a disease in which the carrier state may persist for many years, and may be very difficult to detect because excretion of the organism is intermittent; but when it is detected, it can often be brought to an end by antibiotic treatment. In contrast, carriage of the other members of the genus *Salmonella* seldom lasts for more than a month or two; but attempts to reduce this period by antibiotic treatment may in fact prolong it (p. 116). Hospital outbreaks of wound sepsis and other lesions due to *Staphylococcus aureus* are often traced to nasal or cutaneous carriage of the offending strains by members of the staff (see Chapter 18).

The name *zoonoses* (four syllables) is given to diseases that man acquires from animals—e.g. brucellosis, leptospirosis, rabies.

TRANSFER OF PATHOGENS

Common routes for the spread of microbial diseases are indicated in Table II. The list is illustrative, not comprehensive, and many of the

Table II   Examples of the spread of microbial diseases

Mode of spread	Some infections commonly spread in this way
Fairly direct person to person	
In droplets or droplet nuclei	Most acute respiratory tract infections; tuberculosis; meningitis; measles; rubella; mumps; smallpox
In saliva	Infectious mononucleosis; rabies (from animals)
By the faecal—oral route	Bacterial diarrhoeas; amoebiasis; hepatitis A; poliomyelitis and other enterovirus infections.
By direct contact	Staphylococcal and streptococcal infections; sexually transmitted infections; herpes simplex; ringworm (from humans or animals)
In blood or blood products	Hepatitis B; syphilis; malaria
From mother to foetus in the uterus ('vertical spread')	Rubella; toxoplasmosis; cytomegalic inclusion disease; syphilis
From mother to foetus during birth	Herpes simplex; gonococcal, group B streptococcal and chlamydial infections
In fomites (p 5) or dust	Many infections due to bacteria, viruses or fungi capable of survival outside the patient
Via foods	
Eggs, poultry, meat products	Salmonellosis, campylobacter infections
Unpasteurized milk, dairy products	Salmonellosis, brucellosis, campylobacter infections, Q fever, tuberculosis
Raw vegetables in some hot countries	Amoebic and bacillary dysentery, hepatitis A
In water	
By drinking	Typhoid; cholera
By immersion	Leptospirosis; amoebic meningo-encephalitis; pseudomonas infections of ears or skin
Via showers, humidifiers, etc.	Legionellosis
From soil	Tetanus; gas-gangrene; some systemic fungal infections (deep mycoses)
Via arthropod vectors	
Mosquitoes, fleas, ticks, mites, lice	Malaria; yellow fever; virus encephalitides; bubonic plague; rickettsial infections

infections mentioned can be spread in more ways than we have indicated.

Droplets

'Coughs and sneezes spread diseases'. Even when talking or breathing quietly we constantly emit from our mouths and noses numerous droplets of moisture containing bacteria and viruses. The fate of these droplets depends on their size. The largest of them fall rapidly to the ground, where they dry and the organisms are added to the dust. Small droplets, however, evaporate to dryness in the air, leaving their solid contents as droplet-nuclei. These may remain airborne for long periods and travel considerable distances on air-currents, and they are readily inhaled by other people. Diseases spread largely by means of droplets include most bacterial infections of the respiratory tract, meningitis and many common virus infections.

Faeces

Faecal material, particularly from patients with diarrhoea, is liable to find its way on to toilet seats, or via the hands on to toilet handles, taps, door handles, etc. From all of these places it can find its way on to the hands and so into the mouths of other people ('faecal–oral spread'). Food-handlers who are faecal excretors of pathogens can all too easily transfer them to food unless their personal hygiene and hand-washing facilities are adequate (p. 289). Those who attend to the toilet needs of small children or incapacitated patients are also potential transmitters of infection if they are careless.

Shedding of Staphylococci

Many healthy people carry *Staph. aureus* in their noses and throats and on their skin, and are continually shedding these in very large numbers attached to skin scales—though there is considerable personal variation in rates of shedding. The scales can be transmitted in various ways to other people—mainly in dust or by direct contact. The importance of such *Staph. aureus* carriers is discussed later in connection with surgical ward sepsis (p. 271) and with food-poisoning (p. 285). Those with clinical staphylococcal infections are also important sources of infection to others, but are far easier to detect.

Suggestions for Further Reading

See end of next chapter.

CHAPTER 7

PATHOGENICITY AND HOST DEFENCES

PATHOGENICITY

Pathogenicity is the capacity of a micro-organism to produce disease. There are helpful similarities between our uses of the words 'pathogen' and 'criminal'.

Some people are known to the police as specialists in particular forms of crime; others as more versatile wrong-doers; and others as generally law-abiding citizens who are liable to occasional lapses. To be a known criminal is not to be incapable of any other sort of existence; and to be unknown to the police is not necessarily the same as being innocent.

Similarly, some micro-organisms, such as *Corynebacterium diphtheriae* and *Clostridium tetani*, are known to be responsible for characteristic diseases; others, such as *Staphylococcus aureus* and *Streptococcus pyogenes*, can cause many different forms of disease; and others, such as *Str. viridans*, are usually harmless but in special circumstances may become pathogens. Most known pathogens are capable of existing as harmless commensals; and undoubtedly there are many species with as yet unsuspected pathogenic activities.

To establish beyond doubt that a given organism causes a given disease may be a difficult problem. It is not enough to show that it is constantly present in an appropriate distribution in each case of the disease, for its presence may be a result rather than the cause of the disease. According to the classical criteria of pathogenicity commonly known as Koch's postulates, it should be possible to show that the organism is constantly present as already indicated, to grow it in artificial culture media, and to reproduce the disease in susceptible animals by administering such cultures to them. However, there are many diseases to which these criteria cannot be applied, but which can be confidently attributed to particular organisms. For example, *Treponema pallidum* cannot be grown in culture and does not produce in animals anything closely resembling syphilis, yet its association with that disease is so constant that nobody doubts its causative role.

Even when a particular microbial species is certainly pathogenic, this property is not necessarily, or even usually, shared by all strains of the species. It is common to find bacterial strains that are identical in all measurable characters except that one is pathogenic to certain hosts and the other is not. The term *virulence* is often used in an attempt to quantitate pathogenicity, but caution is needed here. It is sometimes convenient to be able to describe a strain as highly virulent, or of reduced virulence or avirulent; but we can give mathematical expression to virulence only if we define carefully the conditions under which it is measured. We can determine how many organisms of a particular strain constitute a lethal dose (LD) for a mouse, but this information is of little value because mice, like all other hosts, show wide variations of individual susceptibility. We have achieved rather more if we determine the number of organisms which, if administered to each of a large batch of closely similar mice, will kill 50 % of them (the LD 50 for those mice); but even this information is only of value for comparison with the LD 50 of another strain grown under the same conditions in the same medium for the same length of time and administered in the same way to a batch of mice of the same strain which are strictly comparable with the first batch in regard to age, sex, size, nutrition, past experience of infection and any other features that may be relevant. Such a comparison will not necessarily tell us anything about the relative virulence of the two strains for another host species or even for mice of a different breed or age.

Implicit in what we have said about LD 50 measurements is an important concept—that the number ('dose') of organisms taking part in an infection has an important influence on its outcome. In an epidemic, or in an outbreak of common-source illness such as food-poisoning after a party, it is often found that some of those exposed have symptomless infections, some are mildly ill and some are more severely affected. In general such variations are likely to be determined, in part at least, by differences in the doses of pathogens reaching individuals, though other factors such as host immunity can also be important.

The impossibility of comparing virulence without specifying the host is well illustrated by the human and bovine tubercle bacilli (*Mycobacterium tuberculosis* and *Myco. bovis*). Both are pathogenic for man and for guinea-pigs, but cattle and rabbits are far less susceptible to human than to bovine strains. Inoculation of mycobacteria into guinea-pigs provides an indication of their virulence for man; to use rabbits for this purpose would be grossly misleading.

The virulence of a microbial strain for a given host species may decrease progressively when the strain is maintained in laboratory culture or in an unrelated host species; such a strain is described as attenuated. Thus the *Bacille Calmette-Guerin* (*BCG*) is a bovine tubercle bacillus strain attenuated by prolonged artificial culture. When injected into humans it causes only local lesions, but stimulates the development of immunity effective against natural tuberculosis (p. 294).

Characters of Pathogens

In some microbial species pathogenicity is closely associated with recognizable characters of the organisms, and strains without these characters are avirulent. Bacteria are sometimes isolated which have all the properties of the diphtheria bacillus except the ability to form exotoxin. Such strains are known as non-toxigenic *Corynebacterium diphtheriae*, and since it is the toxin which harms the host in diphtheria such strains are avirulent.

Many determinants of pathogenicity are surface components of the organisms (and so are liable to provoke specific immunological responses that protect the host—see the next chapter). Thus *Streptococcus pneumoniae* and various other pathogenic bacteria have thick envelope layers called capsules that protect them against phagocytosis (p. 48), and the virulence and invasiveness of such organisms is directly related both to the amount and to the precise nature of this capsular polysaccharide material. Group A haemolytic streptococci have two components of their fimbriae—lipoteichoic acid, which enables them to bind to host epithelial cells, and M protein, which is antiphagocytic but can provoke production of type-specific opsonins (p. 56). The pilus-like K surface antigens of *Escherichia coli* and the pili of gonococci are included among the substances known as *adhesins*, which promote adhesion of micro-organisms to epithelial cells and so play an important role in the initiation of infections; strains lacking such characters in general fail to establish the initial bridgehead and are non-pathogens. The neuraminidase of an influenza virus can degrade the protective mucus on the surface of an epithelial cell, allowing the haemagglutinin to react with a receptor on that surface and so opening up the way for cell penetration and virus replication.

We can make a number of generalizations about characters that pathogens must have:

1 Apart from a few special cases (e.g. botulism, which is due to the patient's ingestion of a ready-made bacterial toxin; or some of the very superficial fungal skin infections), a micro-organism *must be able to enter the host's body* in order to be able to produce disease. Some (e.g. *Vibrio cholerae, Bordetella pertussis*) attach to the surfaces of epithelial cells and multiply there without entering the cells. Others (e.g. shigellae, coryza viruses) penetrate the epithelial cells but have little or no tendency to spread further. In such 'hit and run' infections microbial multiplication and shedding occur before the specific defences have been mobilized. The many pathogens that penetrate further than the epithelial layers include (for example) *Salmonella typhi*, with its characteristic rapid spread to the blood resulting in enteric fever, and the polioviruses which have to pass through the blood to reach their target cells in the central nervous system. Some viruses and bacteria enter host phagocytic cells which cannot digest them, and then travel around the body inside these (p. 48). In many instances such invasions are prevented by host defences, but the risk of generalized infection is much increased when these are impaired—e.g. by underlying disease or treatment with immunosuppressive drugs.

The term *endogenous* is used to describe infections due to organisms that were previously present as commensals of the same host; and it appears to imply that they are exceptions to our first rule. However, these organisms have of course come originally from outside the host; and their change to pathogenicity usually involves penetration into his tissues or transfer to another part of his body, or results from impairment of his defences.

2 *A pathogen must be able to multiply in or on the host's tissues.* Put the other way round, this means that the host's tissues must supply appropriate nutrients, atmospheric conditions and temperature for the pathogen's growth. Here we can see in broad outline the facts which determine the host ranges of all pathogens, and indeed of all parasites, but we can fill in very few of the details. Similar factors undoubtedly play a large part also in deciding the distribution of parasites within the body of the individual host, and the sites at which pathogens produce their characteristic lesions. For example, the fact that *Mycobacterium ulcerans* and *Myco. marinum* can multiply only in the temperature range 30–33°C presumably accounts for their ability to produce lesions only in the skin of man and not in deeper tissues, and the distribution of leprosy lesions, due to the related *Myco. leprae*, can be similarly explained. So can the restriction of the rhinovirus group of common cold viruses to the upper respiratory tract. Abnormal conditions in the tissues of a host may permit organisms to thrive which could not otherwise grow there. Hence diabetics are unduly susceptible to infections, probably as a result of the high glucose content and other chemical peculiarities of their tissues; and gas-gangrene, caused by anaerobic organisms of the genus *Clostridium*, occurs in tissues which have lost their blood supply and so their source of oxygen. The role of erythritol in localizing brucella infection in bovine abortion is considered on p. 127. In the majority of cases, however, we do not know what determines the localization of organisms of microbial lesions.

3 It is self-evident that to be a pathogen an organism *must be able to damage the host's tissues.* This can happen in many different ways. As we mentioned on p. 24, bacteria may produce local or more remote damage by releasing endotoxins or exotoxins. Viruses invade host cells and divert their synthetic processes to the production of more viruses—sometimes on a small scale, carrying on quietly for long periods without apparent damage to the host cells, but often on such a scale as to disorganize the cells' metabolism, impair their functional efficiency and even cause their rupture and destruction. Malarial parasites also multiply inside host cells, notably red blood cells, and rupture them, causing severe anaemia and other disorders. Tissue damage may be due to host hypersensitivity reactions to the organism rather than to its toxicity. Thus the nerve damage in leprosy is the result of Type IV hypersensitivity (p. 65); and circulating immune complexes, which are found in the blood in many infectious diseases, may well be responsible for such late manifestations of infection as glomerulonephritis and reactive arthritis (Type III hypersensitivity, p. 64).

4 In order to be able to do any of the things mentioned so far, a pathogen *must be able to resist and overcome the host's defence mechanisms.* These we will now consider, continuing to refer at appropriate points to some of the microbial 'answers' to them.

NON-SPECIFIC HOST DEFENCES

As we have seen (p. 43), to be a pathogen an organism needs in nearly all cases to gain access to host tissues. Many of the barriers to achieving this are largely non-specific i.e. effective against wide ranges of organisms.

Superficial Defences
One important defence mechanism that is in operation on mucous membranes as well as in the tissues and the blood stream—phagocytosis—is discussed in the next section (Cellular Defences). The other main defences of the body's various surfaces are as follows.

SKIN This is both a mechanical barrier to micro-organisms and, by virtue of the fatty acid content of sweat and sebum, a death-bed for many of them. However, hair follicles and glands form comparatively weak points in the defences, and by multiplying in these *Staph. aureus* may give rise to pustules, boils and carbuncles. This same bacterial species, being resistant to the bactericidal action of the skin secretions, is commonly present on the surface and may be carried into the subcutaneous tissues by anything which pierces or lacerates the skin. The importance of the skin barrier is emphasized by the high frequency of superficial infections when its efficiency is impaired—e.g. by burning or by vitamin deficiency.

CONJUNCTIVAE These are less of a mechanical obstruction, but they are constantly washed by tears and wiped by the movement of the eyelids. Tears contain an enzyme lysozyme (also present in most other body fluids and in polymorphonuclear leucocytes) which, acting with specific antibodies and complement (p. 60), can lyse bacteria.

MOUTH Saliva contains antimicrobial substances such as lysozyme and lactoferrin. Other defences of the oral cavity are an intact mucous membrane, crevicular fluid, and mechanical flushing that removes bacteria not adherent to epithelial cells or the teeth.

ALIMENTARY TRACT Most micro-organisms are killed or damaged by gastric secretions, particularly the acid component; notable exceptions are *Mycobacterium tuberculosis* and enteroviruses. This barrier can be overcome if a large dose of pathogenic organisms is ingested, and a much smaller dose may suffice to establish infection if acid secretion is reduced. Hence neonates, and also patients who have recently undergone some forms of gastric surgery, have an increased susceptibility to infection with salmonellae and other ingested pathogens; and regular use of antacid tablets has been shown to increase susceptibility to brucellae in contaminated unpasteurized milk. Establishment of infection is also hindered by peristalsis and rapid transit through the intestine, and by the need for the potential pathogens to compete with the resident bacterial flora for attachment to epithelial cells.

RESPIRATORY TRACT   Breathing involves inhalation of very large volumes of air every day, and therefore of considerable numbers of suspended micro-organisms. Larger particles are filtered out in the nose, by impinging on hairs or on the sticky mucous membranes, but smaller particles reach the lower respiratory tract—though only those less than 5 μm in diameter can penetrate as far as the alveoli. The large and complex normal bacterial flora of the upper respiratory tract constitutes an important barrier to colonization by extraneous organisms (see p. 20), and interference with the balance of this population by use of anti-bacterial drugs can have undesirable consequences here, and also on other heavily populated surfaces. In the lower respiratory tract, mucus secretion by the goblet cells and mucus-secreting glands combines with ciliary action of the epithelial cells to provide a remarkably efficient clearance system for inhaled micro-organisms. These are caught on the sticky mucus blanket (where they are exposed to antibacterial substances such as lysozyme and lactoferrin) and are swept upward by the 'mucociliary escalator', to be coughed out or swallowed and dealt with by the gastric secretions. Toxic agents such as cigarette smoke and also some virus infections inhibit ciliary action and so predispose to lower respiratory tract infections. The clearance mechanism is also defective in bronchi damaged by chronic bronchitis or bronchiectasis; and some patients with congenitally defective ciliary function suffer from recurrent or chronic infections of the respiratory tract, paranasal sinusitis or otitis media. Organisms that succeed in reaching the alveoli are usually disposed of by the alveolar macrophages.

VAGINA   Here there is no mechanical cleansing system, but in the adult there is an important hormone-dependent chemical defence mechanism, put into effect by the characteristic normal flora as explained on p. 24. Here, as in the upper respiratory tract and elsewhere, disturbance of the normal flora by antibiotic treatment can allow endogenous pathogens to proliferate—notably *Candida albicans*.

Cellular Defences
Bacteria which get through the outer defences and begin to multiply within the tissues usually provoke inflammatory reactions. The vigour

and pattern of these depend, among other things, on the nature of the organism and on the previous experience of the host. For the first few hours of the inflammatory response there is a phase of increased vascular permeability, with extravasation of plasma and leucocytes—neutrophil polymorphs in the initial stages, followed later by mononuclear cells. Phagocytosis (see below) by these leucocytes, with the assistance of other non-specific local defence factors such as complement and free iron, may result in early elimination of the invading organisms, or in marked reduction of their numbers. During the subsequent phase of decreased vascular permeability, antibacterial drugs may be prevented from reaching the tissues in effective concentrations. Bacteria that survive the local inflammatory response may spread via the lymph to lymph nodes, and if not eliminated there they can reach the blood. *Bacteraemia* means presence of bacteria in the blood stream, which may arise in the way just described or may follow any of a variety of procedures that allow direct access of bacteria from body surfaces into the blood—e.g. dental extraction or even vigorous chewing or use of a tooth-brush; urinary tract catheterization or other instrumentation, especially in the presence of urinary tract infection; and difficult defaecation. When bacteria enter the blood they are as a rule cleared from it rapidly by phagocytes in the liver, spleen and bone-marrow; but virulent organisms may overwhelm this defence mechanism and produce serious, perhaps fatal generalized infections. The term *septicaemia* has been defined in many ways, but is best regarded as the name for a serious clinical condition (including shock) associated with the presence of pathogenic organisms in the blood.

PUS   This common result of bacterial infection is a complex mixture of surviving or dead micro-organisms and leucocytes (neutrophils in acute infections), together with remnants of broken-down host cells, all suspended in tissue fluid.

PHAGOCYTES   The engulfing of micro-organisms by host cells is called *phagocytosis*. An effective mechanism for dealing with the first stages of an infection requires the rapid mobilization of appropriate cells (*phagocytes*). As we have seen, the leucocytes that predominate in early inflammatory exudates are *neutrophils*. These are produced in the bone marrow, and released into the circulation after a two-week maturation process. During this time they develop intracytoplasmic granules that contain enzymes and other factors responsible for mediation of the inflammatory response and for their microbicidal activity. Neutrophils have a short half-life (6–7 hours) in the circulation. During acute inflammation their ability to adhere to and migrate across the vascular endothelium is enhanced—hence their appearance in the exudate. They are therefore in most circumstances the front-line troops that deal with tissue invasion. The other major group of phagocytes are *monocytes* and the larger *macrophages*. These are found free in the blood, free or fixed in the tissues of the lymph-nodes or the spleen, fixed in the liver (Kupffer cells), on the pleural and peritoneal surfaces and in the alveoli of the lungs. As tissue macrophages they have a life of several weeks. They are strategically placed for filtering organisms out of the lymph and the blood, removing them from the pleural and peritoneal fluid, and dealing with those that reach the alveoli. However, some organisms can live and even multiply inside macrophages, using them (like the Trojan horse) to carry infection to other parts of the body.

Phagocytosis begins with *attachment* of the micro-organism to the surface of the phagocyte. This is facilitated by the presence of opsonins (p. 56), which can attach to the surface of the organism and for which there are specific receptors on the surface of the phagocyte. Attachment is followed by *engulfment* by the cell, with formation of an intracellular vacuole, *the phagosome*. The cytoplasmic granules then fuse with the vacuole, discharging their enzymes into it. The mechanism by which phagocytes kill micro-organisms is not yet fully elucidated, but it involves the enzyme myeloperoxidase, a burst of oxidative metabolism and the generation of hydrogen peroxide and superoxide.

Phagocytes migrate to the site of infection in response to chemical stimuli (*chemotaxis*). Products of the micro-organisms themselves may be either directly chemotactic or capable of generating chemotactic stimuli by activating the complement system (p. 61).

Having been attracted to the site, macrophages may be activated in any of three ways: by lymphokines from sensitized T-lymphocytes (p. 62), by immune complexes (p. 64) or through activation of the complement system, especially C3 (p. 60). Activated macrophages liberate substances that also activate biological amplification mechanisms such as the complement, kinin and coagulation systems. Their other products include factors which control generation of neutrophils and monocytes in response to infection; endogenous pyrogen, which acts on the hypo-thalamus to produce fever; thromboplastin, which is important in the development of disseminated intravascular coagulation (p. 62); and interferon (see below).

The importance of the cellular defences is illustrated by patients with quantitative or qualitative phagocyte defects. When the number of circulating neutrophils is reduced below about $500/mm^3$ the risk of infection, particularly by endogenous organisms, is greatly increased; and children with the neutrophil and monocyte enzyme deficiency known as *chronic granulomatous disease*, which results in failure of the phagocytes to kill ingested organisms, have chronic granulomatous discharging abscesses.

Some micro-organisms have special features that protect them against phagocytes. The polysaccharide capsules of bacteria such as pneumococci allow them to escape attachment except in the presence of specific anticapsular antibodies. Those micro-organisms that can survive inside cells can be killed only by the combined action of macrophages and specifically sensitized T-lymphocytes (p. 62). Some organisms have cell-bound or soluble toxins that kill phagocytes (e.g. leucocidins, p. 24).

INTERFERONS These are a group of proteins with broad antiviral activity (within the right host species) and other biological activities. They render host cells resistant to virus infection, and are the first line of defence against viruses, since they are detectable within a few hours of the intiation of infection—whereas protective antibodies do not appear for several days. Type 1 interferons are produced by virus-infected cells and confer protection on neighbouring cells. Type 2 interferons are similar in effect but are lymphokines, produced by stimulated lymphocytes (p. 62).

SPECIFIC IMMUNITY

Specific immunity, which is discussed more fully in the next chapter, is the resistance of an individual to a particular disease as a result of his ability to defend himself against its causative agent. It depends upon his genetic inheritance, his age, his general health and his past experience of micro-organisms. It may be classified as follows:

Innate Immunity

Each individual inherits certain susceptibilities and resistances peculiar to his species, his race and his family, and has his own personal combination of these. Presumably they depend upon his tissue chemistry, his superficial and cellular defence mechanisms, and possibly non-specific humoral agents. As he matures and ages, all of these factors vary through hormonal and other influences, so that immunity changes with age quite apart from the contributions mentioned in the next two paragraphs.

Acquired Immunity

1 *Naturally acquired.* Naturally occurring clinical or subclinical infection commonly provokes responses on the part of the host which enhance his ability to resist the causative organism when he meets it again. These responses involve production of agents that react specifically with the organism or its products—either special proteins called *antibodies* or special sensitized cells (the effect of which is described as *cell-mediated immunity*) or both. Immunity due to the host's own responses is called *active*, whereas immunity conferred by maternal antibodies that enter the infant's circulation via the placenta—or in some animal species via colostrum or milk—is called naturally acquired *passive* immunity because the infant itself has made no contribution to it.

2 *Artificially induced.* Artificial stimulation of specific resistance to infection is called *immunization*, and is discussed more fully in Chapter 20. This also may be *active* or *passive*, in that the subject may be provoked to make his own antibodies or may be given some ready-made.

SOME POSSIBLE RESULTS OF INFECTION

A consideration of all possible outcomes of encounters between pathogens and host defences would be a review of the entire field of microbial diseases. The discussion would be further complicated by the need to take into consideration many different factors in the host's condition and circumstances which may affect the issue—e.g. injuries, anatomical abnormalities, presence of foreign bodies in wounds, nutritional state of the host and effects of treatment with antimicrobial agents or with irradiation, steroid hormones or other agents that impair host resistance. However, it may be helpful to outline and illustrate a few of the situations which develop.

1 *Elimination of the pathogen without any clinical lesion.* This is undoubtedly the commonest outcome of infection by a pathogen, but for obvious reasons it is virtually never observed. If the elimination is not too rapid, it may be possible to demonstrate retrospectively that infection has occurred, because shortly afterwards specific antibodies appear in the host's blood or he develops a specific tissue hypersensitivity.

2 *Localization of the pathogen with production of a local lesion.* This is clearly illustrated by the common small staphylococcal pustule of the skin. There is no impairment of the patient's general health, tissue damage is confined to the immediate vicinity of the pathogen's point of entry, and as a rule the infection is soon eradicated.

3 *Localization of the pathogen with production of distant lesions.* C. diphtheriae is usually itself confined to the throat, but by means of its exotoxin it can produce distant lesions in the heart and nervous system. Cl. tetani, growing as a rule in subcutaneous tissue or muscle, also does serious distant damage by means of a neurotoxin.

4 *Extension of infection to surrounding tissues.* Because it produces hyaluronidase, *Str. pyogenes* is particularly liable to spread rapidly through connective tissue surrounding a primary lesion, causing the diffuse inflammation known as cellulitis. Actinomycosis and caseating tuberculosis spread in quite a different way, advancing slowly through the tissues and causing severe destruction as they go.

5 *General dissemination.* The majority of serious microbial illnesses involve entry of pathogens into the blood stream at some stage. If they are present there in large numbers, they may kill the patient almost at once. If he survives this early septicaemic phase, multiple lesions in various organs may develop, their localization depending largely on the nature of the organism. Complete removal of the organisms from the blood stream by phagocytes, without the development of any secondary lesions, can occur spontaneously, but such an outcome is much more common now that the pathogens may be opposed by lethal or inhibitory concentrations of antimicrobial drugs.

6 *Chronic infection.* Failure of the host's defences to eliminate a pathogen soon after its arrival may result in persistent active disease. Often, however, there is a balance between the pathogen and the defences, and the infection may remain asymptomatic (latent, p. 37) for many years but turn into active disease again when the balance is shifted in favour of the pathogen. Such patterns are further discussed on pp. 67 and 68 and in many places in Chapters 9 to 13.

HERD IMMUNITY

As we have seen, an individual's liability to become ill or to die as a result of exposure to a particular pathogen depends largely on his own immunity. His risk of being so exposed, however, depends largely on the level of immunity of those around him. This in turn depends on the community's experience of the pathogen and of artificial immunization.

The epidemiological story of poliomyelitis is particularly instructive. This virus infection occurs in all parts of the world, but does not take on epidemic form in communities with low standards of hygiene. Extensive studies of virus carriage and of antibody formation in such communities have explained the paradox of the greater susceptibility of more hygienic populations. The virus is excreted in the faeces, and in communities with poor hygiene everyone becomes infected in early life. Some infants get the disease, and a few die, but many first encounter the virus while they are still protected by maternal antibodies, and as this protection wears off continued exposure stimulates them to produce their own antibodies. Virtually all older children and adults are immune, though some continue to carry and excrete the virus, thus passing it on to succeeding generations. As hygienic standards improve, infants are less certain to be infected, until eventually a significant proportion of the population has no experience of the virus and therefore no immunity. In this situation an epidemic may occur, and the victims may include older children and adults. The better the standards of hygiene and the longer the interval since the last epidemic, the greater is the damage likely to be when the next outbreak does occur. This unsatisfactory situation can now be remedied by widespread immunization (pp. 298–9).

In other diseases also there is a danger that partial control may lead to low herd immunity. It is therefore a cardinal principle of preventive medicine that, when a potentially epidemic disease is being brought under control, herd immunity must be kept high by immunization.

Suggestion for Further Reading

The Pathogenesis of Infectious Disease by C. A. Mims, 2nd edn. (Academic Press, London, 1982).

CHAPTER 8

THE HOST'S IMMUNOLOGICAL RESPONSES

Immunology began as the study of that specific resistance to further infection by a particular micro-organism which follows an initial natural or artificial encounter with that organism or with its products, and which we have already described as *acquired immunity* (p. 49). This is now seen to be only part of a more general phenomenon—the initiation of processes in the body, as a result of meeting a foreign substance, which cause the body to react differently when it subsequently meets the same substance or one that closely resembles it. Immunology today concerns itself with all such processes and reactions, regardless of whether they have anything to do with immunity in the strict sense. The modified reactions may be either more or less vigorous than the original; they may be protective or harmful and in some cases they may be both at the same time. Organ transplantation, 'auto-immune' diseases and sundry other immunological topics are full of interest and excitement, but they are only indirectly related to microbiology. In this chapter we briefly review only those areas of immunology which seem most relevant to our subject. In places we present current beliefs and concepts with little or none of the supporting data and without the many qualifications and provisos that would make our account more accurate but longer, less readable and less intelligible. To fill out their knowledge of immunology our readers should consult works such as those recommended at the end of the chapter.

ANTIGENS

An *antigen* is a substance capable of stimulating an immune response in a host. It is recognized as foreign by small lymphocytes that are *immunocompetent* (i.e. capable of mounting immunological responses). The response is specifically directed against particular determinants on the antigen molecule. As the molecular weight of antigen molecules increases, so their *immunogenicity* (i.e. ability to induce immune responses) is also increased. Small molecules which become immunogenic only when coupled to carriers are called *haptens;* although in the uncoupled state they cannot provoke immune responses, they can react directly with appropriate *antibodies* (host proteins with specific affinity for antigens— p. 55). Indeed, most .naturally occurring antigens can be viewed as consisting of carrier portions (usually protein) that render them immunogenic, and haptenic portions (usually non-protein) that determine the specificity of the immune responses.

All but the smallest micro-organisms consist of hundreds or even thousands of antigens, but only a few of these are important in the induction of immunity. Those of greatest importance, and therefore of greatest relevance to our understanding of resistance to infection, are located superficially on the organisms and so are readily accessible to the host's immune mechanisms. They include many determinants of pathogenicity such as those that we considered on p. 43—capsular and other surface polysaccharides; the M proteins of group A haemolytic streptococci; adhesins; and influenza virus neuraminidases and haemagglutinins. Antibodies that react with these substances interfere with their contributions to pathogenicity. Similarly, bacterial toxins provoke the production of specific antibodies (*antitoxins*) that neutralize their toxicity to the host. Virus-infected host cells develop new surface antigens—either virus components or modified host components—that are recognised as foreign and attract the attention of cytotoxic T-lymphocytes (p. 62).

THE BASIS OF IMMUNOLOGICAL RESPONSES

The Lymphoid System

All cells involved in immunological reactions—lymphocytes, granulocytes and macrophages—are derived from a common ancestor, the pluripotent stem cell found in the embryo yolk sac, in the foetal liver and finally in the bone marrow. Immunological responses are initiated by cells that morphologically are small lymphocytes. Some stem cells mature in the *bone marrow* to become *B-lymphocytes*, whereas others migrate to the *thymus* and there mature into *T-lymphocytes*. From these *primary lymphoid organs* the mature lymphocytes move out to the lymph-nodes and spleen—*the secondary lymphoid organs*. Most of them are then in constant migration, from lymph-nodes via the lymph to the blood and back into the lymph nodes through the walls of the postcapillary venules. B- and T-lymphocytes occupy different regions of the secondary lymphoid organs; B-lymphocytes are found in the red pulp of the spleen and in the primary and secondary follicles of the lymph nodes, whereas T-lymphocytes are found in the peri-arteriolar sheaths of the spleen and in the paracortical areas of the lymph nodes. B-lymphocytes are responsible for *humoral immunity*—i.e. that immunity which is determined by antibodies. T-lymphocytes are of central importance in *cell-mediated immunity*; but they can also modulate the activities of B-lymphocytes in ways described on p. 59.

In defence against infection a most important part is played by lymphoid tissues which are associated with mucosal surfaces and so exposed to continual bombardment with micro-organisms and their products. They are responsible for initiating responses to local infections, whereas foreign antigens or organisms that enter the blood are removed by phagocytic cells of the spleen, liver, lungs and blood and the appropriate responses are initiated largely in the spleen.

Specificity and Diversity
Host immunity to infection is based on adaptive responses of the lymphoid system, which eliminate or restrain the infecting organisms. Responses to a particular organism have a specificity that depends on the molecular structure of its surface antigens. Organism-specificity is often not absolute, as cross-reactions can occur with antigens of similar configuration on the surfaces of other organisms and elsewhere. The existence of specificity of response can be explained in terms of the *clonal selection theory*. Each B-lymphocyte or T-lymphocyte has on its surface antigen-binding sites specific for a particular antigenic configuration; in the case of B-lymphocytes these sites are in fact on immunoglobulins. Among the immunologically competent cells of the body there is such diversity of antigen-receptors that any of a wide range of foreign substances can find at least a few cells capable of binding it. Thus such a substance 'selects' its own lymphocytes, and they respond to contact with it by initiating clones of new cells, each clone producing a response that has the same antigen-specificity as the binding sites on the initiating lymphocyte. Because an antigen is bound most avidly by lymphocytes with receptors that give the best 'fit', a small amount of a new antigen will stimulate highly specific responses, but a larger amount will be more than enough for the most relevant lymphocytes and the excess will be available to bind with and stimulate others that are less appropriate.

Although all lymphocytes stimulated by a given antigenic configuration will initiate responses of roughly or more precisely the same antigen-specificity, the nature of those responses may show great diversity in other respects. If both B- and T-lymphocytes are involved, both antibody production and cell-mediated responses will result. Furthermore, each *individual* B-lymphocyte that is stimulated initiates production of antibody of only one Ig class (p. 55); but stimulation of a *population* of B-lymphocytes may well result in production of antibodies of various Ig classes and subclasses. Still further diversity of response to a given antigen molecule results if different areas of its surface can act separately as antigenic determinants.

Immunological Memory
Immunological responses have a built-in 'memory' that is the basis of long-term immunity and of active immunization (Chapter 20). When an antigen (on its own or as part of an organism) is localized in lymphoid

tissue, specific immunocompetent cells are recruited from the recirculating pool (see below). These cease to circulate, and instead they set up an immunological response locally, by dividing and differentiating to form populations of effector cells. In the case of the B-lymphocyte series these are antibody-secreting *plasma cells.* In addition to plasma cells and sensitized T-lymphocytes, such antigenic stimulation also results in formation of *memory cells*—long-lived specifically sensitized recirculating lymphocytes that are responsible for the faster and greater response to the antigen that occurs when it is encountered again.

ANTIBODIES

Antibodies are a distinct family of proteins with specific activity against antigens (p. 52). They are secreted by plasma cells (see above).

Structure

Antibodies are globulins, and are alternatively known as *immunoglobulins* (Igs). Five major classes are distinguished on the basis of physico-chemical, serological and biological properties and of amino-acid sequences; they are designated IgG, IgM, IgA, IgD and IgE. The molecular structure of IgG is illustrated diagrammatically in Fig. 2. Two heavy and two light polypeptide chains, linked by interchain disulphide bonds, form a Y-shaped molecule. Papain cleavage of the molecule divides it into two

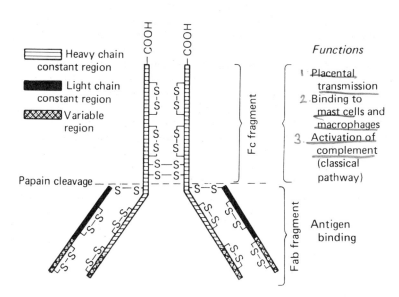

Figure 2 Schematic representation of the 4-chain structure of human IgG (molecular weight approximately 150 000).

Fab (antigen-binding) fragments with identical antigen specificity and an Fc (crystallizable) fragment which contains virtually all structures responsible for the other functions of the antibody. The amino-acid sequences of the N-terminal residues (the antigen-binding sites at the ends of the Fab fragments) vary considerably between immunoglobulin molecules, and determine their antigen-binding specificities; but the remaining parts of the chains are much more constant. IgA, IgD and IgE molecules in the blood are similar in structure to IgG, but secretory IgA found in mucus and other secretions consists of two such units bound to an additional component (see p. 58). An IgM molecule consists of 5 Y-shaped units linked by their Fc regions, so that each such molecule has 10 antigen-binding sites; this structure makes it particularly efficient in binding complement (p. 60). Three-quarters of the total immunoglobulin of normal human serum is IgG, and this is the Ig class that passes most readily from blood into extravascular fluids. Such movement is greatly enhanced during inflammatory processes, when the permeability of blood-vessel walls is increased.

Functions of Antibodies in Protection against Micro-organisms
At various points in this section reference is made to the complement system and its many components (designated C1, C2 etc.). These are explained in the section that begins on p. 60.

OPSONIZATION   Opsonins are substances which combine with surface components of micro-organisms or other particles and increase their susceptibility to phagocytosis (p. 47). Particles with surfaces more hydrophilic than those of the phagocytes are resistant to phagocytosis; and many pathogenic bacteria have surface structures—usually proteins, glycoproteins or polysaccharides—which by virtue of their negative charges make the surfaces hydrophilic. They can be opsonized (by derivation the word means prepared for the table) by attachment of antibodies or complement factors that make their surfaces more hydrophobic. IgG and IgM can each be opsonic, and in each case the antibody molecules first become attached by their Fab portions to their specific antigens on the microbial surfaces. Then in the case of IgG the Fc portions of the molecules become attached to special Fc receptors on phagocyte surfaces. IgM on the other hand, after attachment to its antigen, does not bind directly to phagocytes but fixes and activates complement by the classical pathway (p. 60), generating C3b, which then binds to C3b receptors on the phagocyte surfaces. Binding of the (organism + antibody + complement) complex to the phagocyte surface triggers engulfment, degranulation and a burst of oxidative metabolism (p. 48). The importance of opsonization as a defence against capsulated pathogenic bacteria is illustrated by the high frequency and severity of pneumococcal infections in patients with antibody deficiencies (hypogammaglobulinaemia, pp. 66–7).

BACTERIOLYSIS In some circumstances attachment of antibodies to the surfaces of Gram-negative bacteria is followed by activation of complement components C1–C9 and consequent production of 'holes' in the bacterial cell walls. Complement factors and host enzymes such as lysozyme can enter such a cell, causing damage to the cytoplasmic membrane, loss of its selective permeability and therefore death of the cell. Under the electron microscope, holes similar in appearance and method of production to those in Gram-negative cell walls can be seen in the envelopes of viruses that possess such structures (p. 56). Gram-positive bacteria are resistant to complement-mediated lysis, even though complement is fixed on their surfaces; and capsulate Gram-negative bacteria have decreased susceptibility in proportion to the thickness of their capsules. IgM, having more ability than IgG to fix complement, is more effective in bacteriolysis. The importance of complement-mediated bactericidal systems in protection is illustrated by the increased incidence of severe gonococcal or meningococcal infections in individuals whose serum is congenitally deficient in the late complement components C5–C8 and is therefore devoid of bacteriolytic activity.

TOXIN NEUTRALIZATION As exotoxins are important virulence factors for some bacterial species, so neutralization of such toxins by antibodies (*antitoxins*) is an important defence mechanism. IgG antibodies of appropriate specificity are highly effective for this purpose, but not IgM. Secretory IgA antitoxins are important in protection against toxins released by intestinal pathogens. Antitoxins act by steric inhibition of the reaction between toxins and target cells, and can do no good once the toxin is bound to its target. Consequently, therapeutic administration of antitoxin (p. 292) must be started as early as possible and becomes less effective the longer it is delayed; nor is it effective as soon as it is given intravenously, since it has to pass from the blood into the relevant tissues.

VIRUS NEUTRALIZATION The spread of virus infection can be reduced by the attachment of antibodies to free virus particles—secretory IgA when they are on mucous surfaces and mainly IgG when they are in blood or tissue fluids. Once inside host cells, viruses are protected from such neutralization until they emerge again. Neutralization is effected either by coating the virus particles with antibody or by aggregating them by antibody cross-linking, and so reducing the number of infectious particles. Neutralization is potentiated greatly by the participation of the early components of complement; unlike lysis, this effect does not require components C5–C9.

Placental Transmission of Maternal Antibodies

IgG is the only immunoglobulin class that crosses the human placenta. A neonate has in its blood antibodies that protect it only against organisms to which the mother is immune by virtue of making IgG antibodies. Thus neonates are poorly protected against *Escherichia coli* and other Gram-negative bacilli that stimulate production mainly of IgM; and if removed to special care units or other environments that contain potential pathogens not previously encountered by their mothers, they are particularly liable to succumb to overwhelming infections. Placental transmission of antibodies in humans increases from about the 20th week of pregnancy to reach a maximum in about the 35th week. The length of time for which a neonate is protected against a particular infection depends, among other things, on the level of relevant IgG antibody in the mother's blood in the later stages of pregnancy. Antibody molecules undergo natural degradation, and not much maternal immunity is left by the time that the infant is 3 months old. The importance of the period of transition from passive maternal protection to the establishment of active immunity is illustrated by the account of herd immunity to polioviruses given on p. 51. Congenital defects in the infant's own immunological systems often present themselves clinically as recurrent bouts of infection beginning at about 3 months old. This is also the optimum age for starting some forms of active immunization (see Chapter 20), as presence of maternal antibodies before this time may interfere with the infant's own immune responses to antigens.

The Mucosal Antibody System
As we have seen (p. 54), lymphoid tissue associated with mucous membranes is of particular importance in the defence of the body against microbial invasion. Specialized lymphoid tissue in the intestine (Peyer's patches) and in the respiratory tract is covered with 'microfold' epithelium adapted for taking 'antigenic samples' of the microbial flora of these two regions. B-lymphocytes stimulated by antigen in these areas are transformed into large blast cells which migrate via the lymphatic system to the blood and thence to any of the secretory mucosal tissues in the gut, respiratory tract, salivary and lachrymal glands and lactating breast, and possibly in the urinary tract. They thus provide the basis for a *common mucosal antibody system.* The antibodies are produced by plasma cells derived from the blast cells, and now situated in the mucosal lamina propria. They are IgA molecules, and two such molecules coupled to a secretory piece provided by the epithelial cells constitue *secretory IgA* (p. 56). This is the dominant immunoglobulin in external body fluids, and the degree of surface immunity of an individual correlates with secretory IgA levels rather than with blood antibody levels. It is probable that secretory IgA protects by preventing adhesion of pathogens or binding of toxins to epithelial cells.

New-born babies for the first few weeks produce little IgA but plentiful IgM. Some individuals have a permanent selective inability to make IgA. In both of these situations secretory IgM takes over the role of secretory IgA—and usually plays it very successfully. IgG penetrates to surface secretions only when the mucous membranes are inflamed; it then provides a useful secondary defence system.

Secretory IgA and Breast Milk
Secretory IgA is the dominant immunoglobulin of human milk. It protects the infant's intestinal mucosa against a wide array of pathogens experienced by the mother; for the common mucosal antibody system described above ensures the presence of antibodies reflecting her intestinal and other exposure. This is probably the reason why breast-fed babies have fewer intestinal infections than those fed artificially; and why, particularly in countries with relatively poor standards of hygiene, weaning is often followed by gastro-intestinal infections.

The Role of T-lymphocytes in Antibody Production
Activation of B-lymphocytes by some antigens—e.g. influenza virus haemagglutinins requires 'help' from a special subset of T-lymphocytes called *T helper cells*. Production of IgG, IgA and IgE is particularly dependent in this way on the thymus. In contrast, other antigens—including bacterial capsular polysaccharides and the endotoxins of Gram-negative bacteria—can stimulate B-lymphocytes unaided. The antibody produced is then mainly IgM, and there is little or no memory following a thymus-independent response of this kind. Another subset of T-lymphocytes, *T suppressor cells*, can moderate the intensity of immune responses, and these may be responsible for the immunosuppression (involving both humoral and cell-mediated immunity) seen in many chronic infections.

Time Scale of Antibody Responses
This subject is dealt with more fully on pp. 290–1, in relation to artificial immunization; but for the purpose of understanding the host's immunological responses it is important to appreciate that production of an effective level of antibodies to an antigen not previously encountered by the host almost always takes at least 7–10 days.

Diagnostic Use of Antigen–Antibody Interactions
These interactions are not strictly part of the host's immunological responses—the subject of this chapter—and are discussed in their proper context in Chapter 15 (Immunodiagnosis of Infection). However, the reader needs a brief introduction to them because of frequent references to them in Chapters 9 to 13.

Purposes for which such interactions are studied include (a) detecting and quantifying specific antibodies in serum or other body fluids by means of their reactions with known micro-organisms or their products—usually with the object either of identifying the organism responsible for an infectious illness or of assessing the subject's level of immunity to the organism in question; (b) identifying an unknown organism by means of its ability to react with *antisera* (i.e. sera containing antibodies) of known specificity.

The types of interaction commonly studied for these purposes include: *precipitation* of soluble antigens from solution as antigen–antibody complexes; *agglutination* of suspended micro-organisms into visible clumps by the cross-linking action of antibodies; production in capsulate bacteria of the change in microscopic appearance called *capsule-swelling* and due to the action of specific antibodies; depletion of a known amount of available complement (*complement-fixation*) by its involvement in an antigen–antibody interaction; *attachment of immunoglobulin molecules*— demonstrated by *immunofluorescence* (p. 16) or other means—to the surfaces of micro-organisms or of red blood cells or latex or other particles coated with microbial antigens; and *neutralization, blocking* or *inhibition* of microbial activities by antibodies.

COMPLEMENT AND RESISTANCE TO INFECTION

Though it is often convenient to refer to complement as though it were a single substance (e.g. in the previous paragraph), it is in fact a complex system of some 20 different serum proteins, most of them by now biochemically characterized. Its existence has been known since the beginning of the century, but awareness of the important role played by this complex biological amplification system in the body's antimicrobial defence is far more recent. An orderly sequence of interactions between the protein components of complement leads to the generation of many biologically active substances, and ultimately to the lysis of bacterial or other cells. The possible sequences are indicated in Fig. 3. The system can be activated in either of two ways:

(1) *The classical pathway.* IgM or some IgG antibodies, when combined with their specific antigens, can bind the C1 component, activating it ($\overline{C1}$ in the figure means activated C1, and so on) and so activating the whole sequence.

(2) *The alternative pathway.* A wide range of micro-organisms and their components, and of other substances, can by-pass the early stages of the sequence and activate C3 directly.

In either case the event of central importance in the system is the splitting of C3 into two biologically active components—C3a and C3b. The effects of complement activation which are of greatest importance in defence against infection are:

(a) *Immune adherence.* C3b in particular promotes adherence of micro-organisms or antigen–antibody complexes to phagocytes, as described under Opsonization on p. 56.

(b) *Biological action on host cells.* C3a and C5a both cause release of histamine from mast cells and chemotactic migration of polymorpho-nuclear cells to areas of antigen–antibody interaction, and thus promote

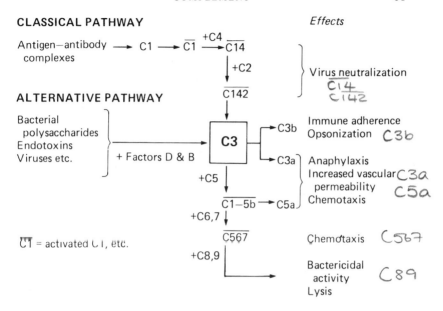

Figure 3 Simplified scheme of complement activation, indicating those effects of complement components that relate to resistance to infection.

both local inflammation and phagocytosis of invading micro-organisms. $\overline{C567}$ is also chemotactic.

(c) *Bacterial cell-wall lesions.* Activation of the complete system through to C9 leads to the formation of 'holes' in cell walls, as described under Bacteriolysis on p. 57. For bacteriolysis to occur, lysozyme is also required.

Complement also enhances virus neutralization by specific antibodies. Much of our information about the activities of complement has come from *in vitro* studies, but patients with deficiencies of individual complement components also throw much light on the role of the complement system in defence against infection. Opsonization, chemotaxis and lysis are all impaired in patients with total C3 deficiency, and they are liable to overwhelming infections with capsulate bacteria such as pneumococci. As we have seen on p. 57, bacteriolysis is much reduced but the other functions are normal in patients with deficiencies of C5, C6 or C8, and they are particularly susceptible to disseminated gonococcal or meningococcal infection.

Two other host mediator systems—the fibrinolytic system and the kinin system—are commonly activated along with the complement system, but homeostatic mechanisms usually limit the intensity of the reaction. However, massive activation sometimes occurs, with serious effects on the patient. Bacterial endotoxins can activate these three systems, with resulting tissue damage, shock and disseminated intravascular coagulation (DIC) and in many cases death of the patient. Such mechanisms probably underlie some of the most serious syndromes associated with microbial infections—acute haemorrhagic adrenal necrosis (the Waterhouse–Friderichsen syndrome, p. 93), 'Gram-negative shock' (p. 25) and the haemorrhages and shock associated with the terminal stages of infection with the haemorrhagic fever viruses (p. 183).

T-LYMPHOCYTES AND CELL-MEDIATED IMMUNITY

We have already considered two of the functional subsets into which T-lymphocytes can be divided—T helpers and T suppressors (p. 59). Other subsets are involved in cell-mediated immunity. Viruses, and some bacteria—notably mycobacteria, brucellae and salmonellae—and various other micro-organisms can cause infections that are relatively resistant to the body's humoral defences (antibodies, complement, etc.) because the infecting organisms are outside their reach, within host cells. Dealing with such intracellular infections is the job of T-lymphocytes of appropriate antigen-specificity. They respond to the antigenic stimulus in a number of ways:

(a) On encountering their specific antigens some sensitized T-cells secrete soluble substances called *lymphokines*. These include chemotactic factors that bring macrophages to the scene of infection; macrophage-migration-inhibiting factor (MIF), that prevents them from going away again; and activators of their cidal activity (against micro-organisms in general, not just against those that stimulated the T-cells). Such 'angry' macrophages themselves secrete other substances that increase the vigour of the inflammatory reaction and its antimicrobial effectiveness. Type 2 interferons are a special class of lymphokines that prevent spread of viruses from cell to cell (p. 49).

(b) Such activities are often accompanied by T-cell-mediated Type IV hypersensitivity reactions to the infecting organisms (see p. 65).

(c) Cytotoxic ('killer') T-cells (p. 53) become detectable 2–4 days after infection with a virus not previously encountered by the host—i.e. several days before such a primary infection has produced any effective antibody response. Thus, while such cytotoxic cells can do nothing to prevent the initial infection, they are of major importance in preventing its further spread and eliminating it. They kill the infected host cells by direct contact, not through the mediation of lymphokines, though lymphokine-producing cells provide valuable help by promoting an inflammatory reaction, stimulating macrophage activity and producing Type 2 interferons.

When the infecting virus is not itself strongly cytopathic, the T-cell response may be more important than the infection in determining the disease manifestations.

Local cell-mediated immunity is independent of its systemic counter-part, and local application of live vaccines is more effective than their parenteral administration in generating local cell-mediated immunity. However, immunity generated in this way is short-lived. Local administration of vaccines consisting of killed organisms or purified microbial products evokes little or no immune response.

Patients with defective T-cell immunity are liable to severe generalized infections, particularly with herpes or pox viruses, mycobacteria or fungi. It is dangerous to give them live vaccines.

HYPERSENSITIVITY REACTIONS

Encounter with a foreign substance sometimes provokes immunological responses that lead to a state of *acquired hypersensitivity* to that substance. Such a state manifests itself in vigorous reactions that occur when the host again encounters the same substance, and such reactions cause damage to his tissues, varying in degree from minor local inflammation to severe illness or even death. Acquired hypersensitivity must be distinguished from *idiosyncrasy*, an abnormal sensitivity to a pharmacologically active compound (e.g. aspirin or morphine) which does not depend on previous experience of the compound and is often familial.

Gell and Coombs have classified hypersensitivity reactions into four main types, differing in their underlying mechanisms.

Type I (Anaphylactic-Type or Immediate Hypersensitivity) Reactions
These reactions depend on special antibodies, known as reaginic or homocytotropic antibodies and belonging predominantly to class IgE; these become attached by their Fc regions to the host's mast cells. Cross-linking of two cell-bound IgE molecules by the sensitizing antigen (*allergen*) leads to release of histamine and other pharmacologically active substances from the mast cells. These substances are responsible for the clinical manifestations of this type of hypersensitivity, which range from mild eczema through hay-fever, asthma and urticaria to acute anaphylactic shock—which is sometimes fatal. Anaphylaxis in man is rare, but can follow injection of foreign serum protein (e.g. antiserum from horses), of vaccines or of drugs (notably, in the microbiological context, of penicillins) in previously sensitized patients.

If a small amount of the sensitizing agent is injected intradermally into an already sensitized subject, a local *immediate-type* reaction consisting of a wheal with surrounding erythema develops within a few minutes. Such a procedure is used in identifying the agent or agents to which a particular patient is sensitized, and also illustrates the course of events which follows natural exposure to such agents. Type I reactions occurring in infected tissues can increase vascular permeability and so aid the protective mechanisms by enhancing diffusion of antibodies and other serum factors to the place where they are needed. In allergic lung disease, on the other hand, preceding Type I reactions are probably important in determining the site of deposition of immune complexes and the consequent local Type III reactions. Thus patients with allergic bronchopulmonary aspergillosis give a dual (Type I + Type III) response to skin or bronchial challenge with aspergillus antigen (p. 204).

Type II Reactions
IgM or IgG antibodies, formed in response to infection, may react either with host-cell surface antigens resembling their 'proper' targets or with micro-organisms or their products that have become attached to host cell membranes. Such a reaction may lead to complement-mediated cell damage or destruction. As an example, most patients with *Mycoplasma pneumoniae* infection develop 'cold agglutinins'—antibodies active only at low temperatures and with an affinity for the I antigen found on adult human red blood cells. These antibodies are useful in the laboratory diagnosis of such infections and are probably responsible for the mild haemolytic anaemia that may occur.

Type III (Immune Complex) Reactions
Formation of antigen–antibody complexes is normally followed by their removal from the circulation by phagocytic cells of the reticulo-endothelial system, and is then beneficial to the host. However, immune complexes formed in the presence of slight antigen excess may circulate widely and be deposited in vascular basement membranes, with harmful effects. Renal glomeruli, the choroid plexus, synovial membranes, the uveal tract and the skin are particularly vulnerable because of their high blood flows and intricate capillary beds. Deposition of complexes can lead to fixation and activation of complement, with chemotactic accumulation of neutrophils that release vaso-active substances and powerful hydrolytic enzymes; local tissue damage results. Common clinical manifestations of such a process are proteinuria, joint pains and skin rashes. The classical example is the *serum sickness* which follows repeated injection of horse antiserum (e.g. for protection against tetanus) and the development by the patient of antibodies to horse serum proteins. Local challenge—e.g. by intradermal injection—with an antigen to which the patient is immune, either actively or passively (p. 49), may produce a local *Arthus reaction*, similar in mechanism to systemic Type III reactions. This takes some 5–8 hours to develop and 24 hours to resolve. 'Farmer's lung' and other forms of allergic alveolitis following repeated inhalation of fine organic dusts were formerly thought to be pure Type III reactions to absorption of antigen through the alveolar lining; but it is now clear that the mini-granulomata of the lungs which are largely responsible for the typical radiological appearances of the chest in this disease are a form of Type IV reaction triggered by the presence of non-degradable complexes of fungal antigen and antibody.

Type IV (Cell-Mediated or Delayed-Type) Reactions

The mechanism of these reactions is as described for cell-mediated immunity (p. 62). The hallmarks of a Type IV hypersensitivity reaction to a skin test—e.g. the tuberculin reaction (p. 253)—are that its development is delayed, taking 48–72 hours to reach the maximum response, and that there is palpable induration, due to lymphocyte and macrophage infiltration of the dermis. It is probable that hypersensitivity of this type arises in all acute and chronic infections, and could be demonstrated by skin tests using appropriate antigens.

FACTORS THAT INFLUENCE IMMUNITY

The various immunological mechanisms that we have considered are influenced by many factors that greatly affect their vigour and effectiveness, including those that we shall now discuss.

Age

The human foetus begins to make antibody (IgM) at about 11 weeks of gestation and immunocompetent T-cells are detectable at about 14 weeks. This is too late to deal with some infections that reach it through the placenta. For example, when a non-immune mother develops rubella during the first trimester of pregnancy, dissemination of the virus in the foetus is unchecked and serious damage may be done to the developing organs. Foetal IgM and maternal IgG appear in the foetal circulation after the damage is done, but the child is born with a congenital rubella infection (p. 175). Presence of IgM in the cord blood (necessarily foetal, as IgM cannot cross the placenta) is evidence of such infection.

From the time of birth the neonate begins to meet innumerable new antigenic stimuli and potentially pathogenic organisms. IgA production is negligible at first and does not reach adult levels till puberty; but the breast-fed infant enjoys protection given by maternal IgA (p. 59), as well as that from placentally transmitted IgG (p. 57). By degrees a pool of memory cells is built up that enables the infant to respond rapidly to subsequent infective challenge; but it seems that the ability to respond to some kinds of antigen takes months or years to develop. For example, bacterial polysaccharides from pneumococci, meningococci or capsulate *Haemophilus influenzae*, encountered naturally or as vaccines, elicit little or no antibody response from children under the age of $1\frac{1}{2}$–2 years—a serious matter in relation to protection against *H. influenzae* type b, a common cause of meningitis and other life-threatening infections in the first year or so of life.

At the other end of life, ageing is associated with increasing susceptibility to many kinds of infection. Impaired blood circulation and consequent tissue anoxia, degenerative changes in vital organs, underlying chronic or malignant disease, and in many cases dietary deficiencies are possible contributors to this situation, giving added emphasis to the decline in efficiency of the defence mechanisms themselves.

Genetics

Resistance to infection, innate or acquired (p. 49), is under genetic control. The nature and size of immune responses to antigenic stimulation are determined by sets of *immune response genes*, and some of these are closely linked to the genes that control the histocompatibility antigens involved in graft rejection. There is an association between possession of some histocompatibility antigens and liability to certain forms of infection—e.g. between possession of antigen HLA-B27 and development of reactive arthritis following salmonella, yersinia or campylobacter infections. The mechanisms of such connections are far from clear, but possible explanations of their existence include (a) bacterial antigens that resemble host HLA antigens and are therefore exempt from host attack (p. 69); or (b) close linkage between the genes determining the HLA antigens and those controlling susceptibility to such infections.

Immunodeficiency and Immunosuppression

Primary immunodeficiencies are congenital or genetically determined defects in immunological defence mechanisms which can be classified as follows:

(1) Deficiency of B-lymphocytes and so of immunoglobulins—hence the name *hypogammaglobulinaemia*.

(2) Thymic hypoplasia and consequent T-lymphocyte deficiency.

(3) Deficiency of the stem cells from which both B- and T-lymphocytes are derived, and thus deficiency of both of these cell types.

(4) Deficiencies of neutrophils and monocytes, resulting in disorders of phagocytosis and killing of micro-organisms.

(5) Complement deficiencies.

The life expectation of patients with these conditions has been considerably increased by treatment with antibacterial drugs and injections of normal human gammaglobulin for (1), with grafts of normal thymus for (2), with grafts of normal bone marrow for (3), with granulocyte transfusions and bactericidal antibiotics for (4), and with plasma infusions for (5).

When discussing the immunological mechanisms we have indicated the types of infection to be expected in patients with any one of these deficiencies. Rather fuller information is given in Table III. Such patients have taught us a great deal about the mechanisms of immunity, but are far less common than patients with *secondary immunodeficiencies* due to malnutrition, underlying malignant or other diseases, or the use of immunosuppressive or cytotoxic drugs. Infections can cause direct immunosuppression. For example, there is a transient suppression of T-cell-mediated immunity in some acute virus infections, notably measles, and this opens up the way for secondary bacterial infections. Extensive use is made in modern medicine of drugs that are intended to achieve immunosuppression (e.g. to prevent graft rejection) or to damage abnormal host cells but at the expense of some damage to normal cells (e.g. the cytotoxic drugs used in treatment of leukaemias and other malignant diseases). Such therapy may unmask latent infection—e.g. with herpes simplex virus; and all patients treated with such drugs are exposed to enhanced risks of exogenous and endogenous infections, even with organisms of little or no virulence to healthy people, and have to be protected accordingly. In special cases of extreme immunosuppression it may be necessary to reduce the patient's microbial population very substantially and to use strict protective isolation, as described on pp. 272–3, to protect him from all extraneous organisms. In less extreme cases it is usually wise to disturb the balance of the patient's normal microbial population as little as possible, and to use antimicrobial drugs for precise treatment of actual infections rather than for diffuse cover against a wide range of potential pathogens; a normal ecological balance may be the patient's best protection, in the absence of humoral and cell-mediated immunity, against external pathogens and even against 'opportunist' activity of normal residents

Table III   Important pathogens in patients with different kinds of immunodeficiency

Disorders of phagocytosis and killing	B-lymphocyte defects	T-lymphocyte defects
Staphylococci	Pneumococci	Measles virus
Klebsiellae	Haemophilus	Varicella virus
Serratia species	influenzae	Cytomegalovirus
Candida	Streptococci	Mycobacterium
albicans	Meningococci	tuberculosis
	Pseudomonas	Legionella
	aeruginosa	pneumophila
	Hepatitis viruses	Candida
	Enteroviruses	albicans
	Mycoplasma	Aspergillus species
	pneumoniae	Pneumocystis
		carini

The use of italics for some of these names is in keeping with the conventions explained on p. 72, and does not indicate special importance.

Hormones
There is a close developmental and functional association between the immune system and the neuro-endocrine network. Even psychosocial factors can alter immunity. For example, it is suggested that stress stimulates the hypothalamic–pituitary axis, causing increased ACTH secretion and a consequent rise in circulating corticosteroid levels. Corticosteroids, produced in excess in this way or given therapeutically, may be immunosuppressive and increase susceptibility to some infections.

Malnutrition

In the world as a whole this is the commonest cause of secondary immunodeficiencies. It operates not only where there is famine but even in such apparently improbable places as the wards of major hospitals, where patients with serious diseases or unable over long periods to take normal diets may develop unsuspected but important nutritional deficiencies. Vitamins and many other dietary components are important to the body's defences, and protein deficiency has an obvious relevance to defence mechanisms that depend on rapid production of immunoglobulins. Malnutrition, impaired immunity and infection can become an inextricable triad, each of which can exacerbate the others. Their interaction can result in a range of clinical conditions similar to those listed in Table III as associated with primary immunodeficiencies. Most immunological defects of nutritional origin can be corrected by providing an adequate diet; but foetal malnutrition may result in long-term immunosuppression. If vaccination of previously malnourished children is to be effective, it must be accompanied by adequate supplementation of their diet. In severe protein-energy malnutrition there is marked involution of the thymus, and consequent lack of T-cell-mediated immunity; this is reflected in the frequency with which children suffering from such malnutrition die of tuberculosis, herpes simplex or measles. Measles in particular is a scourge in these circumstances, and has special clinical features—notably absence of rash, since this is a T-cell-mediated manifestation of the infection, and frequent presence of giant-cell pneumonia caused by the virus.

Chronic Infections

As already indicated, these may result in secondary immunodeficiencies, often by an interplay with malnutrition. The existence of a chronic infection also implies that the host's defences are not adequate to eliminate it. In some such infections the invading organisms themselves induce immunosuppression (e.g. in lepromatous leprosy, p. 135). In others they evade the defences by undergoing changes of their surface antigens (e.g. relapsing fever, p. 143, trypanosomiasis, p. 210), or even— as in the case of herpes simplex virus (p. 185)—by being integrated into the host-cell DNA and so escaping detection over long periods. Some chronic infections are due to organisms that do relatively little harm to host tissues in the short term and are rather weak stimulators of immunity. Examples of this are tuberculosis, leprosy and syphilis; and the interesting variations in immune responses and in consequent clinical manifestations that occur in these diseases are described in Chapter 9.

IMMUNOLOGICAL TOLERANCE AND AUTO-IMMUNITY

When an antigen binds to the surface of a lymphocyte, the usual result is stimulation of the cell and an immune response. Under certain conditions, however, the immunocompetent cell may be switched off or deleted, and *tolerance* of the antigen results. The fact that the body's immunological mechanisms do not normally take action against its own constituents—*self-antigens*—is due to suppression or deletion, during foetal life, of lymphocyte clones with receptors for self-antigens. *Auto-immunity* is a break-down of self-tolerance.

Clone suppression operates mainly against T-lymphocytes. B-lymphocytes with self-antigen specificity circulate in small numbers in the blood of normal adults. They may be stimulated by certain micro-organisms—e.g. the EB virus of infectious mononucleosis—or by microbial products such as endotoxin, since these are liable to stimulate B-cells in general, not merely those with specific affinity for them. Thus patients recovering from infectious mononucleosis may have a wide spectrum of *auto-antibodies* in their blood. Micro-organisms with antigenic components closely resembling those on the surfaces of host cells, and viruses that can alter such host antigens so that they appear to be 'non-self', can stimulate T helper cells, which co-operate with the self-reactive B cells to produce auto-antibodies. Chronic massive tissue destruction, as in leprosy, releases intracellular antigens unfamiliar to the host's immunological system, and also enzymes that alter host-cell surface antigens; such apparently non-self antigens may provoke immunological reactions. The mere presence of auto-antibodies does not necessarily result in *auto-immune disease*. When tissue damage does occur, it is mediated through Type II, III or IV hypersensitivity reactions.

Suggestions for Further Reading

Essential Immunology by I. M. Roitt, 4th edn. (Blackwell, Oxford, 1980).

Basic and Clinical Immunology by H. H. Fudenberg *et al.*, 3rd edn. (Lange Medical Publications, Los Altas, California, 1980).

Clinical Aspects of Immunology by P. J. Lachmann, S. J. Smith and D. K. Peters, 4th edn. (Blackwell, Oxford, 1982).

PART IV

PART IV

MICRO-ORGANISMS OF MEDICAL IMPORTANCE

CHAPTER 9

BACTERIA

BACTERIAL TAXONOMY AND NOMENCLATURE

Bacterial nomenclature can be a source of bewilderment and frustration to medical students, and even to some experienced clinicians. It is, however, a short-hand system of great value to those who learn to read it (and keep up with the changes necessitated by improvements in bacterial taxonomy). When a bacterium has been isolated from a clinical specimen and put through appropriate identification tests, the bacteriologist knows whether it is similar to previous isolates from the same or associated patients, and whether it is likely to be clinically important in the situation from which it was isolated. To communicate this information to his laboratory and clinical colleagues in a few words, he needs a name for the organism. The early device of naming a bacterium according to the disease that it causes—'the typhoid bacillus', 'the tubercle bacillus'—was valid only for those few organisms that are always and exclusively associated with particular diseases. Naming organisms after their discoverers—Koch's bacillus, etc.—was even less useful. Clearly medical bacteriology needed a comprehensive system of bacterial classification and nomenclature—ideally one acceptable in all countries and shared by non-medical bacteriologists.

An obvious choice was the system of orders, families, genera and species, with appropriate Latin (i.e. international) names, used so successfully in other branches of biology. However, vigorous efforts over many years to fit bacteria into such a system have met with limited success, for a number of reasons. Unlike most other biologists, bacteriologists are dealing not with individual organisms but, at best, with what are euphemistically described as *pure cultures*—i.e. populations of individuals all derived from the same single organism, but no longer necessarily identical in genotype or phenotype (see pp. 27–9). The term *strain* is used for a group of pure cultures derived from a common source and thought to be the same—e.g. all apparently identical pure cultures derived from a single clinical specimen, or from different specimens from the same patient, or even from a number of victims of a common-source outbreak of infection. A group of closely similar strains can be said to constitute a *species*, but defining species boundaries among bacteria is a peculiarly difficult problem; cross-fertility, a valuable criterion for this purpose among higher organisms, has no relevance to asexual creatures that are capable of interchange of genetic material between manifestly 'unrelated' individuals (see p. 28). Bacterial species have therefore to be defined according to other criteria, and there has been almost unlimited scope for disagreement as to what these should be. The larger the number of criteria applied, the greater the range of possible permutations becomes and the more apparent it is that the boundaries are in fact artificial. Grouping of species into *genera* also presents problems, and many bacterial taxonomists have given up trying to fit genera into families and families into orders.

An alternative to this approach of selecting *the important* criteria for classification into species and genera is the Adansonian or numerical approach of applying to each bacterial strain the same large range of criteria, all regarded as of *equal importance*; the strain is given a score of + 1 if the character sought by a given test is present, and − 1 if it is absent. This approach has its merits, particularly as a means of sorting large groups of basically similar organisms into clusters of strains of much closer similarity, or as a basis for computer-matching of the properties of an unidentified strain with those of a large number of reference strains; but it has not yet produced an overall system of classification which is of value to the clinical bacteriologist.

Traditional methods of bacterial classification have relied on phenotypic characters as indicators of genotype. A more recent approach, useful in research but not applicable to routine diagnostic bacteriology, is direct analysis of DNA. Determination of the (guanine + cytosine) : (adenine + thymine) ratio in DNA provides useful information—not as a basis for positive classification, since similarity of base-pair ratios is no evidence of overall DNA similarity, but as a means of challenging inclusion in the same species or genus of two strains with markedly differing ratios. Similarities and differences in DNA composition can be demonstrated more precisely by studying homologous segments in DNA extracts. The strands of double-stranded DNA separate on heating and re-associate on cooling. If a mixture of DNAs from two bacterial strains is heated and cooled, the amount of cross-over in the reassociation stage provides an indication of the degree of homology between the two DNAs; prior radio-labelling of one of the two DNAs allows this to be measured precisely. With classification soundly based on such research methods, appropriate simple tests for phenotypic characters can be selected for routine diagnostic work.

Despite all the problems, there is at present a useful level of international agreement about the classification into genera and species of most bacteria of medical importance, and about the standardization of Latin binomials for them. The International Committee on Systematic Bacteriology has made a major effort to tidy up outstanding problems, to put an end to arguments about historical priority of names, and to regulate future changes of names. Scope must of course be left for discovery of new organisms or of new information invalidating the classification of known organisms, but not for the individual bacteriologist to revise names or introduce new ones according to his personal fancy.

Meanwhile the medical student needs a working knowledge of the language. He must reconcile himself to the fact that a Linnean binomial, while it tells the genus (first name, capital first letter) and species (second name, no capital) to which the organism is assigned, may for historical reasons suggest something which is no longer to be believed—e.g. that *Haemophilus influenzae* is the cause of or related to influenza. (Names of humans can be equally inappropriate!) History has created many other nomenclatural problems. For example, the word bacillus, without an initial capital, means any rod-shaped bacterium, and at one time most of these were given the generic name *Bacillus*; now, however, that generic name is confined to aerobic spore-bearing rods (see p. 101), and other rod-shaped organisms (bacilli) are assigned to a large number of other genera. Many species have undergone several changes of name, and some still have alternative binomials in common use, as well as less formal names in many cases. Thus *Streptococcus pneumoniae = Diplococcus pneumoniae* = the pneumococcus. In this book we follow the general custom of using conventional abbreviations for generic names (e.g. *B.* for *Bacillus*, *Br.* for *Brucella*, *S.* for *Salmonella*, *Staph.* for *Staphylococcus*, *Str.* for *Streptococcus*) when the names are being frequently repeated or should have become familiar; and we sometimes employ widely used informal names instead of Linnaean names so that they also will become familiar to our readers. Alternative names are given in brackets following the headings of many sections dealing with individual species.

It is customary to print generic names in italics with a capital first letter when they are used in the singular—e.g. *Staphylococcus* or *Staph.*—but without italics and with a lower-case first letter when they are used as adjectives or in the plural as collective names for organisms belonging to the genus—e.g. staphylococcus (or staphylococcal) strains and staphylococci. Clearly the latter part of the convention cannot be applied to the generic name *Bacillus*.

SPECIAL MORPHOLOGICAL FEATURES

We gave a brief account of bacterial morphology on pp. 12–14, but deferred until this chapter a fuller description of certain special features.

Capsules

A number of bacterial species—e.g. *Streptococcus pneumoniae, Klebsiella pneumoniae, Bacillus anthracis*—characteristically form capsules which surround their cell walls. In most cases these capsules consist of complex polysaccharides, but that of *B. anthracis* is predominantly a polypeptide. Capsules are not satisfactorily shown in preparations stained by ordinary methods, but can be demonstrated by 'negative staining', in which the background between the bacteria is filled with some opaque material such as indian ink; the capsules then show up as unstained holes around the bacterial cells, which can be made more visible by simple positive staining. Capsular development is determined by environmental conditions, and is usually best when the organism is growing in living tissues. The protective value of capsules is discussed on p. 42 and their immunological significance on pp. 48, 56 and 60.

Flagella

These are long, thin thread-like appendages, about 0.02 μm in diameter, which project from the cells of certain bacteria. They have their origin in basal granules in the bacterial protoplast and pass through the cell wall. They are composed almost entirely of protein. The original Latin meaning of *flagellum* is 'a whip', and it is to movements of these appendages that flagellate bacteria owe their motility. Flagella cannot be demonstrated under the light microscope unless they are first considerably thickened by the deposition on their surfaces of special stains. They can be studied more satisfactorily by electron microscopy. Demonstration of motility due to flagella is mentioned on pp. 15 and 109.

Spores

These are round or oval structures formed by bacteria of the genera *Bacillus* and *Clostridium*. Sporulation appears to be in general a reaction to conditions that are unfavourable for normal growth, in particular to deficiency of essential nutrients. The spore has a low water content, its metabolic activity is minimal, and it is surrounded by a thick protective coat which enables it to resist heat, desiccation and other harmful agencies far better than do the vegetative forms (see pp. 31 and 33). Bacterial spores, unlike those of fungi, are not reproductive; one vegetative cell usually produces one spore, which in turn germinates to form a single new vegetative cell. Certain trigger substances (e.g. L-alanine for some species) are needed to initiate the germination of spores.

A spore may be narrower than the bacillus in which it originates, or it may distend it (see Fig. 5, p. 81). Depending on the species, it may be at the end of the bacillus (terminal), near the end (subterminal) or in the middle (central). When mature it is freed from the bacillary cell, which then distintegrates.

Cell Walls, Protoplasts, Spheroplasts and L-Forms

The cell wall is a rigid structure which maintains the shape of the bacterium and prevents it from disrupting under the influence of high internal osmotic pressure. The component responsible for its rigidity is *mucopeptide* (see p. 13). This constitues 50–90 % of the walls of Gram-positive bacteria but only 5–10 % of those of Gram-negative bacteria, which have a thicker outer layer as described on p. 24. Polymers of glycerol phosphate or ribitol phosphate known as *teichoic acids* are found in the cell walls of Gram-positive but not of Gram-negative bacteria. Gram's staining procedure (see p. 16 and 77) had been in use for about 75 years, as an empirical means of dividing bacteria into two major groups, before these differences in cell-wall composition of the groups were demonstrated; the cell wall of Gram-positive bacteria is relatively impermeable to the complex of dye and iodine. Some bacteria are particularly susceptible to the action of lysozymes (enzymes of human, animal or bacterial origin which attack mucopeptide—see p. 45) and by such action they are converted into *protoplasts*. These are complete cells apart from the loss of their cell walls, or at least of important wall components, and consequent loss of rigidity, shape and osmotic resistance. They survive only if kept in suitably hypertonic environments. They are metabolically active and can grow but cannot multiply. Similar structures without cell walls can be produced from suitable organisms by the action of an antibiotic such as penicillin, which prevents mucopeptide synthesis (see p. 35). But many bacteria, under the influence of penicillin or of any of a variety of other agents, *in vitro* or *in vivo*, produce either *spheroplasts* or *L-forms*. Spheroplasts have residual but damaged cell walls and assume bizarre shapes, but when transferred to suitable culture media free from the agent that caused them they may be able to produce orthodox colonies composed of normal individuals. L-forms, on the other hand, are not ordinary bacteria with damaged cell walls, but mutants that do not form cell walls and have been selected out by an environment unsuitable for those bacteria that do form them. As might be expected, these L-forms are delicate and friable, but they differ from protoplasts in being able to multiply. When grown on solid media they form characteristic small 'fried egg' colonies, with central smooth portions deeply embedded in the medium and consisting mainly of minute round forms, and more superficial peripheral zones in which much larger irregular forms are found. Attention has repeatedly been drawn in recent years to the possibility that many kinds of bacteria, when confronted with unfavourable conditions in the body, may persist there as relatively undetectable L-forms and in that state be in some way better able to resist the host's defences.

ISOLATION AND IDENTIFICATION OF BACTERIA

Isolation of an organism as a pure culture is often a necessary preliminary to its identification as belonging to a particular species—though, as we shall see, a great deal of information about identity may be revealed during the process of isolation; but some bacteria can be identified, provisionally or even definitively, by direct examination of the original material. This may be achieved by microscopy of suitable preparations, looking for characteristic morphological features or staining reactions, for capsule swelling (p. 60) or for fluorescent-antibody attachment (also p. 60); or by other methods, such as those mentioned on p. 3. Even so, it is still necessary in most cases to isolate the organism, so as to be able to confirm its provisional identification or to test its antibiotic sensitivities or to acquire other valuable information about it.

The common procedure for obtaining a pure culture of a bacterium is to spread a little of the original material over the surface of a solid culture medium in such a way that individual bacteria, or small clumps of attached and so presumably related individuals, are well separated from one another. On incubation of the culture a distinct pile or *colony* of bacteria is formed by each individual bacterium or clump of attached individuals (in technical language, each colony-forming unit or CFU) that finds the conditions suitable for its multiplication. One of Robert Koch's valuable contributions to bacteriological technique was the use of *agar*, a seaweed derivative, as a means of solidifying media. Added in small amounts (1.5–2 %) to a heated fluid culture medium, this substance causes it to set to a firm jelly when cooled to about 40 °C. This low setting point allows heat-labile ingredients, such as red blood cells, to be added to a medium while it is still fluid. On the other hand, once set the medium will not melt until it is heated to nearly 100 °C, and there is consequently no danger of its liquefying at ordinary incubation temperatures. Agar media are commonly used in circular, flat-bottomed plastic *Petri dishes*, 9 cm or so in diameter, with close-fitting lids. Media and dishes must be sterilized before use (see Chapter 17).

Culture in such a dish (plate culture) can be used to obtain pure cultures from a mixture of bacteria as follows:

(1) The material to be investigated is spread over a segment of the surface of the medium (see Fig. 4, p. 76).
(2) A wire loop, sterilized by heating in a flame and then allowed to cool, is passed several times through the inoculated area on to a fresh area of medium. The bacteria will thus be less thickly spread on this second area than on the first.
(3) Similar transfers are made from the second area to a third and so on until the whole surface of the plate has been used.

In this way, as illustrated diagrammatically in Fig. 4, there is usually at least one area of the plate on which the bacteria are deposited sufficiently

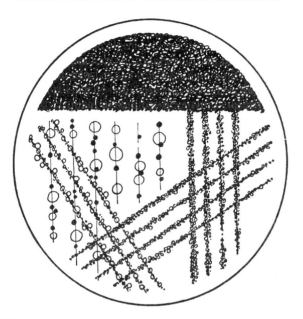

Figure 4 Diagram of plating out of a mixture of bacteria, as described in the text. Note that where the colonies are more widely separated they are larger and more obviously diverse.

far apart to form separate colonies after incubation. In medical bacteriology 37 °C is the usual incubation temperature and most organisms produce colonies large enough for recognition within 18 hours. It is then possible to see whether the original material contained a mixture of bacteria, and to select single colonies for microscopic examination and subculture.

By this stage, we have already learned a lot about the bacterium that is being investigated. We know something about *conditions in which it will grow*, and if we have used several media and various conditions of incubation, we may also know something about conditions in which it will not grow. For example, it may have grown on *nutrient agar*—i.e. a simple broth solidified with agar—but failed to do so on *MacConkey's agar*, which contains bile salts and so is inhibitory to most non-intestinal organisms; or it may have grown on neither of these but on *blood agar*— i.e. nutrient agar to which has been added 5–10 % of blood, commonly horse blood. It may have shown itself to be a strict anaerobe by growing only on plates incubated in an air-tight jar from which all oxygen has been removed; or it may have become clear that it is a strict aerobe or a facultative organism. (Techniques for anaerobic culture are considered on pp. 222–3).

On plates on which the organism has grown, it will have revealed its characteristic *colonial appearances*. In the interpretation of these we have to make allowances for various factors, including the composition of the medium, the conditions and duration of incubation, recent exposure of the organism to antibiotics, and genotypic or phenotypic variations in the organism itself; so that a 'pure' culture may show two or more colonial variants on the same plate and widely different appearances on different media, and may undergo progressive changes of colonial morphology on repeated subculture. Despite all of this, it is possible to describe, for a given species grown under defined conditions on a specified medium, the size, shape, surface appearance, colour, opacity, consistency and other features of typical colonies and of common variants. Bacteriologists have built up a large vocabulary of descriptive terms for this purpose, but these need not concern us here.

We may also have observed *changes in the culture media* produced by the growing bacteria, such as the appearance of clear, colourless zones around and beneath the colonies of many species grown on blood agar; this is due to lysis of the red blood cells (haemolysis). Many culture media contain ingredients specifically intended to detect particular chemical activities of bacteria. For example, MacConkey's medium, mentioned above as containing bile salts, also contains lactose and neutral red, so that colonies of lactose-fermenting bacteria have a red colour on this medium due to acid-production. (From now on, we shall frequently use the term 'fermenting' as synonymous with 'producing acid from', rather than in the strict sense defined on p. 22).

It is likely that we already know something about the *microscopic appearance and staining properties* of our organism, having examined appropriate preparations of the original material. We can now confirm this morphological information by examining the pure culture. By far the most commonly used procedure for this purpose is to suspend a little of the growth in a drop of water on a microscope slide, dry it, fix the organisms to the slide by gentle heat, and then stain them by *Gram's* method. In this, methyl violet or gentian violet is applied first, followed by iodine as a mordant. After such treatment, some organisms, known as *Gram-positive*, resist decolorization by ethyl alcohol or acetone and remain violet or blue in colour. Others, known as *Gram-negative*, readily give up the violet dye and can then be stained red by a counterstain such as neutral red, dilute carbol fuchsin or safranin. This distinction is not absolute, in that faulty technique can give equivocal or wrong results and even in the most skilled hands some strains are difficult to classify. Very young or old cultures may give anomalous reactions. The procedure is open to criticism, in common with any similar staining method, on the grounds that the objects seen down the microscope are distorted artefacts, bearing little resemblance to the original live bacteria. Despite this, Gram's technique provides a division of bacteria, or at least of cocci and bacilli, which is of great practical value, depending as it does on a difference in cell-wall structure that has important effects on various properties of the bacteria (though Gram, who introduced the method in 1884, did not know this).

In the great majority of cases we can now classify our bacterium as a Gram-positive or a Gram-negative coccus or bacillus. Distinction between cocci and bacilli is sometimes difficult if individual cells are studied, but is usually fairly easy if a large number of organisms from the same culture are examined together. Bacterial strains that are classified as cocci may show variation of individual shape from spherical to oval, but never to rod-shaped forms. Bacilli on the other hand may include many very short rods ('cocco-bacilli'), but indisputable rods are nearly always to be found, and filamentous forms may also be present. A culture which shows unusual diversity of size and shape is described as pleomorphic. When all organisms in a particular culture are of indeterminate coccobacillary shape, examination of the same strain grown on a different medium or incubated for a longer or shorter time will usually resolve the doubt.

Table IV shows the classification of some medically important genera of cocci and bacilli according to their Gram-staining reaction. Examination of a Gram-stained film may also enable us to place our organism in its appropriate genus or even species. For example, Gram-positive cocci in definite chains = *Streptococcus*; Gram-positive bacilli with spores = *Bacillus* or *Clostridium* (and the spores of the two genera are usually distinguishable); lactobacilli and some members of the genus *Bacillus* are arranged in chains, whereas corynebacteria lie side-by-side or in bundles. These and other distinctive morphological features are illustrated in Fig. 5 (p. 81). Among the Gram-negative bacilli, all the enterobacteria and members of the genus *Pseudomonas* look much

Table IV   *Some Medically Important Genera of Cocci and Bacilli*

Gram-positive	*Gram-negative*	
COCCI	COCCI	
Staphylococcus	*Neisseria*	
Streptococcus		
	BACILLI	
BACILLI	(a) Enterobacteria	(c) *Vibrio*
Corynebacterium	*Escherichia*	*Campylobacter*
Lactobacillus	*Klebsiella*	(d) Parvobacteria
Bacillus	*Salmonella*	*Haemophilus*
Clostridium	*Shigella*	*Bordetella*
(*Mycobacterium*)[1]	*Proteus*	*Brucella*
	Yersinia	*Legionella*
	(b) *Pseudomonas*	(e) *Bacteroides*

[1] Some mycobacteria, including *Myco. tuberculosis*, are stained only faintly or not at all by Gram's method.

the same in stained films, but are appreciably larger than most of the parvobacteria.

Having obtained our organism in pure culture, examined it by Gram's method and added up all of the evidence already available, we can proceed to further investigations appropriate to the group to which it seems likely to belong. These may include special staining procedures, subculture on other media or under different incubation conditions, tests of carbohydrate fermentation or other biochemical properties, or serological analysis of antigenic composition. Injection into animals may also be necessary, either in order to confirm the identity of the organism or to assess its virulence.

The rest of this chapter deals with groups of bacteria in the following order:

(1) Gram-positive cocci.
(2) Gram-negative cocci.
(3) Gram positive bacilli.
(4) Gram-negative bacilli
(5) Acid-fast bacteria.
(6) Branching bacteria.
(7) Spirochaetes.
(8) Mycoplasmas.

The properties of these organisms in laboratory cultures and also their recognition and isolation from clinical specimens are discussed here, but the collection and handling of clinical specimens is dealt with more fully in Chapter 14. Treatment mentioned in the present chapter is purely antibacterial; no mention is made of the other aspects of the management of patients with bacterial infections.

GRAM-POSITIVE COCCI

The patterns of arrangement of cocci, as seen under the microscope, are a valuable guide to generic distinctions in this group (p. 13). The grape-like clusters from which the genus *Staphylococcus* gets its name are best seen in pus and other body fluids (Fig. 5(*a*), p. 81); films made from cultures may show small clusters and short chains, but as a rule most of the cocci are distributed at random. Sets of 4 cocci in squares and larger geometrically arranged packets are formed by members of the usually non-pathogenic genus *Micrococcus*. Chain-formation is characteristic of the genus *Streptococcus* (Fig. 5(*b*), p. 81).

THE GENUS STAPHYLOCOCCUS

Staphylococci make a very large contribution to man's normal commensal flora and also account for a high proportion of his acute and chronic suppurative lesions. The majority of strains isolated from such lesions produce golden-yellow colonies on common culture media and so they have long been classified as *Staph. aureus*. However, pigment production is a variable property, somewhat at the mercy of conditions of growth, and furthermore some strains which constantly fail to produce pigment are highly pathogenic. The capacity to produce *coagulase* (see below) appears to be a more stable character and is more closely correlated with pathogenicity. The name *Staph. aureus* is currently applied to all strains which are coagulase-positive (i.e. produce coagulase), including a minority which form white colonies. Strains belonging to this species are commonly found as commensals, as well as in lesions, but so far as our present knowledge goes they are all to be regarded as potential pathogens. On the other hand, many of the staphylococci found on the skin and in the upper respiratory tract are coagulase-negative. These almost invariably form white colonies and are at most only low-grade pathogens. They are now classified by taxonomists as *Staph. epidermidis*, though the name *Staph. albus* (originally including all white-colonied staphylococci) is still in common use as an alternative.

Staphylococcus aureus

OCCURRENCE AND PATHOGENICITY   Organisms of this species are common commensals of man. They are to be found on the anterior nasal mucosa of 40–50 % of healthy adults, in the throats of many of them, in the faeces of about 20 % and on the skin of 5–10 %. As well as being carried in these situations they may also multiply profusely there, notably in the nose and on the perineal skin. New-born babies are rapidly colonized by this species, and 90 % or more of those born in hospital carry it in the nose and around the umbilicus within 2 weeks of birth. Droplet spread and shedding of skin scales result in widespread distribution of this species in the human environment, notably in air, dust, clothing and bedding.

Staph. aureus is the commonest cause of pyogenic infections of man. Most infections involve the skin or its appendages—e.g. pustules, furuncles, boils, impetigo, styes and infected surgical or accidental wounds. Abscesses of the subcutaneous and connective tissues are also commonly staphylococcal. Among the other diseases which this species can produce are osteomyelitis, mastitis, bronchopneumonia (mainly in young children or in young previously healthy adults in some influenza outbreaks) and generalized septicaemia. It is also responsible for two forms of intestinal disorder. Staphylococcal food-poisoning is due to the eating of food in which staphylococci have multiplied and produced a toxin (p. 285). Staphylococcal enteritis, on the other hand, is a rare result of broad-spectrum antibiotic treatment that upsets the ecological balance of the bacteria of the intestine and allows *Staph. aureus* to proliferate there; the resulting enteritis may be so severe that it is rapidly fatal unless treated with another antibiotic to which the offending strain is sensitive. (See also p. 82, Toxin Production.)

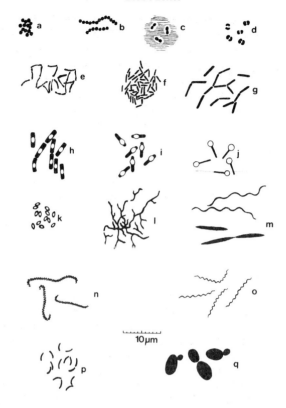

Figure 5 Morphological features of some bacteria.

(*a*) A cluster of staphylococci as seen in pus and tissues.
(*b*) A chain of streptococci.
(*c*) Pairs of capsulate pneumococci as seen in sputum or pus.
(*d*) Pairs of kidney-shaped meningococci or gonococci as seen in pus (where as a rule most of them are inside pus cells).
(*e*) Diphtheria bacilli showing 'Chinese character' arrangement.
(*f*) Enterobacteria.
(*g*) Lactobacilli in branching chains (false branching).
(*h*) Members of the genus *Bacillus*, with spores narrower than the bacilli.
(*i*) Clostridia with subterminal spores wider than the bacilli.
(*j*) *Cl. tetani* with terminal drum-stick spores.
(*k*) Yersiniae showing polar staining.
(*l*) An actinomycete showing true branching and fragmentation.
(*m*) Vincent's organisms (p. 130).
(*n*) Leptospires.
(*o*) Treponemes.
(*p*) Vibrios.
(*q*) A budding yeast for comparison of size.

MICROSCOPY   Staphylococci are Gram-positive spherical organisms, 0.7–1 μm in diameter. Their arrangement is described on p. 79.

CULTURE   *Staph. aureus* grows well on common media under aerobic conditions, but less well anaerobically. Its optimal growth temperature is around 37°C, but it will grow within the range 10–44°C. On nutrient or blood agar, colonies are 2–4 mm in diameter after 18 hours incubation at 37°C, and are smooth, shiny, opaque, yellow to white domes resembling small drops of gloss paint. The ability of staphylococci to grow in concentrations of sodium chloride which are inhibitory to other genera (e.g. 7.5% in nutrient agar or 10% in nutrient broth) is useful for their isolation from faeces and other specimens likely to contain large numbers of other bacteria.

COAGULASE AND DEOXYRIBONUCLEASE PRODUCTION   The thrombin-like enzyme coagulase may play a part in the survival of *Staph. aureus* in the host and enhance its pathogenicity (see p. 25). Production of coagulase and of another enzyme deoxyribonuclease (DNase) are closely associated in staphylococci, so tests for either can be used as the basis for recognition of *Staph. aureus* in the routine laboratory.

In the *tube coagulase test* diluted plasma and a broth culture of the organism are incubated together. Formation of a clot indicates that the organism is coagulase-positive. The *slide 'coagulase' test* is quicker and simpler to carry out, and usually gives the same result as the tube test, though it does not depend on the same mechanism. It is carried out by mixing part of a colony of staphylococci in a drop of water on a clean slide so as to make a milky suspension, and then adding a loopful of plasma. The test is positive if further mixing results in visible clumping of the bacteria, provided that spontaneous clumping (auto-agglutination) does not occur in a comparable suspension to which no plasma has been added. *DNase production* is easily demonstrated by growing the staphylococcus on a nutrient agar made opaque by addition of DNA; the enzyme causes clearing of the opacity around the growth.

TOXIN PRODUCTION   Various *Staph. aureus* exotoxins have been detected and studied in animals. Effects demonstrable include lysis of red cells, leucocidal action (killing of granulocytes and macrophages by lysis of their cell membranes) and vasoconstriction with resultant tissue necrosis. These are probably components of the pathogenicity of *Staph. aureus* to man. Human diseases in which *Staph. aureus* toxins are undoubtedly involved include:

1 *food-poisoning* (p. 285) due to enterotoxin B.
2 *scalded skin syndrome* of young children, due to the epidermolytic toxin (exfoliatin).
3 *toxic shock syndrome* – vascular collapse, fever and a diffuse rash with subsequent desquamation, occurring in some patients with *Staph. aureus* mucosal colonization (notably in the vagina).

PHAGE TYPING   Bacteriophages are virus parasites of bacteria (see pp. 193–5). Many *Staph. aureus* strains carry phages which, when spotted on to plate cultures of other staphylococcal strains as described on p. 194, cause lysis of some of them. This phenomenon makes it possible to divide the species *Staph. aureus* into phage-types—i.e. groups of strains having the same or closely similar phage susceptibilities and resistances. For this purpose a basic set of 2 dozen or so phage cultures is used. These are numbered according to international agreement, and are divisible into 4 groups (I–IV) according to their antigenic composition. Any one strain of *Staph. aureus* is likely to be susceptible to the lytic action of several phages, which often belong to a single antigenic group. The phage type of the strain is then designated by listing the numbers of the phages which can lyse it under specified conditions—e.g. type 52/42B/42C/44A/80/81, notorious for causing outbreaks of hospital sepsis, and commonly given the less precise but more manageable designation 'type 80/81'. A minority of strains are not typable because they are resistant to all of the phages used, but new phages are found from time to time which, when added to the standard set, increase the number of strains that can be typed. Some strains which are not lysed by phages in the dilution routinely employed (Routine Test Dilution or RTD) can be typed by using more concentrated phage suspensions (1000 × RTD).

We shall have more to say about applications of staphylococcal phage typing in connection with hospital cross-infection (p. 274) and food-poisoning (p. 286).

IMMUNOLOGY   Various antibodies are formed in response to staphylo-coccal infection, but their protective value is uncertain and their measurement seldom gives much diagnostic help. *Staph. aureus* strains that have *protein A* as a surface component are resistant to phagocytosis. This is because protein A binds to the Fc region of antibody molecules—i.e. to the end that would otherwise attach to the phagocytic cells (p. 56) but cannot do so in these circumstances. These strains can be coated with antibody molecules specific for other bacteria and can then be used as diagnostic reagents for their detection; mixing of the coated staphylococci and the appropriate other bacteria results in *co-agglutination*. This method is used, for example, in the grouping of β-haemolytic streptococci (p. 87).

ANTIBACTERIAL TREATMENT   Since antibiotics became available, *Staph. aureus* has shown exceptional ability to produce variants which are resistant to them, and consequently have been given their own section of Chapter 21.

Other Staphylococci

Staph. epidermidis resembles *Staph. aureus* in most respects except that it is coagulase-negative, usually forms white colonies, and is generally non-pathogenic. It is found in large numbers all over human skin and on many mucous surfaces. It may play some part in the pathogenesis of acne and in other minor skin lesions, and has occasionally been incriminated as a cause of bacterial endocarditis (as have many bacterial species). In recent years it has achieved greater medical importance as a common cause of bacteraemia associated with intravenous catheters, and of infections around cerebrospinal fluid shunts, artificial heart valves and other prostheses. Such infections often fail to respond to antibiotic treatment and necessitate removal of the prostheses—with the risk, of course, that replacement prostheses may also become infected.

Urinary tract infections due to coagulase-negative staphylococci fall into two main groups. *Staph. epidermidis* strains are commonly responsible for such infections in elderly males, particularly after bladder instrumentation or prostatectomy. In contrast, a common form of acute cystitis in young women—nearly always a sequel to sexual intercourse and often causing severe discomfort, with bladder haemorrhage in some cases—is due to strains which in the diagnostic laboratory can most easily be distinguished from *Staph. epidermidis* by their resistance to the antibiotic novobiocin. After being called *Micrococcus* type 3 for some years, these strains have been reclassified as *Staph. saprophyticus*—a move which leaves the genus *Micrococcus* bereft of importance to the clinical bacteriologist.

THE GENUS STREPTOCOCCUS

Members of this genus are widely distributed in nature, largely as parasites of man and animals. They make a large contribution to the normal bacterial flora of the human respiratory, alimentary and female genital tracts. Certain types belonging to the species *Str. pyogenes* are highly pathogenic, though even these may be carried as harmless commensals. *Str. pneumoniae* is an important pathogenic species but also a common commensal of the healthy upper respiratory tract. Some other commensal streptococci are pathogenic in certain circumstances.

Streptococci are spherical or oval Gram-positive cocci, about 1 μm in diameter, non-motile, non-sporing, sometimes capsulate, and characterized by their tendency to form chains (p. 13 and Fig. 5(*b*), p. 81). Chain-formation is best seen in pathological materials or in fluid cultures—partly because chains are formed more readily in such situations than on solid media and partly because the process of taking part of a colony from a solid medium and suspending it in water to make a microscopic film results in the breaking up of chains. Length of chains also depends upon the species involved. Some form chains containing scores of cocci, whereas at the other extreme *Str. pneumoniae* characteristically appears in tissues and exudates as pairs of cocci (diplococci—Fig. 5(*c*), p. 81).

Streptococci are facultative organisms (p. 22). Those that grow best in *aerobic* conditions include the principal pathogens of the genus, and can be classified (apart from the *enterococci*, discussed separately below) according to their *haemolytic* activities, as follows:

1 *β-haemolytic.* β-haemolysis is the production, around a colony of streptococci (e.g. of *Str. pyogenes*) on a blood agar plate, of a zone of clear colourless medium, in which the red cells have been lysed and the haemoglobin decolorized. This activity may be shown in various degrees by the same strain grown on media containing blood from different mammalian species and is often more pronounced when the plates are incubated anaerobically.

2 *α-haemolytic.* α-haemolysis is the production around the colonies of a zone in which the red cells are partly destroyed (so that the medium becomes somewhat less opaque) and haemoglobin is converted to a green pigment. Such a reaction is produced by streptococci of the viridans group and by *Str. pneumoniae*.

3 *Non-haemolytic.* Many streptococci do not produce either of these forms of haemolysis. A few produce other changes, such as partial destruction of the red cells, with no green pigmentation or a brownish discoloration of the medium, but many have no visible effect on the medium and are described as non-haemolytic. They are as a rule harmless commensals.

β-haemolytic streptococci are divided into Lancefield groups A to H and K to V by means indicated below, in the discussion of the antigenic structure of *Str. pyogenes*. This species name is given to Lancefield group A streptococci, the predominant human pathogens of the genus (see below). Group B·(p. 88) and group D (which contains many of the enterococci—p. 91) are also of medical importance, and strains of other groups (notably C, F, G and R) are occasionally pathogenic to man.

Streptococcus pyogenes (*β*-haemolytic streptococci, group A)

OCCURRENCE AND PATHOGENICITY   Healthy human beings may carry in their throats, or less commonly in their noses, *Str. pyogenes* strains which are potential pathogens; the skin and clothing of such carriers may become heavily contaminated. Strains of this species cause many different human diseases. To some extent the type of disease produced is determined by the portal of entry of the organism. The commonest picture is acute sore throat, often involving suppurative inflammation of the tonsils and cervical lymphadenitis. Its incidence is highest among young schoolchildren, who are exposed to a high risk of infection from other children but have not yet developed a range of antibodies adequate to protect them against the many antigenic types of *Str. pyogenes* (see below). Because streptococcal throat infection cannot be reliably distinguished from a virus infection on clinical grounds, culture of a throat swab is essential for firm diagnosis. A streptococcal throat infection may spread to the middle ears, mastoids and even meninges. *Scarlet fever* is a *Str. pyogenes* infection, usually of the throat, due to a strain which produces erythrogenic toxins (see below). If the patient has no protective antibodies against these toxins, they cause the characteristic skin rash of scarlet fever. *Str. pyogenes* also causes infections of the skin (including impetigo and erysipelas), of the uterus following childbirth (puerperal sepsis) and of many other tissues. Spread into the lymphatic system (lymphangitis and lymphadenitis) and into the blood stream (septicaemia) are common suppurative complications of untreated *Str. pyogenes* infections. The non-suppurative complications—*rheumatic fever* and *acute glomerulonephritis*—are hypersensitivity reactions that develop 2–3 weeks after the initial infection. In rheumatic fever there is immunological cross-reaction between streptococcal group A antigen and cardiac muscle, but it is not yet clear how this causes the myocardial lesions. In acute post-streptococcal glomerulonephritis—which is associated with a limited number of Griffith types of *Str. pyogenes* (see below, under Antigenic Structure)—complexes of streptococcal antigen with antibody produce a Type III hypersensitivity reaction (p. 64) in the kidney. The infection that elicits this complication may be on the skin, whereas rheumatic fever is virtually always preceded by a throat infection.

MICROSCOPY   Chain-formation is usually well marked. The cocci are spherical and conform to the general description given for the genus.

CULTURE   Growth is poor on ordinary nutrient media but better on those containing serum or blood, and is better in aerobic than in anaerobic conditions. The optimal temperature for growth is 37°C, and none occurs below 18°C. Even under optimal conditions on blood agar, colonies are usually only 1 mm or so in diameter after 24 hours; they may be smooth and shiny, but are commonly dry and irregular in contour and outline, especially when they belong to virulent strains. They are greyish-white and opaque or semitransparent. β-haemolysis is best seen if the blood-agar plates are incubated anaerobically, and the zones may then be up to 5 mm in diameter (see below). In fluid cultures there is usually a granular deposit and a relatively clear supernatant, in contrast to the more uniform turbidity of broth cultures of staphylococci and of most other streptococci.

TOXIN AND ENZYME PRODUCTION   (1) *Streptolysin O* is a haemolysin which is oxygen-sensitive and is active only in the reduced state. It is responsible for the larger zones of β-haemolysis following anaerobic incubation. It is powerfully toxic to animals (and presumably to man), acting mainly on the heart.

(2) *Streptolysin S* is also a haemolysin. It is not inactivated by oxygen and is not demonstrably antigenic. It is responsible for the zones of β-haemolysis seen on aerobic blood agar plates. Its action can be blocked by an inhibitor commonly present in human and animal sera.

(3) *Streptokinase*, when released by *Str. pyogenes* into blood or tissue fluid, plays a part in the activation of plasminogen to the proteolytic

enzyme plasmin, which then breaks down fibrin. This process facilitates the spread of the streptococci through the fibrin barrier laid down as part of the host's defence mechanism.

(4) *Hyaluronidase* also facilitates the spread of *Str. pyogenes* by breaking down the hyaluronic acid of the connective tissue cement substance.

(5) *Deoxyribonucleases A, B, C and D* depolymerize DNA and deoxyribonucleoprotein. Since the latter material is largely responsible for the viscosity of purulent exudates, treatment with such enzymes makes them less viscous. Whatever the significance of this may be in relation to streptococcal infection, deoxyribonucleases have been used therapeutically as a means of liquefying pus and so hastening the cleaning up of wounds and abscess cavities. Streptokinase solutions have been used in a similar way.

(6) *Erythrogenic toxins* and their relationship to scarlet fever have been discussed above in connection with the pathogenicity of this species. Production of these toxins depends on a lysogenic relationship (p. 194) between the *Str. pyogenes* strains and bacteriophages. The Dick test for the presence or absence of antibodies to this toxin is described on p. 253.

ANTIGENIC STRUCTURE Lancefield grouping depends on the cell-wall C polysaccharides possessed by most β-haemolytic and some other streptococci. C polysaccharide can be removed from the organisms and obtained in solution by acid, formamide or enzymic extraction, and can then be identified by precipitation tests (p. 241), using antisera for the various Lancefield groups. Many diagnostic laboratories now use simpler and more rapid methods—latex agglutination (p. 242) or co-agglutination (p. 83); the latter has the advantage that it uses streptococcal suspensions and dispenses with the need for extraction. Group A (*Str. pyogenes*) strains can be subdivided into over 60 Griffith types by study of their surface proteins, notably the M proteins which are important contributors to the virulence of the organisms. Such fine subdivision is sometimes useful in studies of the spread of infection, and certain types (notably type 12) are particularly associated with infections that precede the development of acute glomerulonephritis.

IMMUNOLOGY Immunity following natural infection is highly type-specific, and immunization is impracticable because of the large number of types involved. Infection with a strain that produces erythrogenic toxin is followed by the development of immunity to such a toxin. Useful diagnostic information can be obtained by measuring levels of antibodies to extra-cellular products of *Str. pyogenes*—notably antistreptolysin O (ASO) and antideoxyribonuclease B (antiDNase B). The ASO titre invariably rises following *Str. pyogenes* throat infection (but can also do so after infection with group C or G streptococci, since these can produce streptolysin O); but the DNase B titre is a more reliable indicator of recent skin infection. These tests are particularly valuable in confirming or refuting the diagnosis of rheumatic fever or acute glomerulonephritis, conditions which may present clinically when the streptococcus is no longer around.

ANTIBACTERIAL TREATMENT *Str. pyogenes* strains are always sensitive to penicillin, which is therefore usually the agent of choice for the treatment of infections due to them. Patients with *Str. pyogenes* throat infections should take oral penicillin for at least 10 days to minimize the risks of relapse or persistent carriage. *Str. pyogenes* is usually sensitive also to most other antibiotics except the aminoglycoside group, and to the sulphonamides. Tetracycline-resistant strains are now fairly common in many areas.

Group B Streptococci

OCCURRENCE AND PATHOGENICITY These organisms are carried in the female genital tract and in the lower intestinal tract, with carriage frequencies of the order of 5–30 %. During the 1970s it became apparent that they can be important pathogens during the early weeks of infancy. Two disease patterns can be distinguished:

1 *early onset disease*, particularly affecting infants of low birth weight. Infection is acquired from the mother's genital tract during birth, and leads within the next two days to fulminating septicaemia, likely to be fatal if not adequately treated. Such an outcome can be prevented if within two hours of birth 'high risk' infants are given penicillin, which is also the appropriate drug for treatment of infection with these streptococci.

2 *late onset disease*, in which the infection is acquired 1–12 weeks after birth and typically results in meningitis. The source of infection is usually not the mother, and is often not detected. This type of disease is less likely to be fatal.

CULTURE Most group B streptococci are β-haemolytic. Their isolation from the genital and alimentary tracts is made easier by using a medium made selective by adding an aminoglycoside to suppress many other bacterial species. They produce a characteristic orange pigment when grown on serum starch agar.

IMMUNOLOGY Many infants are protected against the risk of group B streptococcal infection by transplacental transmission of relevant maternal antibodies (p. 57), but the mothers of affected infants have no such antibodies. Production of these can be stimulated by immunization with a group B polysaccharide vaccine, and maternal immunization is a possible means of preventing group B streptococcal neonatal infections.

The Viridans Group of Streptococci (*Str. viridans*)

The bacterial flora of the human upper respiratory tract and mouth normally includes large numbers of α-haemolytic streptococci. Some of these may be *Str. pneumoniae* (see below). The rest were formerly lumped together under the name *Str. viridans*, but are now divided into a number of more precisely defined species. However, they are still collectively referred to as 'the viridans group' or 'viridans streptococci'—though in fact some of the new species incorporate non-haemolytic as well as α-haemolytic strains. Some members of the group are important in dental caries—notably *Str. mutans*, which turns sucrose into a sticky layer of dextran on surfaces of teeth. Apart from this the viridans streptococci are rarely pathogenic to man in their normal habitat, the mouth and pharynx, but they are liable to gain access to the blood stream, particularly during dental filling or extraction. They are nearly always eliminated from the circulation without causing any trouble, but in patients with rheumatic endocarditis or congenital heart lesions they may invade the fibrinous vegetations attached to the valves or deformed structures, and they then cause subacute bacterial endocarditis. The species most likely to do this are *Str. sanguis*, *Str. mutans*, *Str. bovis* and *Str. mitis*.

The microscopic appearances of members of this group are in general similar to those described for *Str. pyogenes*. So are their cultural characteristics, except that haemolysis, if present, is of the α type and usually less extensive than the zones of β-haemolysis around *Str. pyogenes*.

The use of antibiotics in prevention and treatment of bacterial endocarditis is discussed on pp. 307, 310–11 and 335.

Streptococcus pneumoniae (*Diplococcus pneumoniae*, the *pneumococcus*)

OCCURRENCE AND PATHOGENICITY This species is both a normal commensal and a common pathogen of the human respiratory tract, and it is therefore difficult at times to assess the significance of its isolation from sputum or other respiratory tract specimens. Its specific name reflects its status as the commonest cause of lobar pneumonia (usually a primary illness in a previously healthy person) and of bronchopneumonia (usually secondary to existing disease or disability). It shares with *Haemophilus influenzae* responsibility for acute suppurative exacerbations of chronic bronchitis. Other pneumococcal infections include pleurisy and pericarditis (usually associated with pneumonia), meningitis, otitis media, paranasal sinusitis and (in girls or young women) peritonitis.

MICROSCOPY In tissues, pus or sputum pneumococci are typically arranged in pairs (diplococci); each coccus is somewhat elongated, and pointed at one end but rounded at the other (lanceolate), and the two members of a pair point away from each other. They are surrounded by a polysaccharide capsule (Fig 5(*c*), p. 81). However, in artificial culture short chains are common and capsules tend to be less evident, so that distinction from other streptococci is not easy on the basis of microscopic morphology.

CULTURE *Str. pneumoniae* resembles the streptococci already described in its nutritional and environmental requirements except that it exhibits more definite enhancement of its growth by the addition of $5-10\%$ CO_2 to the atmosphere in which it is incubated. Its colonies are surrounded by zones of α-haemolysis similar to those of the viridans group, but in general the colonies themselves are larger and more disk-shaped. Typically they have raised edges and concentric ridges on their surfaces which have earned for them the name of 'draughtsmen'. Some strains form moister, more mucoid colonies, whereas others have rough, granular surfaces.

OPTOCHIN SENSITIVITY   Pneumococci are most easily distinguished from viridans streptococci in the routine laboratory by their inability to grow on blood agar in the vicinity of a paper disk containing optochin (ethyl hydrocuprein hydrochloride). Such inhibition may be detectable even in a mixed culture—e.g. a primary plate culture from a sputum specimen.

ANTIGENIC STRUCTURE   Pneumococcal strains form polysaccharide capsules of over 80 immunologically distinct kinds; and on this basis 46 capsular types are recognized, some of them divided into sub-types. Using type-specific antisera, strains can be identified by agglutination or capsule-swelling tests of the organisms themselves or by precipitation of capsular polysaccharide from solution. Surveys in various countries have shown that a dozen or so of the 46 types are between them responsible for the great majority of serious pneumococcal disease, and that the relative importance of individual types varies somewhat according to the disease—e.g. type 1 causes pneumonia more often than meningitis, whereas the reverse is true (in some series, at least) of type 18. Infections due to type 3 tend to have a particularly high mortality rate.

IMMUNOLOGY   Pneumococcal capsular polysaccharide prevents phago-cytosis (p. 43), but anticapsular opsonins (p. 56) overcome this protection and provide the host with type-specific immunity. The appearance of type-specific antibodies in the blood $7-10$ days after the onset on pneumococcal pneumonia was responsible for the 'resolution by crisis' which was the outcome of many such infections in pre-antibiotic days. Type-specific passive immunization, the only effective antibacterial treatment for pneumococcal infections in the 1930s, was abandoned when sulphonamides and penicillin became available, as were attempts to produce a vaccine for active immunization. The continued high mortality of serious pneumococcal infections, despite the *in vitro* sensitivity of pneumococci to penicillin and other antibacterials, prompted renewed interest in active immunization during the 1960s; and this was reinforced by the emergence of antibacterial resistance among pneumococci (see below). Following successful field trials, a 14-type vaccine has been made generally available. It is of particular relevance to patients with hypogam-maglobulinaemia (p. 66) and those who have had splenectomies or whose splenic function is impaired (e.g. by sickle-cell anaemia), since such patients are particularly susceptible to fulminating pneumococcal infections.

ANTIBACTERIAL TREATMENT Pneumococci in Britain are almost invariably sensitive to penicillin, and usually to the sulphonamides and to most antibiotics except those of the aminoglycoside group, though resistance to tetracyclines is now quite common. Strains relatively resistant to penicillin were first reported in 1967 from Australia, and constituted 12% of all pneumococcal strains isolated in a survey in New Guinea, but have fortunately remained rare elsewhere. Strains with a higher degree of penicillin resistance, many of them also resistant to most of the obvious alternative drugs, have been reported from South Africa since 1977, and some have been encountered in Europe.

Carbon-dioxide-dependent Streptococci

From many specimens received in routine diagnostic laboratories two blood-agar plate cultures are set up; one is incubated in air and the other in an anaerobic atmosphere containing $5-10\%$ of CO_2. Given only this choice, many of the streptococci that are common commensals of the vaginal and other mucous surfaces grow only on the second plate—not because they are anaerobes but because they need CO_2 in excess of the amount found in air. Though usually harmless, they can cause puerperal and various other forms of sepsis. *Str. milleri* is increasingly recognized as causing large abscesses in the brain, thorax or abdomen, and some cases of bacterial endocarditis. Some strains of this species are β-haemolytic, and it includes Lancefield group F streptococci, some strains from other groups and some that are not groupable. Penicillin is usually effective against all of these streptococci.

The Enterococcus Group (faecal streptococci)

This is a large and ill-defined group of streptococci which are normal intestinal organisms. As might be expected from this habitat, they differ from other streptococci in being able to grow in the presence of moderate concentrations of bile-salts, for example on MacConkey's medium, on which they form characteristic small colonies of deep magenta colour. They tend to be oval cocci, and to form short chains. On blood agar their colonies are usually somewhat larger than those of *Str. pyogenes*. Some stains are β-haemolytic, some are α-haemolytic, some are non-haemolytic, and some produce a brown discoloration of the medium. They mostly survive heating at $60°C$ for 30 minutes, treatment which is lethal to most other streptococci. Many of them belong to Lancefield group D; such strains are not necessarily β-haemolytic. The specific name *Str. faecalis*, at one time applied to all group D enterococci, now strictly belongs to one of several species into which such organisms are divided.

Enterococci may cause urinary tract infections. They are also occasional invaders of wounds and ulcerative skin lesions and are low-grade pathogens in various other situations; and they may cause subacute bacterial endocarditis which follows gynaecological or genito-urinary instrumentation or surgery in much the same way as endocarditis due to viridans streptococci follows dental operations. This last context gives special importance to the fact that they are resistant to penicillin and often to other antibiotics that are effective against other streptococci (p. 335).

Anaerobic Cocci

There is no satisfactory classification of the Gram-positive anaerobic cocci. Two genera—*Peptococcus* and *Peptostreptococcus*—are recognized, but the group is best considered as a whole. They are commensals of mucous surfaces, notably in the vagina and the large intestine; and are sometimes associated with other anaerobic or facultative bacteria in the production of deep abscesses or of the spreading gangrene around surgical wounds which is known as *Meleney's* or *synergistic gangrene*. The lower abdomen, perineum and external genitalia are the usual sites for such conditions, which may result in extensive tissue necrosis. These organisms can also cause puerperal sepsis and septicaemia, or chronic endometritis. Pus from lesions in which they are involved has an unpleasant smell because they are markedly proteolytic and produce much H_2S. Most strains are sensitive to penicillin, and all to metronidazole.

Gram-negative anaerobic cocci are assigned to the genus *Veillonella*. They are commensals of the mouth and large intestine, but have no known pathogenicity.

GRAM-NEGATIVE COCCI

THE GENUS NEISSERIA

Member of this genus are non-motile and mostly non-capsulate aerobes. They include two important pathogens—*N. meningitidis* or the meningococcus and *N. gonorrhoeae* or the gonococcus—and a number of species that are common commensals of the human respiratory tract. In stained films made from cultures of any of the species, the cocci are usually arranged in pairs, each coccus being somewhat flattened or concave on the side facing its partner. In films of pathological material, such as cerebrospinal fluid or pus, the pathogenic species are characteristically found as pairs of kidney-shaped cocci (Fig. 5(*d*), p. 81), many of which are inside pus cells. The pathogens are more exacting than the commensals in their nutritional, atmospheric and thermal requirements.

Neisseria meningitidis (the meningococcus)

OCCURRENCE AND PATHOGENICITY   This organism is an obligate human parasite. It is the cause of meningococcal (formerly called cerebrospinal) meningitis, a disease of world-wide incidence occurring as sporadic cases or in epidemics. In temperate climates most epidemics have arisen in closely packed communities such as war-time barracks. However, very large epidemics with high attack-rates sweep across extensive areas of Africa in dry weather, and an outbreak in the city of Sao Paulo, Brazil, in 1974 produced more than 13 000 cases in 2 months. Septicaemia, with scattered petechial or larger haemorrhagic lesions of the skin, may accompany the meningitis or may occur without it. The septicaemia sometimes runs a prolonged sub-acute course, but sometimes is fulminating, with sudden death resulting from massive disseminated intravascular coagulation and haemorrhagic damage to the adrenal glands (the *Waterhouse–Friderichsen syndrome*).

CARRIERS   The meningococcus may be carried in the upper respiratory tracts of healthy people. During epidemics more than half of those at risk may become carriers, especially if they are living and sleeping in overcrowded conditions. During the First World War it was claimed that cases of meningitis were likely in barracks when the carrier-rate exceeded 20 %, and that a rise to such a level could be prevented by adequate spacing of beds. Subsequent experience has not confirmed these claims.

MICROSCOPY   See above, in the discussion of the genus. In stained films made from purulent cerebrospinal fluid the meningococcus can as a rule be rapidly recognized and distinguished from other likely causes of meningitis by its characteristic shape, arrangement and predominantly intracellular situation.

CULTURE   *N. meningitidis* will grow on some of the richer varieties of nutrient agar, but does better on blood agar, and better still on a similar medium in which the blood has been heated and which is called *chocolate agar* because of its resultant brown colour. The species is aerobic; its growth is often enhanced by the presence of about 5 % of CO_2 in its atmosphere (p. 223). The optimal growth temperature is about 37°C, but some growth will usually occur anywhere between 25 and 42°C. The colonies formed on a suitable medium are rather small (around 2 mm in diameter after 24 hours), smooth, greyish, semitransparent and devoid of striking positive features. Except on special storage media, cultures usually die within a few days.

Laboratory diagnosis of meningococcal infection usually depends on examination of blood and cerebrospinal fluid (see Chapter 14). It may also be possible to see the meningococci in smears made from skin lesions, and to grow them from such lesions and from nasopharyngeal swabs of cases and carriers (p. 227).

BIOCHEMICAL REACTIONS   In common with most other members of the genus, *N. meningitidis* produces an *oxidase* which can be detected by pouring a 1 % solution of tetramethyl-*p*-phenylenediamine over the culture plate on which it is growing. Neisserial colonies become pink and then purple within a few minutes. This helps their detection in a mixed culture, but in order to survive they must be subcultured as soon as the colour change becomes apparent. A single colony can be tested by transferring part of it to a strip of filter paper that has been impregnated with the indicator; the colour then develops on the paper.

Carbohydrate oxidation by *N. meningitidis* and other neisseriae can be tested by growing them on a specially enriched nutrient agar to which have been added a sugar and an indicator. *N. meningitidis* produces acid from glucose and from maltose but not from sucrose, *N. gonorrhoeae* from glucose but not from the other two, and most of the commensal neisseriae from all three sugars or from none of them.

ANTIGENIC STRUCTURE Seven or more serogroups of this species are currently recognized, but most epidemics of meningococcal meningitis are due to group A strains and most sporadic cases in Britain to those of group B.

IMMUNOLOGY Natural active immunity follows asymptomatic carriage of meningococci, and effective polysaccharide vaccines are available for groups A and C, though infants, the group most needing protection, fail to respond adequately to such stimuli (p. 65). Other aspects of the immune response to meningococci are discussed on pp. 61–2.

ANTIBACTERIAL TREATMENT Penicillin, to which all strains are sensitive, is the treatment of choice for meningococcal disease, but is not effective in prophylaxis. Sulphonamides were highly effective in treatment before bacterial resistance became a problem, and are still of great value as cheap and acceptable prophylaxis in major epidemics due to sulphonamide-sensitive strains. The only other effective prophylactic drug, rifampicin, is not suitable for such widespread use.

Neisseria gonorrhoeae (the gonococcus)

OCCURRENCE AND PATHOGENICITY This is also an obligate human parasite. Its transmission is nearly always by sexual intercourse, and the initial infection is then an acute suppurative urethritis, usually with involvement of the cervix uteri as well in the female. Infection may spread by direct extension to Bartholin's glands, the uterus and Fallopian tubes and the ovaries and peritoneal cavity in the female; and to the prostate, seminal vesicles, epididymis and testes in the male. The rectum is often colonized by direct extension in infected women (some of whom develop a mild proctitis), and is a common site of infection in homosexual males. Colonization of the throat is being recognized with increasing frequency, and there may be a mild pharyngitis. Blood stream spread may lead to suppurative arthritis and to tenosynovitis (infections that are usually very difficult to confirm by isolation of the gonococci), and occasionally to endocarditis or other diseases. Non-venereal transmission is responsible for neonatal ophthalmia of babies born to infected mothers, and for vulvo-vaginitis of young female children; the latter may occur in epidemic form in institutions, being transmitted by towels and other fomites.

CARRIERS   The healthy carrier state probably does not exist, but women with chronic infections, particularly prostitutes, may have no symptoms and play an important part in the maintenance and spread of the disease.

MICROSCOPY   The gonococcus is indistinguishable from the meningococcus by ordinary microscopy, but can be identified by the fluorescent-antibody technique (p. 16). Characteristic intracellular Gram-negative diplococci are to be seen in urethral or cervical pus in the acute stages of gonorrhoea. In chronic infections microscopy often fails to reveal gonococci in material which gives positive results on culture.

CULTURE   The gonococcus behaves like the meningococcus in culture except that it will not grow on nutrient agar, has a more stringent requirement for CO_2 and has a narrower temperature range than the meningococcus, and that its colonies are usually slower to appear and smaller.

Specimens that should be taken for laboratory investigation include purulent urethral discharge (transferred directly to culture plates with a wire loop if possible) or a urethral swab from a patient of either sex, and swabs from the cervix uteri and the rectum of a woman, from the rectum of a male homosexual, and from the pharynx when appropriate. Efficiency of diagnosis is greatly increased by sending swabs to the laboratory in a transport medium that keeps the gonococci alive, and by using special culture media that contain mixtures of antibacterial agents to inhibit more robust bacteria commonly present in the relevant specimens.

BIOCHEMICAL REACTIONS   See under *N. meningitidis.*

IMMUNOLOGY   Immunity does not follow natural infection and cannot be produced artificially. The gonococcal complement-fixation test (GCFT) was widely used, as an 'aid' to the diagnosis of chronic infections, particularly the less accessible ones such as salpingitis and arthritis; but it is unreliable and can be misleading.

ANTIBACTERIAL TREATMENT   Emergence of sulphonamide resistance was much more rapid and widespread among gonococci than among meningococci. The penicillins have remained effective far longer, and in a condition in which treatment failure is often the result of patient default have had the advantage that adequate treatment could be achieved by a single injection of a long-acting preparation or by two oral doses accompanied by probenecid (p. 326) to delay excretion. However, over many years now it has been apparent in various parts of the world that the prevailing gonococcal strains were becoming somewhat less sensitive to penicillins, so that progressively higher doses have been necessary; and more recently frankly penicillin-resistant strains, producing β-lactamase as a consequence of acquiring transmissible plasmids (see p. 318), have appeared in several parts of the world, particularly in Africa and Asia.

Spectinomycin (p. 331) is commonly used as an alternative treatment when such strains are around.

Neonatal ophthalmia need never occur, as it can be prevented by the administration of silver nitrate or penicillin drops to the eyes of all possibly exposed babies as soon as they are born.

Commensal Neisseriae

Other species of this genus—e.g. *N. sicca, N. pharyngis*—make a large contribution to the normal commensal flora of the human upper respiratory tract. They are virtually never pathogenic. They are distinguishable from the pathogenic species by their growth on simpler media and at lower temperatures and by their different sugar reactions. *Branhamella* (formerly *Neisseria*) *catarrhalis*, one of the commonest of nasopharyngeal commensals, occasionally causes low-grade purulent infections of the lower respiratory tract.

GRAM-POSITIVE BACILLI

The genera to be discussed have the following characteristics:

Corynebacterium. Non-sporing; bacilli mostly in palisades or in 'Chinese characters' (see below); aerobic. (*Listeria* and *Erysipelothrix* are similar.)

Propionibacterium. Non-sporing; similar morphology to corynebacteria; anaerobic.

Lactobacillus. Non-sporing; bacilli commonly in chains; mostly micro-aerophilic or anaerobic.

Bifidobacterium. Non-sporing; branched or Y-shaped ('bifid') bacilli; anaerobic.

Bacillus. Sporing, with spores usually not exceeding the bacilli in diameter; aerobic.

Clostridium. Sporing, with spores usually wider than the bacilli; anaerobic.

Their differences in microscopic morphology are illustrated in Fig. 5 (p. 81).

THE GENUS CORYNEBACTERIUM

The genus owes its name to the club-shaped swellings often seen at the ends of the bacilli, especially in old cultures. It includes one important human pathogen, the diphtheria bacillus. Other species cause suppurative diseases of animals. Various non-pathogenic corynebacteria, known as *diphtheroid bacilli*, are normal commensals of human skin, upper respiratory tract, external ears and conjunctivae. Some of these have been given specific names – e.g. *C. hofmanni* and *C. xerosis*. Their properties will only be mentioned incidentally as part of our discussion of *C. diphtheriae*, but they are important to the clinical bacteriologist because they are present in a high proportion of the specimens that he receives.

Corynebacterium diphtheriae (the diphtheria bacillus)

OCCURRENCE AND PATHOGENICITY Diphtheria is now a rare disease in Britain, where widespread immunization against it was introduced in the early 1940s, and in other countries with comparable immunization programmes. However, it remains a common disease in other parts of the world; and rapid bacteriological confirmation of suspected cases is important in countries where it is rare. Its causative bacillus is an obligate parasite, with man as its only natural host. Typically, diphtheria is an infection of the upper respiratory tract, characterized by the formation of a thick adherent exudate or membrane overlying the pharyngeal mucosa; if this extends to the larynx it may cause respiratory obstruction. More remote effects of the disease are due to an exotoxin produced by the bacillus at the site of the infection; this enters the patient's circulation and damages the heart, nervous system, liver, kidneys and adrenals. The severity of the resultant illness depends to some extent upon the toxin-producing ability of the diphtheria bacillus involved. Three biotypes—gravis, intermedius and mitis—can be differentiated in the laboratory and in very general terms are associated respectively with severe, intermediate and mild illnesses.

Occasionally the primary infection is in the skin, a wound or the vagina. In such atypical cases systemic disturbance is usually not severe.

Non-toxigenic and consequently non-pathogenic strains of all three varieties occur (see below); they are most common in the mitis variety.

C. diphtheriae is not naturally pathogenic to animals, but guinea-pigs and rabbits are highly susceptible to injections of toxigenic strains or their toxins, and many other species are less markedly so.

CARRIERS These play an important part in the spread of the disease. Some are convalescent, but many have had only subclinical infections. While the throat and nose are the common sites of carriage, the organism is sometimes carried in an ear or elsewhere.

MICROSCOPY Corynebacteria divide like snapping sticks in which the bark fails to break on one side. In most diphtheroid bacilli the resulting arrangement tends to resemble a stake fence or palisade—rows of bacilli of rather irregular lengths lying side-by-side. The rods of C. diphtheriae are slightly curved, and therefore form less tidy bundles, conventionally likened to Chinese characters (Fig. 5(e), p. 81). An average diphtheria bacillus is of the order of 3 μm by 0.5 μm, and has terminal volutin granules which are clearly visible as metachromatic dots at the ends of the bacilli in films stained by special procedures such as Albert's or Neisser's. Some of the diphtheroid bacilli also form such granules, but rarely in the characteristic bipolar distribution seen in C. diphtheriae.

The diagnosis of diphtheria cannot be reliably confirmed or excluded by microscopic examination of smears from pharyngeal or other lesions. In such situations the appearances of *C. diphtheriae* are not clearly distinguishable from those of commensal corynebacteria, and in any case diphtheria bacilli are often absent from smears made from undoubted cases of diphtheria.

CULTURE   *C. diphtheriae* grows on simple media, but better on those which contain serum or blood. On blood agar its inconspicuous small grey colonies are easily overlooked or mistaken for those of some of the diphtheroid bacilli. Many *mitis* and some *gravis* strains are more noticeable because they are haemolytic.

For the isolation of the diphtheria bacillus from clinical material, two special media are commonly used. *Loeffler's* serum is an inspissated mixture of ox or horse serum and glucose broth. A wide variety of bacteria will grow on it, and colonial differentiation is very poor. However, the microscopic morphology and staining reactions of *C. diphtheriae* after 18 hours incubation on this medium are so characteristic that it can be recognized even in films containing many other organisms. Thus a presumptive diagnosis of diphtheria can often be made in about 18 hours or even less. Confirmation comes from the use of a selective *tellurite* medium, both for primary culture of the original material and for subculture of the Loeffler's serum. This medium is a blood or chocolate agar containing 0.04% of potassium tellurite, which suppresses the growth of most bacteria. It also slows even that of corynebacteria, so that they may take up to 48 hours to produce recognizable colonies. By naked-eye examination of these it is possible to distinguish *C. diphtheriae* from diphtheroid bacilli and from the few other species which are not inhibited by the tellurite. The three varieties of *C. diphtheriae* form colonies of somewhat different sizes and shapes, but all are predominantly dark slate-grey in colour, as a result of metabolism of the tellurite, whereas diphtheroid colonies are usually black, light grey or brown.

BIOCHEMICAL REACTIONS   Grown in a suitable medium *C. diphtheriae* ferments glucose and maltose but rarely sucrose, whereas most diphtheroid bacilli ferment all three or none of these. Only *gravis* varieties of *C. diphtheriae* ferment starch. *C. ulcerans*, an uncommon cause of diphtheria-like throat infection, gives the reactions of *C. diphtheriae* *gravis* in these tests but can be differentiated by other biochemical tests.

TOXIN PRODUCTION   This depends on a lysogenic relationship (see p. 194) between *C. diphtheriae* and a bacteriophage; strains that lack the phage are non-toxigenic. Since pathogenicity of *C. diphtheriae* depends on toxin production, a strain isolated from a typical case of diphtheria can reasonably be assumed to be toxigenic. No such assumption can be made about a strain from a doubtful case or a carrier, and the matter may need to be investigated. The presence of diphtheria toxin in a broth culture can be demonstrated by showing that it produces typical lesions when injected into guinea-pigs, and that these can be prevented by prior administration of diphtheria antitoxin to the animals. An *in vitro* method of demonstrating toxin production is Elek's double-diffusion procedure (p. 241). A strip of filter paper soaked in diphtheria antitoxin is incorporated in a plate of a suitable serum agar, and known and suspected toxigenic *C. diphtheriae* cultures are streaked in single lines across the plate at right angles to the strip. The plates are incubated for 48 hours, during which time antitoxin diffuses out from the paper strip and toxin diffuses out from the growing toxigenic cultures. After incubation, fine white lines of toxin-antitoxin precipitate can be seen in the medium, radiating out from the points at which toxigenic cultures cross the strip. Lines due to antigens other than diphtheria toxin may occur; but a true positive reaction is shown by the fact that the line from the suspected culture, on meeting that from the known toxigenic strain, does not cross it but fuses with it to form an arch between the two cultures (the *reaction of identity*—p. 241).

IMMUNOLOGY   Immunity follows natural infection, often without any clinical illness, and can be detected by studying the patient's response to intradermal injection of a small dose of toxin (the Schick test, p. 252). Antitoxin can also be measured in serum. Active immunization (p. 296) has played a large part in reducing the incidence of diphtheria, as indicated above. Passive immunization—i.e. the administration of serum containing antitoxin—is the only effective treatment for an established infection, and must be given at once to any patient suspected of having diphtheria, without waiting for laboratory confirmation of the diagnosis.

ANTIBACTERIAL TREATMENT   *In vitro* the diphtheria bacillus is sensitive to most antibiotics, but these are of little value in treatment because they cannot deal with toxin already in the patient's body. However, penicillin and other antibiotics can be used to prevent infection and to stop cases from becoming carriers, and are occasionally effective in dealing with established carriers.

THE GENUS PROPIONIBACTERIUM

Anaerobic bacilli, morphologically 'diphtheroid', with propionic acid as the major product of their metabolism, are common commensals of man and animals. They are found in the intestine and on the skin, where *P. acnes* in particular is an important member of man's microflora. This organism breaks down lipid components of sebum, and the acid products of this process are inhibitory to many potentially pathogenic bacteria; but in excess they may be partly responsible for the inflammatory element of acne. Such bacilli are virtually never directly pathogenic, but may colonize artificial heart valves and other prostheses, with serious consequences.

LISTERIA MONOCYTOGENES AND ERYSIPELOTHRIX RHUSIOPATHIAE

These two species, which have many properties in common with one another and with the corynebacteria, are both animal pathogens that occasionally cause disease of man. Both are sensitive to most of the common antibiotics.

Listeria monocytogenes

This aerobic non-sporing Gram-positive bacillus differs from the coryne-bacteria in being flagellate and feebly motile (p. 109), in being agglutin-able by known anti-listerial sera and in causing monocytosis in rabbits. Unlike most parasites of man, it grows well at temperatures down to 4°C; and it is only at temperatures of around or below 20°C that it is motile (in an unusual tumbling style). In humans it causes disease—usually meningitis or septicaemia—in neonates, in the elderly or in those who are debilitated, suffering from malignant disease or on immunosuppressive drugs. Asymptomatic vaginal carriage by the mother is the probable source of most neonatal infections. It is said to cause mild fever in some pregnant women, sometimes followed by abortion or still-birth. Most listeria infections respond to treatment with a combination of ampicillin and gentamicin.

Erysipelothrix rhusiopathiae

This organism resembles *Listeria monocytogenes* but is non-motile and is usually micro-aerophilic. It is widely distributed in nature, causing swine erysipelas and other animal diseases, and it is present on the skin and scales of many kinds of fish. *Erysipeloid*, the human condition for which it is responsible, occurs mainly among those who handle meat, poultry, or fish. The organism enters a skin abrasion, commonly on a finger, and causes a painful purplish local swelling that increases in area by peripheral extension but tends to heal centrally. Penicillin is the drug of choice for treatment.

THE GENUS LACTOBACILLUS

This genus of long Gram-positive bacilli, commonly occurring in chains (Fig. 5(*g*), p. 81), deserves to be ranked as important in medical bacteriology because its members make a substantial contribution to man's normal flora. They are found in the mouth, the stomach, the intestine and the vagina (where they perform an important protective function—see pp. 23–4), and are particularly abundant in the faeces of milk-fed babies. They are mostly anaerobic or micro-aerophilic, some of them will multiply only in an acid environment and they have unusual nutritional requirements. Consequently the average clinical bacteriol-ogist does not grow many of them, and he has little incentive to try to do so, since they are generally regarded as non-pathogens.

THE GENUS BIFIDOBACTERIUM

These anaerobic bacilli have much in common with the lactobacilli, but differ in that their cells are characteristically branched or Y-shaped and that they produce more acetic and less lactic acid. They form a major component of human faeces, where their numbers equal those of *Bacteroides* species (see p. 130) at about 10^{11} organism per gram of wet faeces. They are particularly numerous in the faeces of breast-fed infants where they help to maintain the acetic acid/acetate buffer system and so the acidic pH. They have virtually never been incriminated as pathogens.

THE GENUS BACILLUS

The sporing aerobic bacilli include one highly pathogenic species, *B. anthracis*, and a large assortment of other species that are almost always saprophytic.

Bacillus anthracis (the anthrax bacillus)

OCCURRENCE AND PATHOGENICITY   Mainly a pathogen of herbivorous animals, in which it produces a disease varying from a fulminating haemorrhagic septicaemia to a chronic fever with pustules, *B. anthracis* is an occasional cause of human disease. This may take either of two forms. *Cutaneous anthrax* may occur in farm workers and others in contact with infected animals. In countries such as Britain animal infection is rare and human victims are mostly dockers or factory workers who handle imported hides, bristles, wool or bone meal. A papule at the site of inoculation develops into a blister, then becomes purulent (the 'malignant pustule'), and then becomes a dark-centred necrotic lesion surrounded by oedema, induration and a ring of vesicles. In the absence of effective treatment a severe and commonly fatal septicaemia may follow. The other form of human anthrax, '*wool-sorter's disease*', is a severe haemorrhagic infection of the bronchi and lungs, often accompanied by pleural and pericardial effusions and by septicaemia. It affects only a small proportion of workers who are exposed to the hazard of inhaling anthrax spores in wool or hide factories.

Whereas man does not acquire anthrax readily, cattle and sheep are highly susceptible to natural infection. It also occurs in other herbivorous mammals, including goats, horses and camels. All of these are infected by ingesting spores from contaminated pasture. The organisms then pass from the intestine into the blood stream. Laboratory infections can be produced in mice, guinea-pigs and rabbits by injecting cultures of *B. anthracis*, which cause fatal septicaemia.

MICROSCOPY   Anthrax bacilli are large—4–8 μm long and 1 μm or more wide. Their spores are near the centres of the bacilli, and do not distend them (Fig. 5(*h*), p. 81); they can be seen as non-staining areas in Gram-stained films and can be demonstrated even more clearly by special spore stains. The rods are non-flagellate and, in culture, non-capsulate. They are square-ended and are often arranged in chains.

In smears of vesicle fluid or other pathological material the presence of chains of large Gram-positive rods is strong evidence of anthrax, but not conclusive, since some of the other members of the genus can present similar appearances. In the body of its host *B. anthracis* does not form spores, but usually does have a capsule. Unlike most other bacterial capsules, which are composed of polysaccharides, that of *B. anthracis* contains a polypeptide. It gives a characteristic purple staining reaction with polychrome methylene blue (McFadyean's reaction).

CULTURE   *B. anthracis* grows well aerobically and anaerobically on most common media, but forms spores only in aerobic conditions. Its opaque, greyish-white, rough-surfaced colonies resemble tangles of fine hairs, often with loose curls protruding at the edges ('Medusa-head' colonies).

ANIMAL INOCULATION   The identity of the cultured organism is confirmed by production of the characteristic disease in inoculated mice or guinea-pigs.

IMMUNOLOGY   Pasteur's conclusive and dramatic demonstration, at Pouilly-le-Fort in 1881, of the possibility of immunizing animals against anthrax is one of the milestones of bacteriology. The story is well told in Valley-Radot's biography. Pasteur used a vaccine of *B. anthracis* attenuated by prolonged growth at 42°C or higher. It has not been possible to produce in this way vaccines that are consistently effective and safe enough to be given to man, but dockers, factory workers and others whose work exposes them to special anthrax hazards can now be safely immunized by using a non-living protein antigen which can be precipitated from bacterium-free filtrates of broth cultures of *B. anthracis*.

ANTIBACTERIAL TREATMENT   Passive immunization, using serum of immunized animals, has been superseded by antibiotic treatment. The organism is usually sensitive to penicillin and to several other antibiotics, which are effective if not given too late, though the slow response of the oedema and induration around the primary lesion may cause anxiety to those not familiar with it.

Disposal of animal carcases and other control measures are discussed in Chapter 16.

Other Members of the Genus Bacillus (sometimes called anthracoid bacilli or aerobic spore-bearers)

This is a large and varied group. Its members all form spores and grow better in air than in anaerobic conditions. Many strains are only weakly Gram-positive, often with a characteristic mottled blue-and-red appearance, and a few are frankly Gram-negative. Species differ in the shapes and sizes of their bacilli. The spores are usually narrower than the bacilli, but in a few species are wider and cause distension. Colonial appearances are diverse, and in some cases bizarre. In general, organisms of this group are harmless saprophytes; but they are responsible for very rare cases of meningitis, endocarditis, pneumonia or septicaemia in debilitated patients, and *B. subtilis* occasionally causes severe eye lesions (iridocyclitis or panophthalmitis). *B. cereus* is an important cause of food-poisoning (p. 287). Members of this genus can be troublesome as contaminants of bacterial culture media, blood intended for transfusion, other fluids that should be sterile, specimens from patients, and foods. They can grow in varied conditions, and their spores survive adverse conditions that kill most other bacteria. The bacteriologist can make use of these features in testing the efficiency of methods of sterilization. Heat or irradiation or other physical treatment that can kill organisms of this group—usually represented by *B. subtilis*, the 'hay bacillus', or by *B. stearothermophilus*—is also sufficient to kill all pathogens, including spore-bearers of the next genus to be discussed.

THE GENUS CLOSTRIDIUM

This genus consists of anaerobic Gram-positive bacilli which form spores that in most cases distend their bodies (Fig. 5(*i* and *j*), p. 81). Such organisms are widely distributed in nature as soil saprophytes and as intestinal commensals of mammals. They include the causative organisms of some very serious human diseases—botulism, tetanus, gas-gangrene and several intestinal infections.

Clostridium botulinum

OCCURRENCE AND PATHOGENICITY   This species is to be found in soil in many parts of the world. Botulism is due not to bacterial infection of the victim but to eating food that contains the very powerful neurotoxin of *Cl. botulinum* (p. 287). In man this causes little in the way of alimentary disturbances; the first symptoms are difficulties of vision due to muscle paralysis, and these are followed by progressive bulbar paralysis, frequently terminating in death from respiratory or cardiac arrest. The condition is rare, and can be prevented by proper cooking of food as described in Chapter 19. A different and usually much less severe form of botulism occurs in infants. The organisms are ingested (honey being one recognized source in the USA) and multiply in the large intestine, producing toxin. Since absorption from that site is poor, most of the toxin is excreted in the faeces and the symptoms may be no more than weakness, flaccidity and difficulty in feeding, though some deaths have been reported. Botulism following *C. botulinum* infection of wounds has been described.

There are at least five different types of *Cl. botulinum*, producing slightly different toxins. Types A, B and E cause botulism in man, whereas types C and D cause similar natural diseases of animals. Laboratory animals of many sorts are susceptible to the effects of these toxins given by injection.

MICROSCOPY   The individual bacilli, like those of most clostridia, are intermediate in size between those of the genera *Corynebacterium* and *Bacillus*. They are flagellate and have oval spores which are subterminal in position—i.e. near one end of the rod.

CULTURE   This species is strictly anaerobic (Methods of anaerobic culture are discussed on pp. 222–3). It grows best at temperatures somewhat below 37°C, as is to be expected since it is a saprophyte. It has simple nutritional requirements. Like many other members of the genus, when grown anaerobically on common media it forms diffuse, greyish, semi-transparent colonies of irregular shape.

BIOCHEMICAL REACTIONS   The different clostridial species can be distinguished by their patterns of carbohydrate fermentation (cf. the enterobacteria, p. 110) and by their ability to liquefy coagulated serum and to digest meat.

IMMUNOLOGY   Active immunization is not indicated for a disease that is so rare, and serological diagnosis is out of the question in one that is of such short duration. Antiserum, produced in animals, can be given to counteract the toxin, but its efficacy is low even in those patients who receive it between eating suspected food and developing symptoms. Unless the type of the *Cl. botulinum* strain happens to be known, a polyvalent serum that contains antibodies to the toxins of all types should be used.

ANTIBACTERIAL TREATMENT   Since in the usual adult form of botulism the organism itself does not multiply in the patient's body, there is no indication for using antibiotics.

Clostridium tetani (the tetanus bacillus)

OCCURRENCE AND PATHOGENICITY   Tetanus spores are particularly common in soil to which animal manure has been added. When introduced into the tissues of man, the horse or various other animals, they may cause tetanus, but only if certain conditions are fulfilled. These are imperfectly understood. Interference with the blood supply to at least a small amount of tissue, together with multiplication of other organisms so that all oxygen is used up, appear to be necessary for the production of an anaerobic environment in which the bacillus can grow. Presence of soil in the lesion increases the risk of tetanus, probably because the calcium salts encourage germination of the spores. However, tetanus may follow puncture wounds or abrasions so trivial that they go unnoticed, and it is hard to see how the necessary conditions are then fulfilled. The disease is particularly common in countries in which bare-footed human beings, often with multiple chronic infected lesions of the feet, live in close association with cattle, goats and other domesticated mammals. In such circumstances it is frequently impossible to identify the particular lesion in which the tetanus bacillus is multiplying. Inadequately sterilized dressings or suture materials have often caused post-operative tetanus in the past, and tetanus neonatorum, due to infection of the umbilical stump, is common in communities in which animal dung is used as an umbilical dressing.

Days, weeks or even months after the patient is infected, local multiplication of the organism occurs, with liberation of toxin. This does no harm locally, but travels along peripheral nerves to the central nervous system; here it blocks certain synapses, notably those that modify the effects of limb reflex arcs. Toxin also spreads by the bloodstream to nerves elsewhere in the body and travels up these. The earliest clinical signs are therefore commonly associated with short nerves; trismus ('lock-jaw') is a frequent presenting symptom. The chief clinical features of tetanus are severe muscle spasms and generalized convulsions in response to minimal external stimuli. Patients may die as a result of the direct action of the tetanus toxin on the nervous system, and in the absence of suitable treatment many others succumb to secondary infections, notably of the lungs, by other bacteria.

In the laboratory, most mammals are susceptible to the action of tetanus toxin or to the injection of broth cultures of the organism.

MICROSCOPY In films from cultures or from pathological material *Cl. tetani* has a typical 'drum-stick' appearance, due to the presence of large, round and strictly terminal spores (Fig. 5(*j*), p. 81). However, this appearance can be mimicked by other clostridia, such as the non-toxigenic *Cl. tetanomorphum*, and by some of the aerobic spore-bearers. *Cl. tetani* is usually flagellate and motile (p. 109).

CULTURE A strict anaerobe with an optimal growth temperature of about 37°C, this species grows on ordinary media as a flat, translucent spreading colony with fine finger-like projections. Its ability to swarm over the surfaces of solid media and the heat-resistance of its spores form the basis of procedures for isolating it from the mixture of organisms often present with it in material from lesions. The material, or a suspension or mixed broth culture made from it, is heated to 65°C for 30 minutes, in order to destroy all non-sporing organisms, and is then used to inoculate one side of a plate or the bottom of a slope of blood agar. When the growth begins to swarm across the plate or up the slope the advancing edge is subcultured to another plate or slope. If the resultant growth is still mixed, its advancing edge can again be subcultured, and so on.

It is not surprising that in many typical cases of tetanus the organism cannot be isolated. It may not be possible to identify the relevant lesion, the bacilli may in any case be present only in small numbers, they are often heavily outnumbered in the lesion by other organisms including spore-formers, and it is common for the patient to have received antibiotics before the specimen was collected.

BIOCHEMICAL REACTIONS *Cl. tetani* is unique among medically important clostridia in that it usually fails to ferment any carbohydrates.

TOXIN PRODUCTION   The powerful exotoxin, second in potency only to that of *Cl. botulinum*, can be identified in a broth-culture filtrate by the characteristic spasticity and liability to convulsions that follow its injection into mice and guinea-pigs, and by the neutralization of these effects by specific antitoxin.

IMMUNOLOGY   Immunization is against the toxin, not against the organism itself. Active immunization, sufficiently far in advance and adequately maintained, prevents tetanus. Boosting of active immunity at the time of any appropriate injury, or passive immunization at this stage in those not previously immunized, are of course only applicable to patients whose lesions cause them to seek medical attention. Passive immunization (p. 57) against tetanus has the defect that toxin already fixed in the patient's nervous system cannot be neutralized; all that can be hoped for is the neutralization of any further toxin formed by the organisms. Tetanus immunization is discussed more fully in Chapter 20.

ANTIBACTERIAL TREATMENT   Penicillin and some other antibiotics are effective against *Cl. tetani* in the laboratory, but they have little relevance to the established disease, except in preventing other bacterial infections. However, there is a place for their prophylactic use, along with careful surgical elimination of suitable sites for clostridial germination, in some types of injury, particularly in cases in which temporary protection is needed while active immunity is being induced.

Clostridium perfringens (*Cl. welchii*)

OCCURRENCE AND PATHOGENICITY   This species is commonly present in the intestines of animals and of man and in soil. Together with other organisms of similar habitat, it may gain entry into wounds—from the soil in the case of dirty accidental wounds, but usually from the patient's own intestines, via the skin, in the case of surgical wounds. If there is little or no damaged devitalized tissue in the wound, or if such tissue is promptly and thoroughly excised, clostridial contamination is unlikely to have any ill effects. In the presence of damaged ischaemic tissue, *gas-gangrene* may develop. This condition is due to the multiplication of clostridia (or less commonly of anaerobic streptococci), which produce exotoxins that digest muscle and subcutaneous tissues. In doing this they liberate gas and noxious metabolites, and further reduce the blood supply to the tissues by increasing their internal pressure. Affected wounds have a foul smell, and the surrounding tissues crepitate when handled because of the presence of free gas. Without appropriate treatment the condition spreads and is commonly fatal. Clostridial cellulitis is a less serious infection, often confused with gas-gangrene (clostridial myositis) because there is much gas-formation and crepitation of the tissues, but differing from it in that there is no destruction of muscle.

Numerous *Cl. perfringens* exotoxins have been identified, and strains of this species are classified into six types, A to F, according to the combinations of toxins that they produce. Strains that cause human gas-gangrene belong to type A, and it is therefore with that type that we are chiefly concerned. Types B, C, D and E are all associated with enterotoxaemia in sheep or cattle; types C and F have been reported as occasionally causing a similar disease in man, *enteritis necroticans*; and type C also causes *pig-bel*, an enteritis that occurs in outbreaks following pig-meat feasts in Papua-New Guinea. Finally, certain widely distributed strains which differ slightly from ordinary type A strains (notably in being able to survive prolonged boiling, whereas ordinary strains are killed in about 5 minutes) are responsible for many outbreaks of food-poisoning (p. 286).

Injected cultures of type A strains cause gas-gangrene in guinea-pigs and pigeons, and less readily in mice. Other types vary in their animal pathogenicity.

MICROSCOPY The bacilli are stouter than those of most clostridia, measuring about 4–8 μm by 1 μm. Capsules may be present in films made from pathological materials but are not formed in culture. Most strains fail to form spores in culture, unless fermentable carbohydrate is absent and the medium is alkaline; but small oval subterminal spores are formed freely in natural conditions. The species is not flagellate.

CULTURE A strict anaerobe with an optimal growth temperature of about 37°C, *Cl. perfringens* varies in its colonial appearances, but commonly forms large, round, moderately opaque disks on blood agar, surrounded by zones of haemolysis. The isolation of this and other gas-gangrene organisms from the mixture of bacteria that usually prevails in a gangrenous wound is often a complex procedure, involving a number of special media and techniques which we shall not discuss.

BIOCHEMICAL REACTIONS See under *Cl. botulinum*.

TOXIN PRODUCTION Of the many exotoxins formed by this species, the alpha-toxin is common to all types and is believed to be largely responsible for the toxaemia of human gas-gangrene. It is a relatively heat-stable phospholipase C (p. 24), and is the basis of the Nagler reaction, by which *Cl. perfringens* can be recognized even in mixed culture. Material suspected of containing this organism is streaked across a plate of a transparent medium containing human serum or egg yolk, a small amount of *Cl. perfringens* alpha-antitoxin having first been spread over half of the plate. The plate is incubated overnight, and if *Cl. perfringens* is present in the inoculum a zone of increased opacity will have been produced by the phospholipase in the medium around and beneath the growth on the untreated side of the plate; but on the other side, although the growth is equally good, there is no increased opacity because the phospholipase has been neutralized by the antitoxin. Other phospholipase-producing organisms exist, but only *Cl. perfringens* alpha-toxin and the closely related toxin of *Cl. bifermentans* are inhibited by *Cl. perfringens* antitoxin.

IMMUNOLOGY   In view of the nature of *Cl. perfringens* infections, there is no indication for active immunization. Passive immunization, both prophylactic and therapeutic, using polyvalent sera against the toxins of all of the common gas-gangrene organisms, is possible but of limited value.

ANTIBACTERIAL TREATMENT   Penicillin is the antibiotic of choice for treatment of gas-gangrene, and metronidazole is also effective. Surgical removal of necrotic material, in which anaerobes can multiply and into which antibiotics cannot penetrate, is of fundamental importance, and hyperbaric oxygen treatment may be beneficial.

Other Gas-gangrene Bacilli
Cl. novyi (Cl. oedematiens), Cl. septicum, and, less frequently, *Cl. bifermentans, Cl. histolyticum* and *Cl. fallax* are all capable of causing gas-gangrene similar to that caused by *Cl. perfringens*. In view of the nature of the infection and the similar habitats of the various species, it is not surprising that the same lesion often yields two or more of these species. They are distinguishable by the shapes and sizes of their bacilli, the shapes and situations of their spores, their cultural and biochemical properties and the toxins which they form.

Clostridium difficile
Disturbance of the ecological balance of the intestinal flora by antibiotics—notably lincomycin or clindamycin—or by other factors sometimes permits proliferation of *Cl. difficile*. This species, commonly found in the faeces of healthy neonates but usually hard to detect in those of healthy adults, produces an exotoxin and causes *pseudomembranous colitis* (PMC), which may be severe and can be fatal if not treated promptly and appropriately. The diagnosis of PMC is based on the sigmoidoscopic and histological appearances of the colon and also on demonstration that the patient's faeces contain *Cl. difficile* and that faecal extracts are cytotoxic to cultures of appropriate cells in defined conditions. Oral vancomycin is the antibiotic treatment of choice for PMC, with metronidazole as a less well-tried alternative. Wide variations in incidence of PMC in hospitals with similar prescribing habits suggest that cross-infection with *Cl. difficile* may be important.

Necrotizing Enterocolitis
This is an uncommon but severe and in many cases fatal disease of premature or otherwise compromised neonates. Failure of the intestinal blood supply seems to be its primary component, and is followed by much gas-production in the bowel wall and sloughing of the bowel mucosa. Various clostridia and other anaerobes have been blamed for causing this disease, but their role is by no means certain.

GRAM-NEGATIVE BACILLI: (a) ENTEROBACTERIA

Many species of aerobic, facultatively anaerobic Gram-negative bacilli that ferment (in the strict sense—p. 22) glucose and other carbohydrates and are oxidase-negative (p. 93) are commonly present in the human intestine, usually as commensals but some of them as actual or potential pathogens. Such organisms are also widely distributed in nature. They are collectively known by the informal name *enterobacteria*, though it would have been more logical to call them enterobacilli. The name 'coliform bacilli' is used by some to indicate the same range of organisms, but others use it for only part of that range.

To save repetition, we shall deal with the common properties of the enterobacteria and the chief procedures used for differentiating between them before we discuss the individual genera *Escherichia, Klebsiella, Salmonella, Shigella, Proteus* and *Yersinia*, with brief references to others.

MICROSCOPY Gram-stained films give little or no help in distinguishing between enterobacteria, all of which are medium sized bacilli, about 0.5 μm by 1–3 μm (Fig. 5(f), p. 81), with some (at times many) filamentous forms. Some of the group—notably the klebsiellae and many *Esch. coli* strains—have easily demonstrable capsules. Possession of flagella can be an important criterion for differentiation—e.g. between the genera *Salmonella* (flagellate) and *Shigella* (non-flagellate) or *Klebsiella* (non-flagellate) and *Enterobacter* (flagellate); or between the species *Yersinia pestis* (non-flagellate) and other yersiniae (flagellate). Direct demonstration of flagella by light microscopy is difficult (p. 73), but *motility*, the effect of flagella, is relatively easily detected by direct microscopy of a drop of unstained fluid culture under a microscope, using reduced lighting (p. 15). An alternative non-microscopic method depends on the ability of motile organisms to make their way through a semi-solid medium (0.2 % agar).

CULTURE Enterobacteria grow well over a wide range of temperatures on or in simple media such as nutrient agar or peptone water (a solution containing 1 % commercial peptone and 0.5 % NaCl) under aerobic conditions, but somewhat less well anaerobically. On aerobically in-cubated blood agar, colonies are usually rather large (3–4 mm in diameter after 18 hours) and greyish-white, smooth and moderately opaque; however, dry rough-surfaced colonies, large mucoid colonies and other variants occur. Haemolysis may occur round the colonies, but is not a useful differentiating feature in this group. Having modest nutritional requirements and being tolerant of bile (understandably, in view of their intestinal habitat), enterobacteria grow on MacConkey's agar (p. 76). This medium, frequently used as a means of separating them from a mixture of other bacteria, also provides a useful distinction between the red colonies of lactose-fermenters (the usual behaviour of *Esch. coli* and klebsiellae) and the straw-coloured colonies of non-lactose-fermenters (salmonellae, most shigellae, proteus and yersiniae).

BIOCHEMICAL REACTIONS   Lactose is only one (though the most useful) of a wide range of carbohydrates that can be employed in fermentation tests for the identification of enterobacteria. If such tests are carried out in liquid media, small inverted tubes or other means can be used to detect generation of gas bubbles during fermentation and so to increase the information derived. For example, fermentation of glucose and failure to ferment lactose, sucrose and various other commonly used carbohydrates are properties common to all salmonellae; but *S. typhi* alone in this genus fails to produce visible amounts of gas during glucose fermentation. Fermentation tests using 6 or 8 sugars or alcohols, supported by some of the other biochemical tests mentioned below, permit provisional or even definitive identification of most enterobacteria to species level.

Among other biochemical tests commonly applied to enterobacterial strains are those for the abilities to produce hydrogen sulphide and indole when growing in peptone water; to split urea with liberation of ammonia (the urease test); to multiply in a medium in which citrate is the only carbon source; to decarboxylate various amino-acids; and, when growing in glucose-phosphate broth, to form acetylmethylcarbinol (the Voges–Proskauer test) and to go on producing acid from the glucose until the pH of the medium is lowered to 4.5 or less (the methyl red test).

ANTIGENIC STRUCTURE   Of the many enterobacterial antigens that have been studied, most can be classified according to their location as H (flagellar), O (somatic) or K (capsular or envelope). (The letters H and O are taken from the German terms *Hauch* and *ohne Hauche*, because flagellate proteus strains form spreading films across culture plates, whereas non-flagellate forms are 'without film'.) The relevance of antigenic analysis to our understanding of the various enterobacterial genera is indicated at appropriate places below.

THE GENUS ESCHERICHIA (See also pp. 109–10)

Esch. coli is the only species currently assigned to this genus.

OCCURRENCE AND PATHOGENICITY *Esch. coli* is a normal inhabitant of the intestine of man and animals, but is not always harmless there. In Britain and other temperate countries the commonest form of entero-pathogenicity of this species to man is gastro-enteritis in infants and other young children. Strains of a limited but growing number of O and K serotypes have been found responsible for this, though by no means all strains of those types are potential pathogens. Many of the recognized outbreaks have occurred in hospital nurseries, and there have often been associated deaths, mainly among premature and debilitated babies. The pathogenetic mechanism of these strains (known as 'infantile entero-pathogenic') is still debatable, but strains of other serotypes ('entero-toxigenic') which cause gastro-enteritis in adults as well as children, mainly in tropical countries, do so by producing enterotoxins similar to that of *Vibrio cholerae* (p. 121); and still other strains ('entero-invasive') resemble the shigellae in their ability to invade and destroy intestinal epithelial cells. Such adult infections are rare in Britain, but account for many cases of 'traveller's diarrhoea'. However, despite the increasing amount of information about *Esch. coli* as an intestinal pathogen, its main contribution to human ill-health is made in the urinary tract; here it is responsible for 80 % or more of all infections that occur outside hospital, but a smaller proportion of those acquired in hospital, many of which are due to klebsiellae, proteus, enterococci or other bacteria. *Esch. coli* can also cause biliary tract infections; and it is found, often in association with *Bacteroides* species (p. 129) and other intestinal organisms, in intra-abdominal abscesses and in many infected wounds, particularly those of the abdominal wall. From such sites it may reach the blood-stream, and may cause septicaemia. It is a common cause of meningitis in the first few weeks of life. Its role in the respiratory tract is discussed below, with that of the klebsiellae.

ANTIBACTERIAL TREATMENT   Antibacterial drugs to which entero-bacteria, including *Esch. coli*, are resistant include penicillin, cloxacillin, erythromycin, clindamycin and fucidin. Many *Esch. coli* strains are sensitive to ampicillin and some other penicillins and to the cephalosporins; but strains which produce enzymes (β-lactamases—p. 317) that destroy some of these drugs are increasingly common, especially in hospitals because these provide a selective environment for their propagation. Similarly, many strains of this species are sensitive to sulphonamides, trimethoprim, tetracyclines, aminoglycosides, chloramphenicol and various other drugs; but resistance to one or more is common, especially in hospital strains. When septicaemia or some other serious infection has to be treated urgently, without waiting for results of sensitivity tests on the causative *Esch. coli* strain, a drug to which it is unlikely to be resistant should be used—e.g. gentamicin or one of the newer cephalosporins. Nitrofurantoin or nalidixic acid are sometimes effective in urinary tract infections (p. 326).

THE GENUS KLEBSIELLA (See also pp. 109–10)

Klebsiellae are non-motile, which distinguishes them from the relatively unimportant genus *Enterobacter*. They have polysaccharide capsules, by means of which, like pneumococci, they can be divided into a large number of types. The more pathogenic members of the genus are included in the first 3 types. Type 3 includes the organism, originally known as Friedländer's bacillus, which in some countries (though not in Britain) is a quite common cause of pneumonia, notably of a form characterized by multiple cavitation of the lung; it can also cause meningitis, otitis and sinusitis. Some use the species name *K. pneumoniae* for this organism, and the names *K. edwardsii* and *K. atlantae* for organisms of somewhat similar pathogenicity that belong to types 1 and 2; whereas others include all of these in *K. pneumoniae*. Most other klebsiellae are classified as *K. aerogenes*, a species that includes strains of many serotypes. These are widely distributed in nature, are commonly found in the human intestine, and occasionally cause urinary tract, wound or other infections. Klebsiellae are often present in large numbers in purulent sputum, a situation in which *Esch. coli* and other similar enterobacteria are also quite common, and it is easy to conclude from this that these organisms are common causes of suppurative respiratory tract infections. However, the usual sequence of events is that the patient has already been treated with antibiotics for a lower respiratory tract infection (or for some other reason), that this treatment has disrupted the normal ecological pattern in the respiratory tract, and that enterobacteria resistant to the antibiotics used have taken advantage of the situation—often accompanied by yeasts. In such circumstances further antibiotic treatment aimed at the enterobacteria is likely to complicate the situation still further, whereas stopping all antibiotics usually results in a fairly rapid restoration of the normal bacterial population—except in patients whose defence mechanisms have been severely impaired by serious disease, immunosuppressive treatment, etc., in whom the enterobacteria may be opportunist pathogens (p. 67). Klebsiellae are prominent in this context because resistance to antibiotics, especially to ampicillin and the older cephalosporins, is even commoner in this genus than in *Esch. coli*. (The somewhat similar role of *Pseudomonas aeruginosa* is discussed on p. 120.)

THE GENUS SALMONELLA (See also pp. 109–10)

Virtually all members of this genus are motile, though non-flagellate variants occur. They are all intestinal pathogens. *S. typhi*, *S. paratyphi A*, *S. paratyphi B* and *S. paratyphi C* cause the septicaemic illnesses collectively known as enteric fever, discussed below under *S. typhi*. Other members of the genus occasionally produce a somewhat similar picture, but far more commonly they cause the more localized condition known as gastro-enteritis or food-poisoning (pp. 284–5).

The subdivision of this genus is unusual in that it is based mainly upon antigenic analysis. Most strains can be shown to possess two or more somatic (O) antigens and one or more flagellar (H) antigens. On the basis of O antigens alone the species can be divided into ten major and some minor groups, and even then the members of one group are not identical in their O antigenic structure but simply have one or more antigens in common. Each group can then be subdivided according to the H antigenic structure of its members. In this way over 1800 salmonella types have been distinguished and many have been allotted binomials which suggest that they are species—e.g. *S. typhimurium* and *S. enteritidis*. However, antigenic analysis is a much more delicate means of subdivision than those applied to other genera, and the majority of these different salmonellae, which cannot be distinguished by their microscopic or colonial appearances or, in most cases, by their biochemical reactions, are more reasonably described as *serotypes* rather than as separate species.

Analysis of the H antigenic structure of salmonellae is further complicated by the fact that many types are able to exist in either of two phases differing in their H antigens. Types which are different when in phase 1 may have identical phase 2 H antigens. Thus *S. typhimurium* has the same phase 2 antigens (designated 1 and 2) as *S. derby, S. heidelberg* and a number of other types that are also identical with it in their O antigen composition. When in phase 2, therefore, these types are indistinguishable. However, an apparently pure phase 2 culture nearly always contains a very small minority of phase 1 forms (and vice versa), and there are ways of extricating a pure culture of the minority phase. In phase 1, *S. typhimurium* has antigen i; *S. derby* has f and g; *S. heidelberg* has r; and so on.

What is the point of this fine differentiation of salmonellae, which in some cases can be carried still further by detecting variations of phage sensitivity or of biochemical reactions within a single serological type? It is far from being a purely academic exercise, for it greatly increases the precision and certainty with which the sources and methods of spread of outbreaks of infection can be traced. The finding of a salmonella carrier may or may not be relevant to a particular outbreak; the finding of a carrier of a strain identical with that which caused the outbreak is far more likely to be relevant; and that likelihood increases in step with the accuracy with which the identity of the two strains is established.

Salmonella typhi (the typhoid bacillus)

OCCURRENCE AND PATHOGENICITY   Like all salmonellae, this species is entirely parasitic. It differs from many of the others in that man is its only natural host, and that even in the laboratory it is of low virulence for mice and other animals. Although epidemics are usually spread via water supplies or food (as in the examples quoted on p. 114), the source of the organism is always a human patient or carrier.

In its early stages enteric fever (whether it is true typhoid or due to one of the other salmonellae—see p. 112) is predominantly a septicaemia rather than an alimentary disorder. Having entered the body through the mouth, the organism probably reaches the blood stream via the intestinal lymphatics. After the septicaemic phase it becomes localized, chiefly in the Peyer's patches of the small intestine, in the gall bladder and in the kidneys, but also sometimes in other sites such as the bone marrow, where it may cause osteitis. The clinical picture in the first week of the illness usually consists of progressively mounting fever, headache and severe malaise. Diarrhoea is not common at this stage, and indeed the patient is often constipated. In the second week the nature of the infection is likely to become more obvious with the appearance of the characteristic 'rose-spot' skin eruption and the onset of profuse diarrhoea. Ulceration of Peyer's patches may lead to intestinal perforation or haemorrhage, which are common causes of death in untreated cases. In the convalescent period relapses are common.

CARRIERS   A small proportion of those who recover from typhoid continue to harbour the bacilli in their gall bladders or kidneys, and many excrete them intermittently for many years. Antibiotic treatment often fails to eradicate the organism (see below). Gall-bladder carriers may be rendered innocuous by cholecystectomy, but renal carriage is a more difficult problem. It is highly important that carriers should be aware of their state and should carry out the necessary hygienic precautions. The most famous example of their harmful potentialities is 'Typhoid Mary', a cook who caused at least six small outbreaks in the New York area between 1901 and 1907, and may also have been responsible for a water-borne outbreak that involved 1300 people. She was then kept under strict supervision for a few years, but escaped and became a hospital cook, causing another 25 cases. The 1937 Croydon outbreak, with 34 deaths among 341 known victims, was traced to a carrier who had been employed to repair a well. By a misunderstanding, water from this well was fed into the main water supply without filtration or chlorination. In contrast to these stories, a mysterious occurrence of a solitary case of typhoid in a small baby in London in the 1950s was found to be due to contact with its grandmother, who had had the disease 30 years earlier and was not known ever to have infected anyone else.

CULTURE   Salmonellae, like all enterobacteria, grow well on simple media and are therefore easy to isolate from such specimens as blood or urine. Isolation from faeces is more problematical, because of the large number of other bacteria present; even MacConkey's medium (on which, being non-lactose-fermenters, salmonellae form colourless colonies) is of little use for this purpose, as the salmonellae are often heavily out-numbered by other enterobacteria which grow equally well on this medium. To meet this problem various special *selective media* have been devised, such as *deoxycholate citrate agar* (DCA), which suppresses the growth of most bacteria other than salmonellae and shigellae. When the number of salmonellae in the specimen is very small even such a medium as this may not permit their detection, and the chances of isolating them are then considerably enhanced by using a *selective enrichment medium*, such as *selenite F broth*. In this, the lag phase (p. 29) of salmonellae is considerably shorter than that of other bacteria. From being a very small minority they may therefore become, within a few hours, a considerable proportion of the population, so that they are easily detected when the broth is subcultured.

During the first week of typhoid the organism can usually be grown from the blood. Positive blood cultures are less common as the disease progresses; bone marrow cultures may continue to be positive later in the disease than cultures of peripheral blood, particularly if antibiotic treatment has already begun. Faecal culture, which may be positive at any stage, is more often so in the second and third weeks. The bacillus may also be found in the urine after the second week. Repeated examinations of the faeces and urine of all convalescents make possible the early detection and treatment of those who have become carriers.

PHAGE TYPING   Some dozens of *S. typhi* types have been identified by means of Vi phages, so called because they are effective only against strains that still possess the Vi antigen (see below). The typing procedure is essentially similar to that for staphylococci (pp. 83 and 194) except that it does not depend upon the specificity of naturally occurring phages; phages can be 'trained' to detect strains of particular types.

ANTIGENIC STRUCTURE   *S. typhi* has only a single phase 1 H antigen, which it shares with a few other salmonellae but not with any that have the same O antigens; and it has no phase 2. Freshly isolated strains have a surface antigen, designated Vi (for virulence). Some strains of *S. paratyphi B* and a few other salmonellae have the same Vi antigen.

IMMUNOLOGY   There is no conclusive evidence that useful immunity follows natural infection. Active immunization, using suspensions of killed bacilli (p. 295), causes pronounced antibody responses, but whether it also gives a useful degree of protection has been far more difficult to establish, and depends on the method of preparation of the antigen (p. 296). H, Vi and O antibodies can be measured separately in a patient's serum (the *Widal test*, p. 248). The value of such measurements is discussed on pp. 248–9. In an attack of enteric fever they may give useful diagnostic information from the second week of illness onwards.

ANTIBACTERIAL TREATMENT   Chloramphenicol was the first antibac-terial drug to make a real impact on the treatment of typhoid, being highly effective in controlling the acute illness and greatly reducing the mortality. Unfortunately it fails to eradicate the organism, so that relapse and carriage are common after its use; and in recent years its usefulness has been much reduced in many parts of the world by the emergence of chloramphenicol-resistant strains of *S. typhi*. Alternative drugs for treatment are amoxycillin (which is better than chloramphenicol at eradicating carriage) or cotrimoxazole.

The Paratyphoid Bacilli
S. paratyphi A, B and C, which also cause enteric fever but usually a milder form than that due to *S. typhi*, differ from that species and from one another in their biochemical properties and antigenic structure and in their geographical distribution. *S. paratyphi* B is the only one to occur at all commonly in Britain. Like *S. typhi* it can be divided into many phage-types.

Other Salmonellae
Most of the other salmonella types are primarily animal pathogens which occasionally attack man. Since they are mainly transmitted in food and

cause vomiting and diarrhoea in man, they are further discussed in Chapter 19. *S. typhimurium*, an organism with many other animal hosts besides the mice from which it takes its name, is the commonest cause of human salmonellosis in Britain, but many other types make their contributions, with relative frequencies which vary from year to year as the result of changes in imports of human or animal foods and many other factors. Attempted treatment of salmonella enteritis with antibiotics is seldom beneficial (provided that there is no accompanying bacteraemia); and, probably because it does more harm to the normal intestinal flora than to the salmonella, it is liable to prolong the period of carriage and faecal excretion of the salmonella which commonly follows such an infection.

THE GENUS SHIGELLA (See also pp. 109–10)

OCCURRENCE AND PATHOGENICITY   The dysentery bacilli are obligate parasites, of man or occasionally of chimpanzees or monkeys. They cause illnesses which vary in severity according to the species involved—in the general order *Sh. dysenteriae, Sh. flexneri, Sh. boydi* and *Sh. sonnei*—from severe abdominal pain, fever, prostration and profuse bloody diarrhoea to a mild intestinal upset with little systemic disturbance. In general their pathogenicity is thought to depend on destructive invasion of the intestinal mucosa, but the fiercer onslaught of *Sh. dysenteriae* includes production of a cholera-like enterotoxin. *Sh. sonnei*, the mildest of the four, is the commonest in Britain and causes many epidemics in institutions. Young children are particularly susceptible. In countries with warm climates and poor standards of hygiene, flies are important in transmission, carrying the organisms from human faeces to food; but direct contact and contamination of toilet fittings, door handles and fomites account for the majority of infections in Britain. It has been shown that *Sh. sonnei* can pass through toilet paper and can survive for several hours on fingers.

CARRIERS   Carriage, which is entirely intestinal, is usually of short duration but may persist for years. In most cases excretion is intermittent, but that of *Sh. dysenteriae* may be continuous

CULTURE   Growth on most media is similar to that of other enterobacteria. Isolation of shigellae from mixed cultures is helped by selective media such as DCA (p. 114), on which they form colourless or, in the case of *Sh. sonnei*, pale pink ('late lactose-fermenting') colonies.

TYPING   Being non-flagellate, shigellae have no H antigens, but they can be divided into serogroups and serotypes based on their O antigens. They can also be typed according to their production of *colicines*—antibiotics of a class produced by many enterobacteria, effective only against limited ranges of other enterobacteria, and therefore classifiable by determining the action of each one on a standard set of test strains. (Colicine-typing can also be carried out the other way round, by testing the susceptibility of the unidentified strain to a set of known colicines—a process similar to phage-typing.)

IMMUNOLOGY Immunity following natural infection is type-specific and transitory, and it is therefore not surprising that there are no generally accepted procedures for either active or passive immunization, though success has been claimed for some methods.

ANTIBACTERIAL TREATMENT Many antibacterial drugs are effective against shigellae *in vitro*, but their clinical value is less certain and, widespread use of almost any of them is liable to be followed by rapid emergence of shigella strains resistant not only to the drug used but often to various others as well (see p. 317—transferable multiple antibiotic resistance). Since many cases, especially of *Sh. sonnei* infection, recover spontaneously and completely within a few days, there seems to be a strong argument for restricting attempts at antibacterial treatment to seriously ill or very frail patients and persistent carriers.

THE GENUS PROTEUS (See also pp. 109–10)

The members of this genus are commonly found in faeces, in soil and in many other situations. They resemble *Esch. coli* in their ability to cause urinary tract infections and their involvement in wound infections. Their ability to swarm over the surfaces of many solid culture media, burying the colonies of other organisms, is a constant source of annoyance to the bacteriologist who is trying to obtain those other organisms in pure culture; he has to resort to special inhibitory media or procedures. The genus consists of four species, *Pr. mirabilis, Pr. vulgaris, Pr. morgani* and *Pr. rettgeri*, of which the commonest, in spite of their names, is *Pr. mirabilis* and not *Pr. vulgaris*. They are often resistant to various commonly used antibiotics (the range depending to some extent upon the species), and are therefore liable to persist in wounds and other lesions after treatment has disposed of staphylococci or other primary pathogens.

THE GENUS YERSINIA (See also pp. 109–10)

This genus contains 3 species of medical interest: *Y. pestis* and *Y. pseudotuberculosis* (both previously classified in the genus *Pasteurella*) and *Y. enterocolitica*.

Yersinia pestis

OCCURRENCE AND PATHOGENICITY The causative organism of plague (the Black Death of the Middle Ages, still endemic in many countries) is primarily a flea-borne pathogen of rats and other rodents, among which it causes highly lethal epidemics. Transfer to man occurs when an infected rat-flea (*Xenopsylla cheopis*) abandons the dead body of its rodent host.

Starving because its proventriculus is blocked by multiplying bacilli, it tries to obtain food from a human host. A little blood is aspirated into its proventriculus, mixed with bacilli and then regurgitated into the puncture wound. The human host rapidly becomes ill with *bubonic plague*, developing a marked enlargement or bubo of the regional lymph nodes, usually in the axilla or groin, and then as a rule a septicaemia. If this leads to pulmonary infection, *pneumonic plague*, he becomes a source of droplet spread to other humans. Control of rodents, with particular attention to preventing them from boarding or leaving vessels at ports, has kept Britain and many other countries free of this major scourge for many years.

MICROSCOPY   In tissues and other pathological materials, such as bubo aspirate and sputum, *Y. pestis* is a short, oval, capsulate, non-motile Gram-negative bacillus. With methylene blue and various other dyes it shows bipolar staining—i.e. deeper staining at the ends of the rods than in their centres (Fig. 5(*k*), p. 81). In culture the capsule is lost, bipolar staining is less obvious and the bacilli are often longer and pleomorphic.

CULTURE   This species is unusual among human pathogens in that it grows best at about 27°C (p. 23). In other respects its laboratory behaviour is similar to that of other enterobacteria.

Yersinia pseudotuberculosis and Yersinia enterocolitica
Both of these organisms have been isolated from many species of domesticated and wild animals. In man, *Y. pseudotuberculosis* can cause a fulminating typhoid-like septicaemia, which is fortunately rare; *Y. enterocolitica* can cause enterocolitis, resulting in abdominal pain and diarrhoea; and either of them can cause mesenteric adenitis, occurring mainly in children and young adults and frequently misdiagnosed as acute appendicitis. Yersinia infections are particularly common in Scandinavia. Late sequelae include reactive arthritis (p. 66), Reiter's syndrome and erythema nodosum. The bacteriological diagnosis in such cases can be established either by isolating the organisms (both resembling *Y. pestis* in most laboratory properties) from blood, faeces, lymph nodes or other appropriate material, or by detecting rising levels of specific antibodies in serum. Recovery of *Y. enterocolitica* from faeces is facilitated by 'cold enrichment'—i.e. keeping the specimen for 3 weeks at 4°C, a temperature that suits yersiniae better than most other bacteria present, and culturing it from time to time during that period.

OTHER ENTEROBACTERIA

The organisms classified as *Enterobacter, Citrobacter* or *Serratia* or in various other genera of this group were formerly of interest to the medical bacteriologist only because they are liable to be found in the same situations as potential pathogens and have to be distinguished from them. The position is now less simple, however, as such organisms are sometimes incriminated as pathogens, mainly in seriously debilitated patients in whom they may even cause septicaemia. They are commonly resistant to many β-lactam and other antibiotics.

GRAM-NEGATIVE BACILLI: (b) THE GENUS PSEUDOMONAS

Members of this genus resemble the enterobacteria in microscopic appearance (apart from having polar rather than lateral flagella, a distinction shown only by special microscopic techniques) but differ from that group in being strict aerobes, in oxidizing carbohydrates instead of fermenting them, and in being oxidase-positive (p. 93). Many of them produce fluorescent pigments. They are widely distributed, and include plant pathogens and many saprophytic species. With the exception of the one species described below they are rarely pathogenic to man or of any other interest to the medical bacteriologist.

Pseudomonas aeruginosa (*Ps. pyoćyanea*)

OCCURRENCE AND PATHOGENICITY   This species, commonly present in the human intestine, has the ability to grow in almost any moist situation over a wide temperature range, needing only oxygen and a modest supply of nutrients. Consequently it can multiply in such preparations as eye-drops, ointments, lotions or even weak disinfectant solutions, and so be applied in large numbers to patients' surfaces or wounds. In such circumstances it can cause serious local or even systemic infections. (See p. 42 for the importance of numbers in bacterial infections.) Similarly, it can multiply in the warm moist conditions prevailing inside baby-incubators or ventilating machines and so be inhaled in large doses and colonize the patients' respiratory tracts. Here it usually does little or no harm, but it sometimes causes a necrotizing pneumonia, which may be fatal. Its resistance to most of the antibiotics available for clinical use adds to its capacity for causing trouble, as it is liable to take over when the primary causes of infection in wounds, burns and many other situations have been eliminated by treatment. Its behaviour is much the same in the severely damaged airways of patients with bronchiectasis or cystic fibrosis who have received antibiotics for treatment of more orthodox respiratory tract pathogens. Again, it is usually harmless there but may cause pneumonia. A curious feature of such invasion of the lower respiratory tract is that any strain of this species which has established itself there is liable to undergo a change that causes it to form mucoid colonies on plate cultures. In the urinary tract, pseudomonas infection is a common and often intractable complication of neurological or other conditions that interfere with bladder emptying. *Ps. aeruginosa* is frequently present in inflamed external auditory canals, and may be pathogenic there, particularly in swimmers and divers. Outbreaks of pseudomonas skin and ear infection sometimes occur among users of swimming pools and heated whirlpool baths with inadequate chlorination.

CULTURE   As already indicated, this species grows well on simple media under aerobic conditions. Typically its colonies are rough and irregular (but see the previous paragraph), and are recognizable also by their green pigment (p. 25), which diffuses into the medium and colours it green also. (This pigment-production accounts for the characteristic blue-green colour of pus due to this organism, which is the origin of the older specific name *pyocyanea*; and colonies and pus share also a distinctive musty smell.)

TYPING   This species may subdivide by *pyocine typing* (analogous to colicine typing—p. 116), by serotyping or by bacteriophage typing.

IMMUNOLOGY *Ps. aeruginosa*, an opportunist pathogen (p. 38), can cause severe infections in immunocompromised (notably neutropenic) patients. The normal flora and antibodies to antiphagocytic polysaccharides and extracellular products—e.g. exotoxin—are the basis of host resistance. Immunization with polyvalent (i.e. many-strain) vaccine may give some protection to patients with extensive burns. Neutropenic patients with *Ps. aeruginosa* infections may require granulocyte transfusion (p. 66).

ANTIBACTERIAL TREATMENT   Widespread resistance is the rule in this species. Antibiotics of the polymyxin group are usually effective in the laboratory but often less so in the patient. The penicillins ticarcillin and azlocillin and the aminoglycosides gentamicin and tobramycin are the most useful drugs currently available, but resistance to them is not uncommon. Some of the cephalosporins now being developed may improve the situation. The shortage of reliable drugs for treating them makes it all the more important to minimize the frequency of serious pseudomonas infections, by avoiding the situations that were described above as giving rise to them and by taking care not to transmit pseudomonas strains (especially those that are unusually resistant) from one patient to others. Relatively minor superficial infections should be treated by local application of disinfectants, as use of antibiotics may encourage development of resistance to them. Removal of *Ps. aeruginosa* from the respiratory tract can seldom be achieved by a direct antibiotic attack, but in selected cases withholding of all antibiotics may permit other more manageable bacteria to displace the pseudomonads.

GRAM-NEGATIVE BACILLI: (c) VIBRIOS AND CAMPYLOBACTERS

Vibrio resembles enterobacteria in being aerobic, facultatively anaerobic Gram-negative bacilli that ferment carbohydrates (cf p. 110). They resemble pseudomonads in having polar flagella and in being oxidase-positive (cf p. 93). They differ from both in other respects, notably in that their rods are typically not straight but comma-shaped (Fig. 5(*p*), p. 81). They are widely distributed in nature. The species of medical importance are *V. cholerae* and *V. parahaemolyticus*. The closely related organisms now called *Campylobacter* were formerly classified in the genus *Vibrio*.

Vibrio cholerae

According to current nomenclature this species includes, in addition to the organism responsible for cholera, a large number of biochemically identical or closely similar vibrios that are found in fresh or brackish (but not salt) surface waters in many parts of the world, including Britain. The true cholera vibrio has its own distinctive O antigen, designated O1. The other *V. cholerae* strains have been called 'non-agglutinating vibrios' because they are not agglutinated by O1 antiserum; but they are agglutinable by sera to their own O antigens, and in this way can be divided into numerous O serotypes. It is better to call them 'non-cholera vibrios' (NCVs), though even this is not entirely correct, as some of them cause diarrhoea when ingested by man and on rare occasions this is severe enough to resemble cholera.

True cholera follows ingestion of adequate numbers of cholera vibrios, usually in water or food. They multiply in the intestine and produce an enterotoxin. This stimulates adenylcyclase activity in the intestinal epithelium and so provokes a sustained outpouring of water and electrolytes, manifested clinically as a profuse watery diarrhoea. The consequent dehydration may be rapidly fatal, but with prompt, adequate and properly balanced fluid and electrolyte replacement the prognosis is good, since the organism does not invade the host's tissues or blood and its pathogenicity is entirely due to the local action of its toxin. As the 'rice-water stools' are little more than fluid cultures of *V. cholerae*, it is easy to see how the disease can be transmitted directly onto the hands and so into the mouths of attendants, or via food or water supplies if the standards of hygiene and sewage disposal are not good.

Having been endemic in the Indian subcontinent for many centuries, cholera spread around the world in a series of devastating pandemics during the 19th and early 20th centuries, but was then restricted in range again until 1961. Up to that date it was predominantly due to what is now called the 'classical' cholera vibrio, which produces severe disease in a large proportion of those infected but is not able to establish a stable relationship with its host—i.e. it is excreted by those incubating or suffering from the disease and for perhaps a few weeks after infection but persistent carriage does not occur. The eltor biotype of *V. cholerae*, named after the Sinai village of El Tor where it was first identified in 1906, became established as a cause of a rather mild form of cholera in and around Indonesia during and after the second world war, and then from 1961 onwards it spread westward across Asia into Africa and Europe. Cholera was unknown in Britain from 1909 to 1970; but in that year a holiday-maker returned from North Africa infected with the eltor vibrio, and another 25 such cases had been recognized by 1980. The eltor vibrio produces severe disease less frequently than the classical strain. Its 'success' in spreading so rapidly and so widely can be attributed to the fact that many of those infected are only mildly ill or symptomless but are nevertheless vigorous excreters of the organism.

In the laboratory, cholera vibrios can sometimes be recognized by microscopy of the fluid stools, as slightly curved rods with characteristic darting motility; but diagnosis in this way is unreliable except in cases of severe and clinically obvious cholera. Isolation of the vibrios is made easier by their ability to grow in alkaline peptone water (pH 8.0 or more) and to form yellow colonies on TCBS (thiosulphate citrate bile salts sucrose) agar. Their identity is confirmed by agglutination with specific O1 antiserum, and the biotypes are distinguished by an assortment of other tests.

Natural immunity to *V. cholerae* depends on secretory IgA, which prevents adherence of vibrios to the intestinal epithelium and also binding of enterotoxin to cell receptors. Immunization with killed *V. cholerae* has been widely practised but is of little value. Prevention depends on good general hygiene, with particular reference to protecting water supplies from faecal contamination.

Vibrio parahaemolyticus

This salt-water vibrio is a cause—in Japan a common cause—of acute gastro-enteritis that comes on some 10–20 hours after eating raw or inadequately cooked sea-food and lasts for a day or two. In Britain the organism has been isolated from locally bred oysters, but imported sea-foods such as prawns are more likely sources. Its isolation from foods, vomitus or faeces is helped by its ability to grow in media containing 3% NaCl and to form green colonies on TCBS agar (as used for *V. cholerae*).

Campylobacter jejuni and Campylobacter coli

The clinical importance of these two species has become apparent since the publication in 1977 of a simple method by which diagnostic laboratories can isolate them from faecal specimens. It uses the fact that they differ from other *Campylobacter* species and from most other bacteria of the human intestine in being 'thermophilic' (in the loose sense of that term indicated on p. 23). They will grow, forming distinctive colonies, on plates containing selective antibiotics and incubated at $43°C$ in an atmosphere containing $10\% CO_2$. They are oxidase-positive Gram-negative bacilli that resemble vibrios in their microscopic appearances and motility. In Britain they are now recognized as causing gastro-enteritis at least as often as salmonellae, mainly among young adults and among children up to 5 years old, whereas in some other countries most of the patients are infants. The illness usually starts with fever and acute abdominal pain, followed by watery and often bloody diarrhoea. Recovery usually occurs spontaneously in a few days, but can take several weeks; erythromycin may be helpful if symptoms persist. A few patients have developed septicaemia. The epidemiology of this disease still includes large areas of uncertainty. The thermophilic *Campylobacter* species are carried in the intestinal tracts of many animals, especially birds, and many isolated cases or small outbreaks of infection have been associated with eating contaminated poultry or other meat. Large water-borne or milk-borne outbreaks have been described. Pet dogs or cats may suffer from and transmit the disease. Human carriers are rare in Britain, but high carriage-rates have been reported from warmer countries. It is not yet clear how much *C. jejuni* and *C. coli* differ in clinical significance and epidemiological behaviour. Measurement of antibodies after the infection may be helpful for retrospective diagnosis or to identify the factor that precipitated a reactive arthritis (p. 66).

GRAM-NEGATIVE BACILLI: (d) PARVOBACTERIA

Whereas the enterobacteria are a group of essentially similar genera, the name 'parvobacteria' has no sound taxonomic basis; we retain it merely as a convenient collective term for a rather heterogeneous group of aerobic Gram-negative bacilli that differ in a number of respects from those described so far. They are smaller, usually 0.3–0.4 μm in width, and are often cocco-bacillary. They are not intestinal parasites. They are generally exacting in their nutritional requirements, forming much smaller colonies on blood agar than do the enterobacteria. With a few exceptions they also differ from the enterobacteria in failing to grow on MacConkey's medium. Included among them are a number of important pathogens.

THE GENUS HAEMOPHILUS

Members of this genus are characterized by, and classified according to, their need to be supplied with X and V factors (haemin and nicotinamide-adenine dinucleotide, p. 23). Both factors are absent from some forms of nutrient agar, and strains can therefore be tested for their requirements by growing them on such a medium in the presence of filter-paper disks soaked in one or both factors. On blood agar, which contains X factor and a little V factor, enhanced growth of V-factor-requiring organisms occurs around colonies or streaks of *Staph. aureus* and various other species which liberate V factor into the medium—a phenomenon known as *satellitism*. Heating of blood agar to produce chocolate agar destroys a substance in the red cells which is inhibitory to V factor, and the amount of this factor present is then sufficient to support a good growth of all haemophilus species.

Haemophilus influenzae (Pfeiffer's bacillus, the influenza bacillus)

OCCURRENCE AND PATHOGENICITY The species occurs purely as a parasite of man, and is very commonly carried in healthy nasopharynges. Most of these 'respiratory' strains are not capsulate, but a small percentage of healthy people carry capsulate strains, divisible into six types (a to f). Type b strains are of great clinical importance, being responsible for many cases (in some countries, notably the USA, for the great majority of cases) of bacterial meningitis in young children, and for various other serious acute infections, mainly in the same age-group. These include two conditions virtually always due to *H. influenzae* type b: epiglottitis, a disease that is likely to be rapidly fatal unless promptly and appropriately treated; and a characteristic cellulitis, usually on the face and neck or on a limb. Other forms of infection that may be due to *H. influenzae* type b or to other bacterial species include otitis media, suppurative arthritis and lobar or segmental pneumonia. Capsulate strains of the other five types are much less often incriminated as pathogens. Non-capsulate strains are the principal cause of suppuration, either persistent or intermittent during acute exacerbations, in the bronchi of patients with chronic bronchitis or bronchiectasis (pp. 229 and 339).

The name of the species is derived from the claim of its discoverer, Pfeiffer (in 1892) that it was the cause of influenza. This suggestion was not finally discredited until the influenza virus was discovered (1933).

CARRIERS   When a child has meningitis or any of the other acute illnesses caused by *H. influenzae* type b, there are commonly several nasopharyngeal carriers of this organism among his family or other close contacts; and secondary cases of illness occur during the next few weeks or months in a small minority of such situations.

MICROSCOPY   Members of this species are small non-flagellate, non-sporing and usually non-capsulate Gram-negative bacilli. Films from young cultures grown under favourable conditions usually consist of cocco-bacilli; pleomorphism with filament formation is commoner in cultures on less adequate media.

CULTURE   Factors X and V are both required for growth. Colonies on blood agar after 24 hours' incubation vary according to the quality of the medium from minute pin-points to translucent domes approximately 1 mm in diameter. In mixed cultures, satellite clusters of colonies around V-factor-producing colonies of other species are characteristic, and routine addition of a staphylococcal streak to blood agar cultures of respiratory tract specimens can be used as an aid to rapid recognition of the species. Chocolate agar is also a useful primary medium, since colonies formed on it by *H. influenzae* are considerably larger than those formed on blood agar. Capsulate strains can be recognized by growing them on a suitable transparent medium (e.g. *Levinthal's agar*), on which their colonies exhibit iridescence when examined by strong, obliquely transmitted light.

ANTIGENIC STRUCTURE   The six capsulate types have distinct polysaccharide capsular antigens, and with the aid of type-specific rabbit antisera they can be recognized by capsule-swelling tests, by agglutination of the bacilli or by precipitin tests using aqueous extracts of the bacilli.

IMMUNOLOGY Antibodies to somatic and capsular antigens are common in the blood of adults, and it is thought that acquired immunity is responsible for the restriction of acute infections due to type b strains almost exclusively to young children. Because of the significant mortality from infections with type b, and the disturbingly high rate of permanent disabilities following haemophilus meningitis, active immunization is desirable, but so far the otherwise promising type b polysaccharide vaccine has the major defect that it fails to stimulate antibody formation in children under $1\frac{1}{2}$ to 2 years old.

ANTIBACTERIAL TREATMENT Chloramphenicol is the agent of choice for treating haemophilus meningitis and other life-threatening *H. influenzae* type b infections; its action against this species is bactericidal, it has proved highly effective in such situations, and chloramphenicol-resistant haemophili are as yet rare. Ampicillin, which has been much used for these infections, had proved somewhat less reliable even before the emergence, from 1974 onwards, of penicillinase-producing *H. influenzae* type b strains against which it is liable to be disastrously ineffective. 'Third generation' cephalosporins such as cefotaxime and moxalactam seem likely to be useful, especially if strains resistant to both chloramphenicol and ampicillin are encountered. As yet no antibiotic has proved fully effective for treating carriers of *H. influenzae* type b or protecting children at risk of infection with this serotype. Long-term prevention or control of haemophilus infections in chronic bronchial disease is a difficult problem; amoxycillin, the tetracyclines and cotrimoxazole are the main weapons for this purpose.

Other Haemophilus Species
H. aegyptius (the Koch–Weeks bacillus), an organism which was incriminated as a cause of outbreaks of acute conjunctivitis in Egypt and elsewhere before Koch described his 'influenza bacillus', resembles *H. influenzae* very closely.

H. para-influenzae differs from *H. influenzae* in not requiring X factor. It is a common mouth organism, and (like many other species, especially mouth commensals) it causes occasional cases of bacterial endocarditis. There is some evidence that haemolytic variants of this species (*H. parahaemolyticus*) may sometimes cause acute pharyngitis.

H. ducreyi, the causative organism of the human venereal disease chancroid, requires X but not V factor, but it also has other special nutritional needs.

THE GENUS BORDETELLA

Bordetella pertussis (the whooping cough bacillus)

OCCURRENCE AND PATHOGENICITY Purely a human parasite, this organism causes a well-known febrile respiratory tract infection of childhood, characterized by paroxysms of coughing that end in loud inspiratory whoops. The disease is potentially lethal in infancy, or may leave the child with serious brain damage. Adults are sometimes affected. The infection is a superficial one of the trachea and bronchi, with epithelial damage and impairment of the normal ciliary clearance mechanism. Some cases of clinical 'whooping cough' are due not to *Bord. pertussis* but to adenoviruses or myxoviruses.

MICROSCOPY   The bacilli resemble cocco-bacillary cultures of *H. influenzae*.

CULTURE   Ordinary media do not suffice for primary isolation; for this purpose charcoal blood agar is used, or the medium containing glycerol, potato extract and 50 % horse blood which has been widely used ever since Bordet and Gengou described it in 1906. Inclusion of a low concentration of penicillin makes these media more selective. Several days of aerobic incubation at 37°C are necessary before the typical 'bisected pearl' or 'aluminium paint' colonies of *Bord. pertussis* appear. Once grown in this way, the organism can be transferred to serum agar or blood agar.

Specimens are collected by pernasal swabbing of the nasopharynx (p. 227), sometimes supplemented by holding a culture plate in front of the mouth of the coughing patient ('cough plate').

IMMUNOLOGY   Natural infection is followed by lasting immunity. Active immunization is discussed on p. 295. Agglutinating and complement-fixing antibodies can be detected in the blood from the third week of the disease.

ANTIBACTERIAL TREATMENT   Although *Bord. pertussis* is sensitive *in vitro* to numerous antibiotics, these drugs have little effect on the disease once symptoms have developed—presumably because after that it is too late to prevent epithelial damage. Erythromycin given during the incubation period may be of value; and antibiotics have an important role in dealing with secondary invasion of the lower respiratory tract by other bacteria, which may result in bronchopneumonia.

THE GENUS BRUCELLA

OCCURRENCE AND PATHOGENICITY   The three closely related members of this genus which cause undulant fever in man—*Br. melitensis, Br. abortus* and *Br. suis*—are primarily pathogens of goats, cattle and pigs respectively. The human disease, of which *Br. abortus* is virtually the sole cause in Britain, derives its name from the recurrent bouts of fever which are its principal feature. Fatigue, sweating, malaise, headache, anorexia, pains in joints and muscles and persistent depression are other common components of a clinical picture that often causes difficulty in diagnosis. The organism is widely distributed throughout the body, including the blood stream. Multiple small granulomatous nodules and micro-abscesses are found in affected tissues, the bacilli being mainly intracellular. Human infections with *Br. melitensis* occur chiefly in the Mediterranean area (Malta fever), Africa, and parts of the Far East and America. *Br. suis* is found in the USA and in Denmark. Ingestion of unpasteurized cows' or goats' milk or of milk products may disseminate infection widely, but in Britain today infection is mostly restricted to those in close contact with farm animals, notably veterinary surgeons, abattoir workers and farm workers and their families.

Contagious abortion of cattle due to *Br. abortus* is one of the very few microbial diseases in which the localization of the pathogens can be explained. Unusually high concentrations of erythritol are present in certain layers of the bovine placenta and in the foetal fluids, and are believed to account for the vigorous multiplication of *Br. abortus* in precisely these sites which is a feature of contagious abortion.

MICROSCOPY The bacilli are small and usually short. They are non-flagellate, non-sporing, non-capsulate (except possibly in some fresh isolates) and Gram-negative.

CULTURE *Br. abortus* requires $5-10\%$ CO_2 in its atmosphere for primary isolation (p. 223). Otherwise all three species are aerobes, with an optimal growth temperature of $37°C$. They are not particularly exacting in their nutritional requirements, but grow slowly, producing translucent and undistinguished colonies. Various special media, including selective media, are available. Isolation from patients is usually attempted by culture of large amounts of blood (up to 40 ml) added to a suitable broth. Appropriate atmospheric conditions must be provided if growth of *Br. abortus* is expected, and incubation should be continued for at least three weeks. Even with these precautions, repeated attempts to isolate *Br. abortus* are often unsuccessful; the other two species are easier to recover from blood. Culture of aspirated bone marrow is sometimes successful when blood-culture has failed. The organism may also be isolated by inoculating the buffy coat from centrifuged blood into a guinea-pig. Similar culture procedures and guinea-pig inoculation are used in isolating brucellae from milk and other animal materials.

SPECIES DIFFERENTIATION For epidemiological reasons it may be important to be able to identify brucella isolates precisely. Recognition of species, and of biotypes within species, is based on biochemical tests (mostly different from those used for other genera), on susceptibility to a bacteriophage specific for *Br. abortus* and to the inhibitory action of low concentrations of dyes in culture media, and on agglutinability by antisera specific for one or other of the two main antigenic components of the members of this genus. Using these criteria *Br. abortus* can be divided into 9 biotypes and *Br. melitensis* and *Br. suis* into 3 each.

IMMUNOLOGY   Some immunity follows natural infections. An attenuated *Br. abortus* strain has been widely used in Russia for immunization of humans exposed to high occupational risks of brucella infection. Measurement of antibody levels in the blood of patients for diagnostic purposes is discussed on pp. 249. Skin hypersensitivity following infection or immunization can be detected by using an extract of bacilli—*the brucellin test*—but this test is of little diagnostic value.

ANTIBACTERIAL TREATMENT   Probably because of the intracellular situation of the organisms, antibacterial treatment must be continued for several weeks to have a good chance of success, and the course may have to be repeated. The most commonly used drugs are the tetracyclines (sometimes with streptomycin, on empirical grounds) or cotrimoxazole. If these fail, a course of gentamicin may be beneficial.

PREVENTION   Transmission of brucellae in milk can be prevented by efficient pasteurization (p. 282). Eradication of the disease has been, or is near to being, achieved in some countries. It depends on vaccination of young animals of appropriate species, and slaughter of animals with serological or other evidence of brucella infection. It is costly, in money terms, but far less so than persistence of infection among cattle, which causes abortions, still-births, infertility and reduced milk yield, and inevitably results in transmission to some humans, in whom it produces long periods of obscure ill-health and impaired working capacity.

THE GENUS PASTEURELLA

Among the organisms (small Gram-negative bacilli, mostly oxidase-positive and unable to grow on MacConkey's agar) that remain in this genus after the departure of those now classified as *Yersinia*, there are some that cause haemorrhagic septicaemia and other infections in a wide range of animal hosts. They have had a diversity of names, but are now all included in a single species *P. multocida*. Such organisms are sometimes found in dog and cat bites of human beings, having come from the animals' mouths. The wounds may fail to heal until pasteurellae are eliminated by suitable antibiotic treatment—usually penicillin. Organisms of this and other *Pasteurella* species occur in the sputum of patients with chronic bronchial disease, but their significance there is uncertain.

FRANCISELLA TULARENSIS (*Pasteurella tularensis, Brucella tularensis*)

This small Gram-negative bacillus is an insect-borne pathogen of rabbits and other rodents in many countries, notably in the western USA and in Russia and Siberia. In such hosts it causes a plague-like illness known as tularaemia. Occasionally humans who handle infected animals are themselves infected, through skin abrasions, and develop a brucellosis-like illness which responds to tetracycline therapy. In the laboratory the organism resembles a pasteurella in some of its properties and a brucella in others.

LEGIONELLA PNEUMOPHILA

In 1976 there were 183 cases of pneumonia or other respiratory illness, some of them severe and 29 fatal, among over 3500 delegates to an American Legion convention in Philadelphia. A previously unrecognized small bacillus was shown to be the cause of this 'legionnaire's disease' or legionellosis, and is now known to have caused numerous other outbreaks and sporadic cases of illness in many countries, both before and since 1976. It is called *Legionella pneumophila*. It is Gram-negative, though it hardly stains at all unless the method is suitably modified; and it was difficult to grow until special media were devised. There is an obvious paradox about an organism that is now known to be widely distributed in water—e.g. in water-tanks, in shower-heads and in the cooling towers of air-conditioning systems—and yet is difficult to grow in the laboratory; the explanation may well lie in its dependence on other organisms, such as amoebae, found in its natural environments. Most of the recognized outbreaks of the disease have been associated with large buildings, such as hotels and hospitals. Illness presumably follows inhalation of the organism in droplets, and is characterized by fever, unproductive cough, headache, confusion, gastro-intestinal symptoms and in some cases renal failure. Mild illness is common, and *L. pneumophila* is certainly not the deadly killer that reporting by news media has suggested. The diagnosis can be made by using immunofluorescence to demonstrate the presence of the organism in sputum or bronchial secretions, or in biopsy or autopsy material. The organism can be grown from such specimens, either directly on a selective medium or following passage through a guinea-pig. Detection of specific antibodies in the patient's blood is currently the simplest way of establishing the diagnosis, but they often take several weeks to appear there. Erythromycin has been the most successful antibiotic for treatment of legionellosis, but has given disappointing results in some series of cases.

GRAM-NEGATIVE BACILLI: (e) THE BACTEROIDES GROUP

The genera *Bacteroides, Fusobacterium* and *Leptotrichia* consist of Gram-negative anaerobic bacilli that do not form spores and are mostly non-motile.

OCCURRENCE AND PATHOGENICITY These organisms are obligate animal parasites, forming part of the intestinal flora of all animals from termites to primates. In man, *B. fragilis* and related species are as numerous in faeces as bifidobacteria (p. 101); *B. bivius* and *B. melaninogenicus* are normal inhabitants of the adult vagina; and members of the *B. melaninogenicus/oralis* group and of the other two genera are found in the mouth, colonizing the gingival crevice and forming part of dental plaque. These Gram-negative anaerobes are frequently involved in necrotic or gangrenous lesions, with a distribution related to their normal habitats. *B. fragilis* is the one most commonly found in pus from intra-abdominal lesions, or in abdominal wound infections. *Bacteroides* species are frequently associated with septic abortion, post-partum uterine infection, Bartholin's abscess or other purulent infections of the female genital tract. Oral species, notably *B. oralis*, *B. melaninogenicus* and fusobacteria take part in infections of the head or neck, such as cerebral, dental or soft tissue abscesses. Also the fusiform bacillus now known as *Leptotrichia buccalis* is usually present in large numbers, along with the anaerobic spirochaete *Borrelia vincenti* (p. 143), in the oropharyngeal ulcerative condition called *Vincent's angina*, and these two have long been called 'Vincent's organisms' and suspected of causing the condition; but it now appears that *B. melaninogenicus*, also present in large numbers but less conspicuous in stained smears, is chiefly responsible for the inflammation and tissue destruction. *B. asaccharolyticus* and *B. ureolyticus* (*B. corrodens*) are commonly involved in necrotic or gangrenous lesions of the perineum, genitalia, lower abdomen or lower limb, especially in diabetics. Gram-negative anaerobes are seldom isolated in pure culture from septic lesions; they are usually accompanied by aerobic or facultative organisms, notably *Esch. coli* (p. 111), and in many cases by other anaerobes. Various forms of synergy between these different organisms have been postulated, but the anaerobes are probably responsible for most of the tissue damage. Discharges from lesions in which they are involved characteristically have a foul, putrid smell. In the absence of adequate antibacterial treatment Gram-negative anaerobes are liable to spread from the original lesions via the blood to give serious generalized infections.

MICROSCOPY *Bacteroides* are in general small round-ended bacilli, sometimes uniformly cocco-bacillary but often plemorphic; they are as a rule clearly Gram-negative. Bacilli of the other two genera are commonly long and tapered at both ends ('fusiform'), and may be difficult to see in Gram-stained films.

CULTURE Many Gram-negative anaerobes are rapidly killed by exposure to oxygen or by desiccation. They survive much better in pus than on swabs (p. 220); if there is no pus and swabs must be used, they should be sent in a transport medium (p. 221). Most strains from human sources grow well on blood agar if incubated anaerobically (p. 222); presence of $5-10\%$ CO_2 enhances the growth of many. The *B. fragilis* group produce small non-descript colonies overnight as a rule, but other species may take several days to do so. *B. melaninogenicus* and *B. asaccharolyticus* colonies on blood agar turn brown or black on prolonged incubation through accumulation of altered haemoglobin.

ANTIBACTERIAL TREATMENT   Removal of pus and necrotic tissue is an essential part of treatment of infection by anaerobes; appropriate antibacterial treatment is important, but of little avail on its own in many cases. Gram-negative anaerobes are resistant to many commonly used antibiotics, notably to the aminoglycosides—an important point when gentamicin is used for treatment of septicaemia associated with intestinal lesions or surgery. The most commonly pathogenic species, *B. fragilis*, is also penicillin-resistant. Metronidazole, to which virtually all of these organisms are sensitive, is currently the treatment of choice, and its prophylactic use has greatly reduced the frequency of infective complications following intestinal or female genital tract surgery (p. 308).

ACID-FAST BACILLI

THE GENUS MYCOBACTERIUM

The tubercle bacilli (*Myco. tuberculosis* and *Myco. bovis*), the leprosy bacillus (*Myco. leprae*) and the other members of this genus are distinguished by their acid-fast staining—i.e. their resistance, after being stained with hot carbol fuchsin, to decolorization with acid (p. 132). This property is at least partly dependent upon their high content of certain lipids, notably mycolic acid, but this is not the whole explanation. Mycobacteria are Gram-positive, but some of them are difficult to stain at all by Gram's method or by most other common procedures.

Mycobacterium tuberculosis and Myco. bovis (the tubercle bacilli)

OCCURRENCE AND PATHOGENICITY   Although these two species have different primary hosts (human and cattle), they have much in common and it is convenient to retain the name 'tubercle bacilli' as a means of referring to them collectively. Both are pathogenic to man, but they differ in their pathogenicity to other species as indicated on p. 42. Man acquires infections with *Myco. tuberculosis* from his fellow human beings, usually by inhalation, and the resulting disease commonly involves the lungs. The risks of airborne infection are considerably increased by the ability of *Myco. tuberculosis* to survive for months outside the host—e.g. in dust and in books. Human infection with *Myco. bovis* usually results from drinking milk. It has been almost eliminated from this and many other countries by pasteurization of milk and control of tuberculosis in cattle. Because it enters the human body by the alimentary tract, *Myco. bovis* characteristically causes cervical and mesenteric adenitis rather than pulmonary lesions. Either species may travel via the blood to attack the meninges, bones, joints, skin and almost any other part of the body, and full discussion of the many possible forms of the disease is beyond our present scope.

It is important, however, to grasp the difference between *primary* and subsequent (variously known as *post-primary*, *secondary* or *adult-type*) infections. Infection of a subject who has no previous experience of tubercle bacilli results in a mild acute inflammatory reaction at the point of entry, with carriage of the bacilli to the local lymph nodes. Here a more vigorous reaction occurs, with enlargement of the nodes, which often undergo the caseous necrosis typical of tuberculosis. The small local lesion and the enlarged lymph nodes are together known as the *primary complex*, or, in the case of a lung lesion with mediastinal lymph node enlargement, as a *Ghon focus*. The infection may be arrested at this stage, the bacilli remaining alive for many years inside the lymph nodes, which become fibrotic and calcified. Alternatively, by travelling further along the lymphatic system or by the rupture of a caseous node into a blood vessel, the bacilli may enter the blood stream and be scattered throughout the body. It is likely that such blood stream dissemination occurs on a small scale in many cases, but results only in widespread minute lesions which, like those in the lymph nodes, undergo fibrosis and calcification. Even in the absence of treatment it is only in a small minority of patients that blood stream spread on a larger scale takes place, resulting in small progressive lesions of many organs. This condition is known as *miliary tuberculosis*, and commonly includes meningitis as its principal feature. Before the introduction of streptomycin it was almost invariably fatal within a few weeks.

Quiescent lesions left over from the primary infection may be reactivated later in life, often as a result of some other illness which lowers the patient's resistance. Alternatively, post-primary infection may be exogenous. In either case, the pattern of response is now quite different from that to the first infection. Because of a hypersensitivity reaction (Type IV, p. 65) to tuberculin and probably also of other less well recognized immunological responses to the primary infection, the bacilli are no longer permitted to travel through the tissues to the lymph nodes. they are prevented from doing so by a chronic granulomatous reaction. Slowly progressive lesions result, often involving extensive tissue destruction. Even this form of tuberculosis may lead to rapid miliary dissemination if the advancing lesion erodes the wall of a blood vessel and discharges its contents into it.

MICROSCOPY Mycobacteria do not form flagella, capsules or spores. Bacilli of this genus are best seen in films stained by the Ziehl–Neelsen (ZN) method. In this they are stained with hot carbol fuchsin for 5 minutes and then decolorized. Most mycobacteria other than *Myco. leprae* (p. 135) are resistant to decolorization by 20% sulphuric acid and are therefore called *acid-fast*, but the tubercle bacilli have the distinctive property of being also *alcohol-fast*—i.e. they cannot be decolorized by 95% ethyl alcohol. (As an alternative to using these two reagents separately, *acid-alcohol-fast* bacilli can be detected by washing the stained preparation with 3 % hydrochloric acid in 95 % ethyl alcohol.) Films are counterstained with methylene blue or malachite green, which stain micro-organisms that have not retained carbol fuchsin and also host cells and other structures, providing a suitable background against which to see the red mycobacteria. In pathological materials such as sputum and pus, tubercle bacilli are fine, slightly curved bacilli, measuring about 3 μm by 0.3 μm, and often appear beaded. As a rule they are scanty in such preparations, so that a prolonged search may be necessary before they are found. The auramine method (p. 16) is better than the ZN method for their rapid detection, though less good for demonstrating their morphology. Films from cultures usually show shorter, straight bacilli arranged parallel to one another in 'cords' or 'ropes'.

The finding of tubercle bacilli in pathological material signifies that the patient has an active tuberculous infection. If they are found in sputum, they also indicate that his lesion is 'open'—i.e. is discharging into his respiratory tract—and that he is a danger to those around him; and similar deductions can be made from their presence in any other excreted or discharged material. Because they are of such great significance, and also because they may be present only in very small numbers in a specimen, they must be searched for carefully in the smears. Smears from a concentrate of the specimen (see below) may give positive results when no bacilli are to be seen in those from the untreated specimen. It is very important to appreciate that *acid-alcohol-fast bacilli found in smears of pathological material are not necessarily tubercle bacilli.* Their identity must always be confirmed by culture and appropriate further tests.

CULTURE Tubercle bacilli are strict aerobes with a rather narrow range of growth temperature around 37°C, are exacting in their nutritional requirements and will not grow on ordinary media. The widely used *Löwenstein–Jensen medium* is made from eggs, glycerol, asparagine, potato starch and mineral salts; it also contains malachite green which inhibits other organisms and colours the medium so that the slightly yellow, dry, wrinkled colonies of *Myco. tuberculosis* are more easily detected. Solid and fluid culture media of simpler composition are also used. Even on optimal media growth is very slow, and colonies take ten days at least, and more commonly several weeks, to become visible.

Most pathological materials to be examined for the presence of tubercle bacilli contain them in small numbers, irregularly distributed throughout the specimen and mixed with larger numbers of faster-growing organisms. Various *concentration methods* are used to overcome these problems. They homogenize and liquefy such materials as sputum, so that the tubercle bacilli can be concentrated into a small volume by centrifugation; and they also kill virtually all of the other bacteria present. For this they rely upon the high resistance of tubercle bacilli to various forms of chemical treatment, but there is rather a narrow margin between the minimum treatment that will achieve the desired ends and that which will also kill all of the tubercle bacilli. The problem is enhanced when a specimen (e.g. faeces) contains bacteria of many species, including spore-formers.

Myco. tuberculosis can be distinguished from *Myco. bovis* in culture by differences in its colonial appearance, by its enhanced growth in glycerol-containing media and by its ability to synthesize niacin.

GUINEA-PIG INOCULATION   This procedure was in general use for many years as the most sensitive way of detecting the presence of tubercle bacilli in clinical specimens, and also for distinguishing between tubercle bacilli, which cause typical tuberculosis in guinea-pigs, and other mycobacteria, which fail to do so. Improvements in *in vitro* techniques have been such that guinea-pigs are now rarely used except for specimens thought likely to contain tubercle bacilli in very small numbers.

IMMUNOLOGY   Immunity to tuberculosis is cell-mediated, and depends largely on interaction between sensitized T-lymphocytes and macrophages (p. 62). Patients present a spectrum of clinical, bacteriological and immunological features ranging between states of low and high resistance. At one extreme, in miliary tuberculosis, cell-mediated immunity and tuberculin hypersensitivity are absent, and mycobacteria are numerous. At the other extreme, when there is a healed localized tuberculous lesion, cell-mediated immunity and tuberculin hypersensitivity are strong, and bacteria are few or absent. Patients may swing between these extremes—e.g. waning of immunity from age or disease may be associated with reactivation of disease, whereas successful drug treatment is correlated with increased cell-mediated immunity and elimination of the mycobacteria. Active immunization, using an attenuated bovine strain (BCG), is discussed on pp. 294–5, and the tuberculin test on pp. 253–4.

ANTIBACTERIAL TREATMENT   The prognosis of tuberculous infections, especially of progressive primary infections, was revolutionized by the introduction of streptomycin; but using it alone commonly resulted in the development of resistance to it by the tubercle bacilli, and the treatment then became ineffective. Present-day drug treatment of tuberculosis is discussed on pp. 338–9.

Mycobacterium leprae (the leprosy bacillus, Hansen's bacillus)

OCCURRENCE AND PATHOGENICITY   This organism was first described by Hansen, as early as 1874. It is an obligate parasite of man. It causes leprosy, a disease now largely restricted to tropical countries, where the total number of patients is of the order of 10 millions and is probably still rising. The disease has been difficult to investigate because it has only recently become possible to grow *Myco. leprae* in non-living culture media, and until 1960 there was no known means of infecting animals. Contrary to popular belief, human infection does not occur readily, and depends on prolonged exposure; skin-to-skin contact is probably less

important than was once thought, infection being mainly by inhalation of
bacilli shed from the noses of patients with lepromatous disease (see
below). The name leprosy is today restricted to *Myco. leprae* infections;
but as used in the Middle Ages and in English translations of the Bible it
must have included a range of other diseases.

The diverse clinical manifestations of infection with *Myco. leprae*
cannot be described here. Much of the diversity depends on differences in
immunological response, both between patients and at different times in
the same patient (cf. tuberculosis, p. 132). There is thus a spectrum of
disease, running from *lepromatous* through *borderline, dimorphous* or
intermediate to *tuberculoid* leprosy. In lepromatous disease bacilli are
numerous in the lesions and are shed in large numbers in nasal and other
discharges; the host seems to offer little resistance to the infection, which
is progressive and has a bad prognosis in the absence of treatment. At the
other end of the spectrum, tuberculoid leprosy is characterized by cell-
mediated immunity and by a Type IV hypersensitivity response in the
lepromin test which is somewhat analogous to the tuberculin test. Bacilli
are scanty in the lesions of tuberculoid leprosy, and there is a strong
tendency towards spontaneous healing as a result of the cell-mediated
response, but at the cost of a good deal of tissue and nerve destruction.
The main value of the lepromin test is that a positive result indicates a cell-
mediated response and hence a good prognosis. A negative result
indicates a poor prognosis in the absence of suitable treatment.

MICROSCOPY   *Myco. leprae* resembles *Myco. tuberculosis* in its morphology, but it is not alcohol-fast and is less strongly acid-fast. Five
per cent sulphuric acid is therefore substituted for 20 % in the decolorization of ZN films aimed to detect this organism. It is Gram-positive.

For diagnostic purposes, smears are made from scrapings of the nasal
mucosa of patients with lepromatous disease, and from subcutaneous
material obtained by making small skin incisions into actual lesions and
at a number of standard sites such as the ear-lobes and forehead. Staining
and microscopy of such smears is useful not only for establishing the
diagnosis but also for assessing the effectiveness of treatment, since a
satisfactory response is indicated by granularity and fragmentation of the
bacilli.

ANIMAL INOCULATION AND CULTURE   During the past 20 years it has
become possible to propagate *Myco. leprae* in the laboratory in various
ways: (1) in the foot-pads of mice, where it produces granulomatous
lesions, followed by 'borderline' lesions in other parts of the body after
many months; (2) in thymectomized irradiated mice, which develop
'lepromatous' disease; (3) in armadillos and hedgehogs, which have
appropriate body temperatures (see below); (4) in human nerve tissue
culture; and (5) in artificial media. In any circumstances the organism
grows very slowly, with an optimal temperature of 30 °C.

IMMUNIZATION   In Uganda in 1960–64 BCG vaccination of children was found to give a degree of protection against leprosy comparable with that which it gives against tuberculosis. Subsequent reports from other countries have been less encouraging.

Other aspects of the immunology of *Myco. leprae* infection have already been discussed above, because they are inextricably linked with the diversity of clinical presentation.

ANTIBACTERIAL TREATMENT Dapsone (diaminodiphenylsulphone), continued for 2–4 years, has been the mainstay of antibacterial treatment for leprosy. However, dapsone resistance has become an increasingly serious problem, and has necessitated multiple-drug treatment as in the case of tuberculosis (pp. 338–9). Rifampicin and clofazimine are currently added to the dapsone regimen. Rifampicin has been shown to be bactericidal to *Myco. leprae* and so to eradicate the infection in mice, but so far has not been shown to achieve total cure of human lepromatous leprosy.

Other Mycobacteria

Some cases of tuberculosis-like illness in man are due to organisms that have been given the unsatisfactory collective name *atypical mycobacteria*. Their chief clinical importance is that primary (i.e. pre-treatment) resistance to some of the standard antituberculous drugs (pp. 338–9) is common among them. Unlike tubercle bacilli, which have a narrow range of growth temperatures around 37°C, some of these other mycobacteria can grow at 25°C, some at 42 or even 45°C and some throughout the range 25–45°C. Some produce orange-pigmented colonies, but only when growing in light (*photochromogens*) and some do so in light or in darkness (*scotochromogens*). Some are fast-growing by myco-bacterial standards, forming visible colonies in a few days. With the possible exception of *Myco. ulcerans*, the atypical mycobacteria are not transmitted from man to man but are derived from environmental sources—including in some cases birds, fishes or amphibia.

The photochromogenic *Myco. kansasi* is the mycobacterium that most often causes lung lesions resembling those of true tuberculosis; but it can also cause disease of lymph nodes or elsewhere. Conversely, the non-chromogens cumbrously called the *scrofulaceum/avium/intracellulare* group (because they are less easily divisible into 3 species than was once thought) are now responsible for most cases of mycobacterial cervical lymphadenitis in children in Britain, but can also attack the lungs. *Myco. ulcerans*, which grows very slowly with little or no pigment and only within the range 31–34°C, has been shown to cause skin ulcers in Africa, Australia and elsewhere, and may prove to be rather closely related to *Myco. leprae*. *Myco. marinum*, a photochromogen with a preference for low temperatures, is a pathogen of fish and amphibia but also causes 'swimming bath granuloma' in man. Fast-growing mycobacteria are widely distributed in man's environment and are mostly non-pathogenic to him; but *Myco. chelonei* can cause abscesses (e.g. at injection sites) or even disseminated infections, usually in patients with impaired defence mechanisms.

BRANCHING BACTERIA

Some bacillary species form branched chains, but the branching occurs at the meeting-points of bacilli, not within individual bacilli. True branching, in which the branches are parts of the same cell, is shown by the filamentous fungi (Fig. 6(*b*), p. 197) and by certain bacteria known as *higher bacteria* (Fig. 5(*l*), p. 81). These include the genera *Streptomyces*, *Actinomyces* and *Nocardia*. The first genus is important to us because its members include many of the important antibiotic-producing organisms (see Chapter 21). The genera *Actinomyces* and *Nocardia*, sometimes referred to collectively as the actinomycetes, include a number of pathogenic species. They are non-motile, non-capsulate, non-sporing Gram-positive filamentous organisms. The filaments, which are much narrower than those of filamentous fungi, tend to fragment into conventional bacilli when grown in artificial cultures.

THE GENUS ACTINOMYCES

Members of this genus are micro-aerophilic or virtually anaerobic, though their metabolic pathways are not those of strict anaerobes. They are obligate parasites, and, unlike some Nocardia species, are not acid-fast. *A. israeli* causes human actinomycosis, and the closely related *A. bovis* causes 'lumpy jaw' in cattle. The non-pathogenic *A. naeslundi* can cause confusion, since it is found in human mouths and resembles *A. israeli* in many ways, but it is recognizable by its ability to grow aerobically.

Actinomyces israeli

OCCURRENCE AND PATHOGENICITY   The normal habitat of this species is the human mouth. It can be found around the teeth, gum margins and tonsils of many healthy individuals as well as in the lesions and discharges of actinomycosis, but has not been isolated from sources outside the body.

Actinomycosis is an acute, sub-acute or chronic granulomatous infection, often progressive if not treated. It is characterized by the formation of abscesses which drain to the surface of the body through sinuses that become surrounded by much fibrous tissue. The disease is believed to be endogenous, the *A. israeli* normally commensal in the mouth becoming pathogenic in circumstances which are only partly understood. Trauma, such as dental extraction or fracture of the jaw, may precede the onset of the disease, allowing implantation of *A. israeli* in damaged tissue, and it has been suggested that some form of sensitization to the causative organism may also play a part. Intra-abdominal actinomycosis follows inflammation or perforation of the appendix or large bowel. A small Gram-negative bacillus, dignified with the disproportionately long name of *Actinobacillus actinomycetemcomitans*, is sometimes found in large numbers in closed actinomycotic abscesses, together with *A. israeli*, but its significance is unknown.

The cervico-facial region is involved in over 50 % of cases of actinomycosis, the abdomen in 20 %, the thorax in 15 % and other parts of the body in the remaining few cases. Infection may remain localized, may spread through the tissues in a continuous manner, or may on rare occasions be disseminated through the blood stream. Lymphatic spread apparently does not occur. Colonization of intra-uterine contraceptive devices by actinomycetes is being recognized with increasing frequency, and is sometimes followed by infection of the uterus and adnexae.

MICROSCOPY   On close naked-eye examination of actinomycotic pus small yellow bodies—'*sulphur granules*'—can often be seen. These are in fact colonies of *A. israeli*, and if one of them is crushed between two microscope slides and stained, it can be seen to consist of a tangled mass of Gram-positive branching filaments. This appearance differs from that of a film made from a culture only in that short 'V' and 'Y' forms (a few of which are shown in Fig. 5(*l*), p. 81) are common in the latter. In Gram-stained sections of actinomycotic tissue, colonies resembling the sulphur granules are to be seen, surrounded by radiating 'clubs' of Gram-negative lipoid material produced by the host's tissues, probably as a form of protection.

CULTURE   *A. israeli* cannot grow in air. Some strains are micro-aerophilic and others require anaerobic conditions. The addition of 5–10 % CO_2 to the atmosphere often stimulates growth. The optimal growth temperature is 37°C, and growth does not occur at temperatures much below this. Raised, irregular, opaque colonies become visible after 3 or 4 days' incubation on blood agar or serum agar. They adhere firmly to the medium. Good growth also occurs in cooked meat medium (p. 222) and the other fluid media for anaerobic growth mentioned on p. 223, or in a glucose agar shake culture. This last is set up by inoculating the organism into a tube of melted medium at 50°C and dispersing it throughout the medium by shaking. When it has set, the medium is incubated for several days at 37°C. Colonies of *A. israeli* develop best about 10–15 mm below the surface, and also in the depths of the medium, but not near the surface, where the oxygen tension is too high.

For isolation of this species from pus, sulphur granules should be used as the inoculum. The pus is shaken up with water, and the granules are allowed to sediment. The diluted pus is then removed and the granules are repeatedly washed by shaking them up with more water, in order to rid them of accompanying bacteria.

ANTIBACTERIAL TREATMENT   The prognosis of abdominal and thoracic actinomycosis, formerly often fatal conditions, was radically altered by the advent of antibiotics, to many of which *A. israeli* is sensitive. Penicillin is the agent of choice, but prolonged high dosage may be required, since in chronic cases extensive deposition of fibrous tissue may restrict the amount of antibiotic which reaches the lesion and inadequate dosage may result in the development of antibiotic resistance by the organism. Good results have also been obtained with the tetracyclines, erythromycin or clindamycin.

THE GENUS NOCARDIA

These organisms differ from those of the genus *Actinomyces* in that all of them are aerobes, many are acid-fast and the majority are soil saprophytes. A few species are pathogenic to man, causing chronic granulomatous lesions.

Nocardia asteroides
This causes a rare pulmonary infection which may be mistaken for tuberculosis, particularly as acid-fast bacillary fragments may be found in the sputum. The disease may be carried to the brain or the skin via the blood stream. Sulphonamides may be effective if given early in the disease, which is otherwise usually fatal and unaffected by antibiotics.

Nocardia madurae
This is one of the causative agents of the chronic granulomatous, sinus-forming disease of the human foot known as *Madura foot* or *mycetoma*. Other forms of the disease are caused by fungi (notably those of the genus *Madurella*), other actinomycetes and streptomycetes. It occurs in tropical areas, particularly in South India and parts of Africa, where feet are often bare and liable to repeated minor trauma. The form due to *N. madurae* is characterized by the presence of white or yellowish granules in the pus, and responds to treatment with sulphonamides or with dapsone (p. 136). Such treatment has no effect on the forms due to fungi, which produce black granules.

SPIROCHAETES

The bacteria included in this group differ markedly in structure from any of the others that we have described. They consist of spiral filaments, in many cases too slender to be seen by ordinary microscopy of stained preparations (see below). They have no flagella, but are motile—often vigorously so—by means of whip-like flexion movements of their bodies or by screw-like rotation around their long axes. Partial digestion and electron-micrography have revealed the presence of one or more fine axial fibrils intertwined with the coils of their bodies. It seems likely that these are contractile and are responsible both for maintaining the spiral shapes of the organisms and for the movements that result in locomotion.

The spirochaetes of medical importance belong to the genera *Treponema*, *Leptospira* and *Borrelia*.

THE GENUS TREPONEMA

Treponema pallidum

OCCURRENCE AND PATHOGENICITY   Apart from experimental infections of apes, monkeys and rabbits, this organism is purely a pathogenic parasite of man. It is transmitted almost exclusively by sexual intercourse or by intra-uterine infection, and causes *syphilis*. The typical ulcerating primary lesion of extra-uterine infection, the *chancre*, appears several weeks after exposure, usually on the skin or mucosa of the genitalia but sometimes around the mouth or anus or elsewhere. It is not certain whether the spirochaete can penetrate unbroken skin or mucosa or depends upon trivial surface lesions for its entry. *T. pallidum* is present in profusion in the exudate from an early chancre, and also in the red macular skin lesions, the moist peri-oral and ano-genital papules (*condylomata*) and the 'snail-track' mouth and throat ulcers of the secondary stage of syphilis, which generally follows within a few weeks of an untreated primary lesion. It is less profuse, but often demonstrable, in the granulomatous lesions of many organs (*gummata*) which characterize the tertiary stage and in the arterial and nervous system lesion of late syphilis. Congenital syphilis, transmitted through the placenta in the latter half of pregnancy, involves many tissues and may kill the foetus.

MICROSCOPY   The organism consists of a delicate thread only about 0.15 μm thick, which is wound into a neat spiral 5–15 μm long and 1–5 μm wide with a 'wavelength' of about 1 μm (Fig. 5(*o*), p. 81). Being difficult to stain and of low refractility, *T. pallidum* is best seen by dark-ground microscopy (p. 16). A clinical diagnosis of primary or secondary syphilis can be confirmed by examining exudate from the lesion or lesions in this way; *T. pallidum* can be distinguished from the non-pathogenic treponemata (see below) and from other spirochaetes by its delicate structure and by its leisurely motility, which involves flexion and rotation. In dried smears or sections its presence can be demonstrated by the silver-impregnation methods of Fontana and Levaditi, but these methods obscure fine structural detail. Fluorescent-antibody staining is a better way of demonstrating the morphology of *T. pallidum* and also establishes its identity (p. 16).

CULTURE   It is doubtful whether *T. pallidum* has ever been grown in laboratory cultures. Spirochaetes have been isolated from lesions and maintained in culture, but these were almost certainly contaminating saprophytes. Nelson devised a medium in which *T. pallidum* can be kept alive for several days, but it does not multiply during that time. It can also survive for several days in refrigerated blood, and could therefore be transmitted by blood transfusion. It can be propagated in the laboratory by intratesticular inoculation of a rabbit and transfer to a new rabbit every 3 weeks or so.

IMMUNOLOGY   The natural history of syphilis, including long periods in which the organism remains latent in the tissues, indicates that some form of partial immunity does develop. Furthermore, reinfection of a person whose tissues already contain live *T. pallidum* does not result in a fresh primary lesion. However, immunity seldom, if ever, progresses to the stage of spontaneous eradication of the organism, and resistance to reinfection disappears following adequate bactericidal treatment of the first infection. Whereas the cell-mediated immunity of tuberculosis (p. 132) or leprosy (p. 135) develops early in the disease but may fluctuate, causing a 'horizontal' spectrum of disease manifestations, that of syphilis develops slowly but progresses, producing the 'vertical' spectrum (i.e. progressive sequence) of manifestations described above. Gummata represent further increase in the immune response, whereas neurosyphilis is a manifestation of an ultimate lowering of host resistance with proliferation of spirochaetes. Immunization is not practicable. The serological diagnosis of syphilis is discussed on pp. 249–52.

ANTIBACTERIAL TREATMENT Chemotherapy with arsenical compounds, introduced by Ehrlich in 1910, was effective but tedious and not without dangers. It has been entirely replaced by antibiotic treatment. Penicillin is the drug of choice because *T. pallidum* is always sensitive to it and because the possibility of giving a single injection of a long-acting penicillin preparation has overcome the great problem of continuance of treatment at venereal diseases clinics. Other antibiotics can be used for patients who are hypersensitive to penicillin.

Other Treponemata

Yaws or *framboesia* (an ulcerative skin disease occurring in hot countries and affecting mainly those of negro race) and *pinta* (also a disease of dark-skinned races, with non-ulcerative skin lesions and later cardiovascular and nervous system involvement) are caused by spirochaetes respectively named *T. pertenue* and *T. carateum*. Like the causative organism of *bejel* (a highly infectious skin disease occurring in Arabia), they are indistinguishable from *T. pallidum* in their morphology, in the serological reactions that they evoke and in their response to treatment. Since they also cannot be grown in culture, it is impossible to say whether they ought to be regarded simply as variants of *T. pallidum*. The diseases are non-venereal, being transmitted by direct contact or by insects. In addition to their pathological effects, they give rise to problems of serological diagnosis and can cause difficulties for would-be immigrants into countries whose laws exclude those with positive serological tests for syphilis.

Non-pathogenic treponemata are found in the mouth and around the genitalia, but usually differ in morphology from *T. pallidum* and stain more easily by ordinary methods.

THE GENUS LEPTOSPIRA

OCCURRENCE AND PATHOGENICITY   Like the salmonellae, these organisms have been divided serologically into a large number of types. These are now all classified within the single species *L. interrogans*, which is subdivided into 2 complexes. The biflexa complex includes saprophytic strains, which are numerous and widely distributed, particularly in water (even in domestic supplies); and the interrogans complex, consisting of some 130 serotypes arranged in 16 serogroups, includes most of the pathogenic and parasitic strains. These occur throughout the world, but many individual serotypes are geographically restricted. Many are pathogens of animals—e.g. rats (serotype *icterohaemorrhagiae* and many others), mice (*grippotyphosa, hebdomadis*), dogs (*canicola*), and cattle and pigs (*pomona*)—but can survive for long periods in neutral or alkaline (but not acid) water. Their ecology is exceptional, in that they continue to exist by means of living and multiplying in the urinary tracts of convalescent or unaffected carrier members of their various host species. Excreted in the urine, they enter new hosts through skin abrasions or mucous membranes. Man becomes infected in many different ways. In sugar-growing countries, which provide a large proportion of the world's total of cases of human leptospirosis, infection often results from workers scratching their legs and feet on cane-stubble on which rats have urinated. *Icterohaemorrhagiae, canicola* and a number of other serotypes occur in Britain, mostly with rodents as their principal hosts, though *canicola* affects dogs and pigs. Human infection in this country occurs particularly in agricultural workers, fish-farm workers and meat handlers, and can also follow accidental or recreational immersion in some rivers, lakes, etc. *L. canicola* infection most commonly occurs in those who have been caring for sick dogs, usually puppies. The former relatively high incidence among sewer workers, miners and fish-cleaners is no longer seen. The clinical picture produced in man depends to some extent upon the serotype responsible. Thus *icterohaemorrhagiae* infection typically results in classical *Weil's disease* with fever, jaundice, haemorrhage and renal failure and a high mortality, and *canicola* infection typically produces a milder disease of which the main feature is lymphocytic meningitis. However, many leptospiral infections produce nondescript pyrexial illnesses and some mimic conditions usually associated with other organisms.

MICROSCOPY   The tightly coiled fine spirals, similar in length to those of *T. pallidum*, are often bent into hooks at one or both ends (Fig. 5(*n*), p. 81). The organisms are vigorously motile, spinning so rapidly around their long axes that the hooks often have the appearance of closed loops.

CULTURE   Leptospires usually grow well just below the surfaces of various fairly simple fluid or semi-solid media. The optimal temperature for growth is about 30°C.
Blood culture, by adding a few drops of patient's blood to a few ml of

one of the fluid media, is often successful in isolating the organism during the first week of the illness. It can profitably be supplemented by intraperitoneal injection of blood into a young guinea-pig or hamster. If leptospires are present they can be recovered in pure culture a few days later by cardiac puncture of the animal, which also goes on to develop the characteristic and fatal haemorrhagic disease. Leptospires can sometimes be recovered from urine in the second or later weeks of the illness by such animal inoculation, but rarely by culture.

IMMUNOLOGY   Immunity to many or all serotypes follows recovery from natural infection. Artificial immunization has been used successfully in Japan. Complement-fixation tests and various other serological procedures are used in diagnosis.

ANTIBACTERIAL TREATMENT   Treatment with penicillin (in high doses) or one of the tetracyclines is sometimes helpful if used early in the disease but is valueless later on.

THE GENUS BORRELIA

These large, motile spirochaetes with only a few loose, irregular waves are distinctly Gram-negative.

Borrelia vincenti and *Leptotrichia buccalis* (Vincent's organisms—see p. 130 and Fig. 5(*m*), p. 81), are present in large numbers in smears from the lesions of *Vincent's angina*—an ulcerative condition of the lips, mouth or throat. Both organisms are also found in small numbers in normal mouths and throats. Both are strict anaerobes, difficult to isolate in pure culture, and the laboratory diagnosis of Vincent's angina is usually based entirely upon their abundant presence in the smears. Dilute carbol fuchsin stains them well. Their role in the pathogenesis of the disease is doubtful. Vincent's angina is in most cases preceded by malnutrition, debilitating disease, poor oral hygiene, injury or mouth lesions due to virus infections; these conditions somehow lead to abnormal multiplication of various anaerobic bacteria, of which *Bacteroides melaninogenicus*, though not the most conspicuous, is probably the most important (p. 130). However, the clinical picture associated with the presence of Vincent's organisms in large numbers is a distinctive one and almost always responds rapidly to treatment with metronidazole or penicillin.

A similar combination of organisms is also frequently found in material from lung abscesses, and in superficial ulcerating and necrotic lesions, especially those related to mucocutaneous junctions and sometimes known as *noma*.

Borrelia recurrentis and *Borrelia duttoni* cause relapsing fever in Europe and in West Africa respectively. Closely related organisms have been described as causing the same disease in other parts of the world. They are transmitted from rodents to man or from man to man by lice or ticks. They can be recognized in the peripheral blood as long, coarse spiral threads, and can be grown in blood-containing media under anaerobic conditions. The relapsing nature of the disease is thought to be due to repeated cycles in which antibody production temporarily checks the progress of the infection but then allows the selective multiplication of antigenic variants of the spirochaete which are unaffected by the antibodies so far produced. The organisms are sensitive to penicillin and tetracyclines *in vitro*, but the erratic and unpredictable behaviour of the disease makes treatment difficult to assess.

MYCOPLASMAS

These are very small bacteria that do not form cell walls (see p. 12). They closely resemble L-forms of more orthodox bacteria (see p. 74), and it has been repeatedly suggested, but never confirmed, that they are stable derivatives of these. All mycoplasmas are exacting in their nutritional requirements, and the parasitic species (see below) can be grown only on very rich media that must contain sterols, usually supplied by incorporating 20 % or so of blood or serum in the medium. Even on such media they grow very slowly, taking weeks rather than days to produce their typical minute 'fried-egg' colonies.

Saprophytic mycoplasmas are found in soil and sewage and elsewhere. Parasitic species can be isolated from plants and from moist mucosal sites in animals. Many human beings carry them in their respiratory and genito-urinary tracts. The only species undoubtedly pathogenic to man is *Mycoplasma pneumoniae*. This was first isolated (and described as a virus) in 1944 from patients with *primary atypical pneumonia*—a condition so called largely because it differed from 'typical' (pneumococcal) pneumonia in its failure to respond to penicillin treatment. *M. pneumoniae* infection of humans is common in many parts of the world, and estimates for many different communities suggest that it causes 10 to 30 % of all acute lower respiratory tract infections. In most places it is the most common cause of the primary atypical pneumonia syndrome, which occurs both as sporadic cases and in local (often seasonal) outbreaks; other causative organisms include respiratory viruses, *Chlam. psittaci* (p. 252), *Cox. burneti* (p. 150) and *Leg. pneumophila* (p. 129). In about half of the cases due to *M. pneumoniae*, and also in some due to other agents, the patient's blood contains 'cold agglutinins', which agglutinate human red cells at refrigerator temperatures. The most definite serological evidence of *M. pneumoniae* infection is the development, during the course of the illness, of antibodies which give complement-fixing reactions with suspensions of *M. pneumoniae*. The organism can be cultured (in due course) from pharyngeal swabs, sputum or blood in some cases. Since mycoplasmas have no cell walls, they are resistant to β-lactams (penicillins and cephalosporins), but treatment with tetracyclines or erythromycin is usually effective in controlling *M. pneumoniae* infections.

Other mycoplasmas frequently isolated from man include *M. hominis*, and strains formerly called T-strains (because they form particularly tiny colonies) and now known as *Ureaplasma urealyticum* (a name based on their characteristic urea-splitting activity). Both species frequent the human genital tract of either sex, are transmissible by sexual intercourse, and are frequently found in association with genital tract infections. However, it remains uncertain whether they play a part in producing or maintaining these infections.

Suggestions for Further Reading

Bacteriology Illustrated by R. R. Gillies and T. C. Dodds, 4th edn. (Churchill Livingstone, Edinburgh, London and New York, 1976) and books mentioned in the Preface.

Table V   Summary of the More Important Bacterial Causes of Human Disease

	Principal diseases
GRAM-POSITIVE COCCI	
Staphylococcus aureus	Pustules, boils, abscesses, wound infections and various acute or chronic infections, including septicaemia; food-poisoning
Streptococcus pyogenes	Pharyngitis, tonsillitis, scarlet fever, erysipelas, and other acute infections, including septicaemia
Group B streptococci	Neonatal meningitis and septicaemia
Viridans streptococci	Subacute bacterial endocarditis
Str. pneumoniae	Pneumonia, otitis, sinusitis, meningitis, infection of damaged bronchi
Enterococci	Urinary tract and wound infections, subacute bacterial endocarditis
GRAM-NEGATIVE COCCI	
Neisseria meningitidis	Meningitis, septicaemia
N. gonorrhoeae	Gonorrhoea
GRAM-POSITIVE BACILLI	
Corynebacterium diphtheriae	Diphtheria
Bacillus anthracis	Anthrax
Clostridia	Botulism and other food-poisoning, tetanus, gas-gangrene, pseudomembraneous colitis
GRAM-NEGATIVE BACILLI	
Escherichia coli	Urinary tract and wound infections, infantile gastro-enteritis, neonatal meningitis
Klebsiellae	Urinary tract and wound infections, pneumonia, meningitis, sinusitis, otitis
Salmonellae	Enteric fever, gastro-enteritis
Shigellae	Bacillary dysentery
Proteus	Urinary tract and wound infections

(Table cont. overleaf)

Table V (*contd*)

Pseudomonas aeruginosa	Infections of wounds, burns, urinary and respiratory tracts
Vibrio cholerae	Cholera
Campylobacters	Gastro-enteritis
Haemophilus influenzae	Meningitis, epiglottitis, infection of damaged bronchi
Bordetella pertussis	Whooping cough
Brucellae	Brucellosis (undulant fever)
Legionella pneumophila	Pneumonia
Bacteroides	Intra-abdominal and other abscesses, wound infections, gangrenous lesions
ACID-FAST BACILLI	
Mycobacterium tuberculosis	Tuberculosis
Myco. leprae	Leprosy
BRANCHING BACTERIA	
Actinomyces israeli	Actinomycosis
SPIROCHAETES	
Treponema pallidum	Syphilis
Leptospires	Leptospirosis (including Weil's disease)
MYCOPLASMA	
Mycoplasma pneumoniae	Primary atypical pneumonia

CHAPTER 10

RICKETTSIAE, COXIELLA AND CHLAMYDIAE

The rickettsiae, *Coxiella burneti* (the sole species in that genus) and the chlamydiae belong to the borderland between the bacteria and the viruses, though they are closer to the former. They resemble bacteria in containing both RNA and DNA, in having muramic acid in their cell walls, in having enzymes and demonstrable metabolic activities, in multiplying by binary fission, and in their sensitivities to many antiseptics and antibiotics. Their main point of resemblance to viruses is that, with *R. quintana* as the only known exception, they are obligate intracellular parasites, unable to reproduce themselves without the aid of host cells. Consequently, virological rather than bacteriological procedures are used in the laboratory for their isolation and culture. Being similar in size to the smallest bacteria and the largest viruses, they are visible by light microscopy. Unlike viruses they can be stained by Gram's method. However, the reactions are weak (Gram-negative except for *C. burneti*—see below) and they are better stained by other methods, such as those of Giemsa, Castaneda or Macchiavello. They are killed by heating to 60°C for 30 minutes (except for *C. burneti*—see below), or by low concentrations of phenol or formalin. Many of them can survive for long periods outside their hosts at usual atmospheric temperatures. They are sensitive to many antibiotics, but in general only the tetracyclines and chloramphenicol are sufficiently potent against them to be of therapeutic value, and these drugs are merely inhibitory. The sulphonamides inhibit growth of chlamydiae but enhance that of rickettsiae. The latter are inhibited by *p*-aminobenzoic acid (p. 34).

RICKETTSIAE

These organisms, which cause typhus and related diseases, are named after Dr. H. T. Ricketts, who died of typhus while investigating its cause and transmission. They are primarily intestinal parasites of bloodsucking arthropods, such as ticks, mites, rat-fleas and lice, to which they are not usually harmful and indeed may in some cases be necessary for survival. They are pathogenic to man, and to many animals in the laboratory though their natural host ranges are restricted. Man becomes infected by direct inoculation into bites, by contamination of bites or scratches with arthropod faeces or by inhalation of dried arthropod faeces.

MICROSCOPY   Rickettsiae range from 0.3 to 1.5 μm in length and from 0.25 to 0.5 μm in breadth. They are pleomorphic, forming cocci, bacilli and filaments. They can be stained as described above.

ISOLATION AND CULTURE   These procedures are restricted to specialized laboratories because they are technically difficult and because of the high infectivity of rickettsiae for man. Material suspected of containing rickettsiae is injected into guinea-pigs, rats or mice (the choice depending upon the organism expected), and these animals are examined for clinical changes, for development of specific antibodies, and for the presence of rickettsiae (visible microscopically or transmissible to other animals or to chick embryo yolk-sacs) in their tissues. Tissue culture, as for viruses, has also been used. Yolk-sac culture is used for production of vaccines and of antigen preparations for the more specific serological tests.

SERODIAGNOSIS

1 *The Weil-Felix reaction.*   This is the mainstay of rickettsial diagnosis. Its discovery was the result of a fortunate accident. In 1916 Weil and Felix found that certain *Proteus* strains recovered from the urine and the blood of patients with typhus were agglutinated by the patients' sera. This is now known to be due to the sharing of carbohydrate antigens by the causative organism of typhus (*Rickettsia prowazeki*) and the *Proteus* strains, of which the most strongly agglutinated was named *Proteus* OX 19. The technique of the test is similar to that of the Widal test (p. 248). The antigenic suspensions are made from non-flagellate variants of the proteus strains since the relevant antigens are of O (somatic) type. By the end of the first week of an attack of epidemic typhus it is usual for the *Proteus* OX 19 suspension to be agglutinated by a 1 : 100 or greater dilution of the patient's serum, and much higher titres are reached by the end of the second week; a suspension of *Proteus* OX 2 is agglutinated only by low serum dilutions or not at all. The findings in endemic typhus are similar. In Rocky Mountain spotted fever and related tick-borne rickettsial infections both *Proteus* OX 19 and *Proteus* OX 2 are strongly agglutinated; in scrub typhus negative results are obtained with both of these strains but a third, *Proteus* OX K, which gives negative results in the other diseases, is strongly agglutinated (Table VI, p. 150).

    Since the antigenic suspensions for the Weil–Felix test are easily prepared and distributed, its use is not confined to specialized laboratories.

2 *More specific serological tests.*   Patients with rickettsial infections also form species-specific and even strain-specific antibodies, and so it is

possible by use of genuine rickettsial antigens to distinguish between the individual members of the groups of diseases detected by the Weil–Felix reaction. However, the difficulty of preparing rickettsial antigens limits the use of such tests.

THE INDIVIDUAL RICKETTSIAL DISEASES

Epidemic Typhus (classical, famine or European typhus)
This is purely a human disease, due to *R. prowazeki* and transmitted by the human body louse. After being ingested in human blood by the louse and multiplying in its intestine, the organism appears in large numbers in its faeces and enters the body of the next human victim by contamination either of a louse-bite or of the scratches which he inflicts on himself in response to the bites. A severe febrile illness follows, characterized by a widespread rash and cerebral disturbances. The death-rate in the absence of antibiotic treatment is high, especially in older patients.

Louse infestation is a product of overcrowding and poor hygiene, and typhus epidemics are consequently associated with war and famine. Spread can be prevented by 'delousing' threatened populations, their clothing and their bedding by spraying them with an insecticide. A formalin-killed yolk-sac culture of *R. prowazeki* has been widely used as a vaccine for active immunization, but there are few indications for its use at present, as typhus persists in only a few areas and can be treated satisfactorily with chloramphenicol or a tetracycline.

Brill's Disease
This is a recrudescence of typhus in a mild atypical form in a patient in whose tissues *R. prowazeki* has remained dormant, sometimes for many years, following a previous typical attack. The Weil–Felix test may give negative results in this condition.

Endemic Typhus (murine typhus)
This is primarily a disease of rats, due to *R. typhi* (*mooseri*) and transmitted by the rat-flea and the rat-louse. Sporadic cases of human infection occur throughout the world in places where the rat population is high. The resultant disease is much less severe than epidemic typhus.

The Spotted Fevers
These are tick-borne diseases of man, horses, dogs and rodents. The ticks themselves are the main reservoirs for the causative organisms, passing them on from generation to generation via their eggs. All of the human diseases are characterized by fever and rashes, but they vary in severity. Rocky Mountain spotted fever, caused by *R. rickettsi*, has a mortality comparable to that of epidemic typhus, whereas at the other extreme Mediterranean fever or 'fièvre boutonneuse', caused by *R. conori*, is a mild illness.

Scrub Typhus (tsutsugamushi fever)
This occurs in Japan, Malaya and the Pacific area. The causative

organism, *R. tsutsugamushi*, is transmitted to man by mites, which become infected by biting field mice, rats and other rodents, and which then pass on the infection to succeeding generations of mites. Mite larvae are common on scrub in low-lying damp areas; human beings who walk there are liable to be bitten unless they wear protective clothing and use insect repellants. The resultant disease resembles epidemic typhus with the addition of a local black-scabbed ulcer or eschar at the point of entry of the organism.

Rickettsialpox
Yet another mite-borne disease transmitted to man from rodents is caused by *R. akari*. There is again an eschar at the point of entry, but the disease is mild. It occurs in Russia, Korea and America.

Trench Fever
This louse-borne disease of grossly overcrowded and dirty populations gained its name during the first world war and was prominent again in some areas during the second world war. Its main contemporary interest is that its causative organism, *R. quintana*, which has never been isolated from any host except man and the louse, has been shown to be capable of extracellular multiplication in the lumen of the louse gut and has been grown on non-living culture media.

Table VI   Summary of the rickettsial diseases and Q fever

Diseases	Organism	Reservoir	Vectors	Weil-Felix reaction OX 19	OX2	OXK
Epidemic typhus	*R. prowazeki*	Men	Lice	+ + +	(+)	–
Brill's disease	*R. prowazeki*	—	— Usually	–	–	–
Endemic typhus	*R. typhi*	Rats	Fleas, lice	+ + +	+	–
Spotted fevers	{ *R. rickettsi* { *R. conori etc.,*	Men, horses, dogs, rodents	 Ticks	+ +	+ +	–
Scrub typhus	*R. tsutsugamushi*	Rodents	Mites	–	–	+ + +
Rickettsialpox	*R. akari*	Mice	Mites	–	–	–
Trench fever	*R. quintana*	Men	Lice	–	–	–
Q fever	*C. burneti*	Various animals and birds	Ticks, droplets, dust, milk	–	–	–

COXIELLA BURNETI

An influenza-like febrile illness, with variable manifestations that usually include patchy pneumonic consolidation, was first recognized as an entity in 1935 in Queensland, Australia. It was named Q fever, not because of its place of origin but because of the original query about its aetiology. When the causative agent was identified, it was named *Rickettsia burneti*. However, it differs from the rickettsiae in being more resistant to heat, desiccation and antiseptics; in staining positive by some variants of

Gram's staining method; in its base-pair ratio (p. 71); in its mode of transmission to man (see below); in the pattern of illness that it produces; and in various other respects. It therefore now has its own genus. It is found throughout the world, and affects various birds and wild animals as well as the domesticated goats, sheep and cattle from which man usually acquires his infection. It is carried between animals largely by ticks, but human infection is usually by inhalation of dust or droplets contaminated from the excreta or other products of infected animals, or by ingestion of infected milk. Its spread is therefore greatly assisted by its resistance to desiccation, and by its ability to survive heat treatment only slightly less than that generally recommended for the pasteurization of milk. Slaughterhouse men and farm workers are among those most at risk, and there have been instances of accidental infection of laboratory workers. There is serological evidence that subclinical infection is common in rural communities, in Britain and elsewhere. An important but fortunately uncommon sequel of clinical or subclinical infection is chronic endo-carditis, usually superimposed on existing heart-valve abnormalities and resembling the bacterial endocarditis produced by viridans streptococci.

Q fever can be diagnosed by isolating the organism from the patient's blood, sputum, urine or cerebrospinal fluid; or by inoculation of such material into the peritoneal cavities of guinea-pigs or into chick-embryo yolk-sacs. However, agglutination and complement-fixation tests on the patient's serum are the mainstay of laboratory diagnosis. For the complement-fixation tests two different antigenic preparations of *C. burneti* are used—phase 1, grown in arthropods, and phase 2, from yolk-sac culture. In acute Q fever there is a rise only of antibodies to phase 2, whereas in Q fever endocarditis there are usually high titres of antibodies for both phases.

Tetracyclines are the most useful antibiotics for treatment of Q fever, but their effects are unreliable, especially in endocarditis. Addition of either lincomycin or cotrimoxazole is said to enhance their efficacy.

CHLAMYDIAE

Some of the properties of these organisms have been mentioned in the first paragraph of this chapter. They share a common antigenic component not found in rickettsiae; they are not arthropod-borne; and they also differ from rickettsiae in being spherical, with no bacillary or filamentous forms, and in having an unusual type of predominantly intracellular developmental cycle. The infective forms (elementary bodies), about $0.3 \mu m$ in diameter, are phagocytosed by host cells and develop within them into larger forms (reticulate bodies) up to $2 \mu m$ in diameter. More reticulate bodies are formed by binary fission during the next 20 hours or so, but by about 40 hours these have become reorganized into large numbers of elementary bodies. Rupture of the host cells 48–72 hours after infection releases the elementary bodies, which can then infect new host cells. Intracellular clusters of chlamydiae can be seen as basophilic inclusion bodies in Giemsa-stained smears, whereas those formed by viruses (p. 162) are acidophilic. Two *Chlamydia* species are recognized. Strains belonging to *C. psittaci* (formerly Subgroup B) are primarily bird pathogens, but sometimes infect man or animals. *C. trachomatis* (formerly Subgroup A) includes the *lymphogranuloma venereum* (LGV) and *trachoma and inclusion conjunctivitis* (TRIC) agents and also the strains involved in various genital-tract infections as indicated below; so far as is known members of this species are natural parasites of man only, though primates have been infected in the laboratory and closely related organisms have been isolated from rodents.

DIAGNOSTIC MICROSCOPY   Intracellular chlamydial inclusions can be made visible by Giemsa or similar staining, by use of fluorescent antibodies or by electron microscopy. These techniques can be applied to appropriate clinical material—scrapings from eye lesions, bubo pus or lymph-node biopsy material from cases of LGV—and are also used to demonstrate infection in cultures (see next paragraph).

ISOLATION   Chlamydiae can be isolated from clinical material by yolk-sac or tissue culture (pp. 158–9) or by inoculation into mice. *C. psittaci* can be isolated from the patient's blood in the first week of the illness or from sputum at any stage. Tissue culture is the most sensitive means of detecting the presence of *C. trachomatis* in the various situations, indicated below, in which it may occur.

SERODIAGNOSIS   Complement-fixation tests based on a heat-stable lipoprotein–carbohydrate antigen common to all chlamydiae is useful in diagnosis of the systemic chlamydial infections psittacosis/ornithosis and LGV; it does not distinguish between them, but this matters only when the antibodies may be due to some past infection, since there is no danger of clinical confusion between these two conditions at the time of active infection. Superficial ocular and genital chlamydial infections do not as a rule provoke sufficient humoral antibody response for complement-fixation tests to help in their diagnosis. More sensitive fluorescent antibody and other tests are available, but the results are difficult to interpret.

ANTIBACTERIAL TREATMENT   The tetracyclines are the most effective agents for treatment of all sorts of chlamydial infections. *C. psittaci* is resistant and *C. trachomatis* is sensitive to sulphonamides—a fact more relevant to making the distinction between the species than to treatment.

Chlamydia psittaci

Psittacosis in the strict sense is an infection of psittacine birds (parrots, etc.), or of man with chlamydiae derived from such birds. Similar infections of many other kinds of birds, including pigeons, ducks, turkeys and gulls, are collectively known as *ornithosis*; when transmitted to man they tend to produce illnesses milder than psittacosis. Human infection usually results from inhalation of dust containing dried droppings from infected birds (which may be apparently healthy or only mildly ill). Less commonly it follows a bite from such a bird, or is acquired from a laboratory culture. Droplet transmission between human beings is possible. Human infection may be subclinical, or may produce pictures varying from a mild influenza-like illness to a severe and sometimes fatal pneumonia. Respiratory tract carriage of the organism may persist long after recovery from the disease.

Since the reintroduction in 1976 of controls on the importation of psittacine birds, the number of human cases of *C. psittaci* infection in Britain attributable to exposure to such birds has fallen; but the overall number of reported human cases of ornithosis has risen. It is not clear how much of this rise reflects a real increase in infection from other sources and how much is due to more efficient investigation of relevant patients.

Chlamydia trachomatis

(a) Lymphogranuloma Venereum (LGV)

This is purely a human disease, transmitted as a rule by sexual intercourse, though non-venereal infection can occur—e.g. through the conjunctiva. It is largely confined to tropical and sub-tropical countries. In its common form it produces ulcerative genital lesions with regional lymph-node suppuration (called 'climatic bubo' when the inguinal glands are involved). Generalized dissemination follows, with fever and diffuse aches and sometimes with conjunctivitis, arthritis or encephalitis. Chronic infection leads to anal and genital strictures and elephantiasis.

The *Frei test*, a test for hypersensitivity similar in principle to the tuberculin test (pp. 65 and 253), is no longer in common use for the diagnosis of lymphogranuloma, since its antigen (a heat-inactivated suspension of lymphogranuloma agent) is difficult to prepare and standardize.

(b) Trachoma and Inclusion Conjunctivitis (TRIC)

Trachoma is a form of conjunctivitis in which formation of fibrous tissue in the conjunctiva and cornea commonly leads both to lid deformities and to blindness; indeed, it is the world's commonest cause of blindness. It is a disease of communities with poor hygiene, especially in the Middle East and in Africa. It is mainly transmitted by direct and close contact—e.g. mother to baby—or by flies.

Inclusion conjunctivitis is a similar but milder condition, of worldwide distribution. The strains of *C. trachomatis* that cause it are indistinguishable in the laboratory from those causing trachoma, but have their primary habitat in the human genital tract rather than in the eye (see below). Neonatal conjunctivitis ('inclusion blenorrhoea') is a result of contamination of the infant's eyes, during delivery, with chlamydiae from the mother's genital tract. 'Swimming bath conjunctivitis' is a similar condition in older children or adults, believed to be due to transmission of the organism from the genitalia of one bather to the conjunctivae of another via the water.

Carriage of *C. trachomatis* in the human genital tract can be asymptomatic, but it has a frequent and probably causal association with the common sexually transmitted disease that is known (because of earlier lack of any positive indication of its cause) as 'non-gonococcal urethritis' (NGU) or 'non-specific urethritis' (NSU). Similarly, *C. trachomatis* is commonly isolated from patients with urethritis that persists after adequate penicillin treatment of gonorrhoea and is consequently called 'post-gonococcal urethritis' (PGU); presumably there was a double infection, of which the penicillin cured only the gonococcal component. There is also evidence incriminating *C. trachomatis* in cervicitis, salpingitis and other genital tract infections; Tetracyclines are the most appropriate treatment for these conditions. Infants born to mothers who are carrying *C. trachomatis* may develop neonatal pneumonia; in such a case both infant and mother should be treated with erythromycin because tetracyclines are contra-indicated (p. 332).

Suggestions for Further Reading
See Preface.

CHAPTER 11

VIRUSES

Before reading this chapter it may be helpful to look again at the summary of the properties of viruses given on p. 14. Since viruses have no metabolism of their own and cannot reproduce themselves, it is arguable whether they should be described as living organisms. For this reason, viruses which are able to invade host cells and to replicate there are often described as *active* rather than alive, and those which have lost the ability to do these things are then described as *inactivated* rather than dead.

STRUCTURE AND GROUP CLASSIFICATION

Increased knowledge of virus structure has made possible their logical classification, and although there is not complete agreement as to the best system, the one on which Table VII is based is widely accepted. The characters used in delineating the main groups include:

1 *The nature of the nucleic acid in the genome.* This is either RNA or DNA but not both.

2 *The symmetry of the capsid.* This is determined by the shapes and mutual attractions of the units, called *capsomeres*, of which the capsid is composed. In some virus groups these protein 'building bricks' are such that the capsid is an icosahedron—a hollow near-spherical structure with 20 identical triangular faces. Such a capsid is said to show *cubic symmetry*, and the classification of these viruses into groups is based on the numbers of capsomeres that they possess. In other groups the capsomeres arrange themselves in a spiral thread, forming a hollow cylinder, and such a capsid is said to show *helical symmetry*. In either case, if the virus is intact the genome is inside the capsid. Some virus groups have more elaborate structures not classifiable as either cubic or helical, and are described as *complex*. Since analysis of capsid structure depends on interpretation of fine details in two-dimensional electronmicrographs, it is understandable that even among virus groups that are of medical interest there are some of which the capsid designs are as yet incompletely understood or unknown. The complex tadpole-like design of many bacteriophages is described on p. 193.

3 *The presence of an envelope.*   In some virus groups the *nucleocapsid* (i.e. nucleic acid core + capsid) is surrounded by a loose membranous envelope consisting of lipids, proteins and carbohydrates. Some of these components closely resemble those of host cells, and are believed to be derived from host cell membrane as the virus is liberated from the host cell. Many enveloped viruses are described as *ether-sensitive* because they are inactivated by treatment with ether (or with other lipid solvents). Presumably this means that lipid components of their envelopes are

Table VII   Classification of the more important viruses affecting man

Nucleic acid	Capsid symmetry	Enve- lope	Group	Approx. size (nm)*	Members of the group	Principal diseases caused
RNA	CUBIC	−	PICORNAVIRUSES	24–35	Enteroviruses: polioviruses coxsackieviruses echoviruses —>	Poliomyelitis Aseptic meningitis Aseptic meningitis Hepatitis A
					Rhinoviruses	Common cold
		−	REOVIRUSES	60–80	Reoviruses Rotaviruses	Gastro-enteritis
		+	TOGAVIRUSES	40–70	Alphaviruses Flaviviruses —>	Encephalitides Yellow fever, dengue Rubella (German measles)
	HELICAL	+	ORTHOMYXOVIRUSES	80–120	—>	Influenza
		+	PARAMYXOVIRUSES	100–120	Parainfluenza viruses —> —> Respiratory syncytial virus	Croup, other respiratory infections Mumps Measles Bronchiolitis
		+	RHABDOVIRUSES	80 × 180	—>	Rabies
		+	CORONAVIRUSES	80–130	Coronaviruses	Common cold
		+	ARENAVIRUSES	110	—> —>	Lymphocytic choriomeningitis Lassa fever
	UNCLASSIFIED				Marburg virus Ebola virus	Viral haemorrhagic fevers
DNA	CUBIC	−	PAPOVAVIRUSES	50	Papilloma virus	Warts
		−	ADENOVIRUSES	80		Respiratory infections, Conjunctivitis
		+	HERPESVIRUSES	120	—> Varicella-zoster virus Cytomegalovirus Epstein-Barr virus	Herpes simplex Chickenpox, shingles Cytomegalic inclusion disease Infectious mononucleosis
	COMPLEX	−	POXVIRUSES	230 × 300	Variola Vaccinia —>	Smallpox Cowpox Orf
	UNCLASSIFIED −			42	—>	Hepatitis B

* Most viruses are roughly spherical, except rhabdoviruses (bullet-shaped) and poxviruses (brick-shaped)
—> = virus(es) named after the disease listed in the right-hand column—e.g. hepatitis A virus, rubella virus.

necessary for their activity. Closely associated with the envelopes of the myxoviruses are numerous projecting spikes, and these are connected with haemagglutinating activity of these viruses. Viruses that do not have envelopes are described as *naked*.

4 *Particle size.* Viruses are measured in nanometres (nm—see p. 14). The size of virus particles used to be determined by filtration through membranes of known pore-size, by measuring their rate of sedimentation in a high-speed centrifuge, or by density-gradient centrifugation; though the last of these, which involves finding the depth to which the particles can be centrifuged through a fluid that increases in density from top to bottom, is primarily a means of measuring the specific gravity of particles rather than their size. All of these procedures are still useful as means of purifying virus preparations, but for the determination of virus particle size they have been superseded by electron microscopic comparison of the particles with structures of known size.

REPLICATION

Viruses do not reproduce themselves; they are replicated by host cells. The essence of this process is that the virus nucleic acid enters a host cell and uses its nucleic acid and protein synthesis mechanisms, diverting them to production of virus components. In the laboratory such a take-over can be achieved by nucleic acid alone, free from capsid or envelope. Indeed, the host range of such naked nucleic acid may be far wider than that of intact virus; e.g. intact polioviruses can infect only primate cells, whereas poliovirus RNA, freed from its capsid protein, can be made to infect chicken cells and to cause them to manufacture complete polioviruses—which, being now complete, cannot invade further chicken cells. The capsid protects the nucleic acid when it is not in the host cell, and in the case of a naked virus makes possible its entry into the fresh host cells and determines the range of hosts into whose cells such entry can be made. (It also largely determines and is the main target for the host's immunological responses to the virus.) Entry of enveloped viruses into host cells is determined by the envelope. The first step towards invasion of fresh host cells is attachment and *adsorption* of viruses to their surfaces. For some and possibly for all groups of animal viruses adsorption depends on interaction—chemical in some cases and electrostatic in others—between parts of the virus surface and receptor areas on the surfaces of the host cells; hence the limitation of host range imposed by the outer coat of the virus, and probably also the fact that the various tissues of a host differ in their susceptibility to a given virus. Much remains to be discovered about adsorption mechanisms, but some facts are clearly established. It is known, for example, that adsorption of myxoviruses is a function of projections associated with their envelopes (p. 176) and that their host-cell receptors are mucoproteins, whereas receptors for polioviruses are lipoproteins. Once adsorbed, viruses gain admission to animal cells by a process resembling phagocytosis if they are naked or, if they have envelopes, by fusion of these with host-cell membranes (in contrast to the self-injecting mechanism of bacterio-phages—p. 193). The nucleic acid loses its capsid and is released into the cells. At this stage and for some hours afterwards no infective virus can be recovered from the host cells, and the virus is said to be in *eclipse*. During this period the take-over is proceeding, and the cells, acting on instructions given by the invading nucleic acid, are forging enzymatic tools with which to make new viruses. Where these viruses are made and assembled depends upon the group to which the virus belongs. Some are made within the host nucleus and some within the cytoplasm. Some viruses appear to be made entirely in one part of the cell, whereas for others the nucleic acid core is made in one site and capsomeres are transported ready-made from other sites (within the same cell). The degree of disturbance of the host cell's metabolism also varies, as does its fate. For example, orthomyxoviruses are released from the cell surface by a budding process, acquiring their envelopes as they emerge, and the cell can continue to produce and release them for a long period; whereas polioviruses accumulate inside the host cell, kill it and are released in large numbers when it bursts.

CULTURE

Laboratory Animals
In earlier days the isolation and recognition of viruses depended on the availability of suitable laboratory animals. Thus the proof that influenza is a virus disease had to await the discovery that it is transmissible to ferrets. Animal inoculation still has a place in the investigation of virus diseases, as is indicated in later sections of this chapter, but wherever possible it has been replaced by the methods described below, which are simpler and more economical of time, space and money, and which often give more useful information.

Chick Embryos
Fertile hens' eggs are fairly readily available, require a minimum of attention and have the advantage over laboratory animals that their reaction to viruses is not complicated by the possession of acquired immunity. They must be only a few days old when incubation begins, and are inoculated with virus a week or so later, provided that inspection by bright transmitted light ('candling') confirms that the embryos are still alive. After a small hole has been drilled in the shell of an egg, viruses are introduced, according to their nature, into the allantoic or amniotic cavity or on to the chorio-allantoic membrane. The amniotic cavity is used for primary isolation of influenza and mumps viruses, but for subsequent cultures of influenza viruses that have adapted to growth in the egg it is technically easier and generally satisfactory to use the allantoic cavity. When grown on the chorio-allantoic membrane, the pox viruses and some

herpes viruses produce characteristic lesions which, like bacterial colonies on a plate culture, permit the identification and the enumeration of the organisms in the inoculum. (Hens' egg yolk sacs are used for growing rickettsiae, *C. burneti* and chlamydiae—pp. 148, 151 and 152; multiplication of these organisms in this site may lead to the death of the embryos.)

Tissue Culture

When it became possible to grow mammalian tissues in test tubes, a new method was available for artificial propagation of viruses. However, it was at first of limited value because the cells were in the form of tissue particles suspended in fluid and were therefore difficult to examine. Furthermore, their susceptibility to virus infection was hard to predict. It then became possible to grow tissues as *monolayers* (sheets of single-cell thickness) attached to the inner surfaces of the glass or plastic of culture tubes or bottles, where they can be examined microscopically at any stage without being disturbed. Furthermore, standard 'cell lines', mostly of human or simian origin and in many cases derived from neoplastic or foetal tissues, have been developed and distributed throughout the world, so that different laboratories can use tissue cultures of comparable and predictable virus susceptibilities. Monolayers need nourishment, and this is usually supplied by bathing them in nutrient fluid. However, it is then virtually impossible to separate out pure virus lines from a mixture, just as it was difficult to obtain pure bacterial cultures until solid media were introduced (p. 75). The virological equivalent of plating out bacteria to obtain separate colonies is to seed a monolayer with virus inoculum and then cover it not with fluid but with a nutrient agar. Any one virus particle and its progeny are then restricted to the cell originally entered and those in its immediate vicinity. If these cells are damaged (see below, CPE), a visible plaque of degeneration may appear in the monolayer. As with a bacterial colony, the appearance of the plaque may be characteristic of infection with a particular virus, and subculture from a single plaque is likely to yield a pure strain.

The replication of virus in tissue culture can be detected by:

(1) *cytopathic effect* (CPE)—i.e. degenerative changes in the infected cells which can be seen when a monolayer is examined microscopically. Viruses of many different groups produce such effects, and to some extent the nature of the virus can be deduced from the type of change which occurs in the cells;

(2) functional changes in the cells which can be detected by tests of such metabolic activities as acid production;

(3) the presence of detectable antigens, *haemagglutinins* (see below) or other virus components or products in the fluid bathing the cells;

(4) acquisition by the cells of the power to adsorb red blood cells on to their surfaces (*haemadsorption*). This results from infection by some of the myxoviruses, and the consequent formation of virus-containing buds on the surfaces of the infected cells;

(5) resistance of the cells to infection by other viruses (*interference*—see below);

(6) attachment of virus-specific fluorescent antibodies to virus particles or virus antigens within the cells.

Though monolayer culture has many useful features, simple suspensions of cells in suitable nutrient fluids may suffice for virus propagation and for carrying out tests that depend on changes in cell metabolism.

Organ culture is another form of tissue culture that has given valuable results (p. 172). Portions of intact ciliated epithelium from the respiratory tract of a human embryo can be kept alive on a culture medium for several weeks, and their cilia continue to beat. Some respiratory-tract viruses that cannot be grown in any other form of tissue culture (as well as many that can) are able to infect such portions of epithelium and demonstrate their presence by damaging the cells—notably by stopping their visible ciliary activity. It seems probable that the development of similar cultures of other intact tissues will lead to the discovery of other new viruses. As well as being useful for primary isolation and subsequent maintenance of viruses that cannot be grown in other ways, organ cultures of respiratory epithelium have made possible some most elegant studies of precisely what viruses do when they infect tissue that was functioning normally prior to their arrival.

HAEMAGGLUTINATION

Orthomyxoviruses and members of several other virus groups have the ability to agglutinate red blood cells of various species. This property, which in some cases at least is related to the organism's method of entering host cells (p. 157), has the following laboratory applications:

(1) Such viruses can be detected in fluids by their ability to agglutinate human or other suitable red cells.

(2) Some of them endow infected tissue culture cells with the power of haemadsorption, as indicated above.

(3) The haemagglutinins are antigens, and infected hosts are stimulated to form antibodies. These can be demonstrated and measured by their specific inhibition of the *in vitro* haemagglutinating activity of the responsible virus, and their presence in a patient's serum is evidence of infection with that virus (p. 169, haemagglutination-inhibition test).

There are 3 kinds of virus haemagglutination:

(*a*) Orthomyxoviruses attach themselves, by means of some of their projecting spikes (p. 176), to mucoprotein receptor areas on the cell surfaces, and since each virus may adsorb on to several cells, the cells are agglutinated into masses. In the course of a few hours neuraminidase released from other surface projections of the virus (p. 176) destroys all the mucoprotein substrate and the agglutinates disintegrate. The red cells cannot be further agglutinated by fresh viruses of the same kind, but the original viruses are still able to agglutinate fresh red cells.

(*b*) The poxviruses and some others produce lipoprotein haemagglutinins which are distinct from the viruses themselves and can be separated from them by centrifugation.

(*c*) The haemagglutinins of the togavirus group, like those of the influenza group, are integral parts of the organisms, but they do not permanently alter the surfaces of red cells and their attachment can be repeatedly broken and renewed.

INTERFERENCE

Host cells infected with one virus may be resistant to infection with a second virus. This phenomenon of interference does not depend on the two viruses being closely related, and in some cases it is not even necessary for the first virus to be active; after inactivation by heating or by exposure to ultra-violet light it may still protect the host cells containing it from subsequent infection by an active virus. Interference is sometimes due to an activity of the host cells—production of *interferons* (pp. 49 and 62). These do not prevent the second virus from entering host cells, but they do prevent it from diverting host-cell ribosomes into making the proteins essential for its replication. In other cases interference is a direct result of the activities of the first virus; it may have destroyed all of the receptor areas on the surfaces of the cells so that further viruses are unable to attach themselves, or it may have taken complete control of the enzyme systems of the cells and directed them to its own reproduction, so that a second virus may enter the cells but finds no available enzymes. However, it is possible for two viruses to exist and multiply together in the same cell—e.g. herpes simplex and vaccinia, in the nucleus and the cytoplasm respectively.

It is easy to see in theory the possible relevance of the interference phenomenon to the prophylaxis of virus diseases, but its possibilities have not yet been widely exploited. Oral administration of live poliovirus vaccine can be rapidly effective in preventing spread of an epidemic, because the vaccine virus established itself in the recipient's intestine to the exclusion of wild poliovirus strains (p. 298). Conversely, pre-existing natural enterovirus infections may impair the success of such oral vaccination with live poliovirus.

TRANSMISSION AND PATHOGENESIS OF VIRUS INFECTIONS

Most of the viruses pathogenic to man are primarily human parasites, but some have other animal species as their principal hosts. Transmission is in accordance with the general outline given in Chapter 6. Droplet infection is of pre-eminent importance: it is the common mode of spread of diseases which involve the respiratory tract predominantly (e.g. the common cold and influenza) or in addition to other parts of the body (e.g. measles), and also of many diseases which have no apparent connection with the respiratory tract (e.g. smallpox). Infection with a poliovirus or other enterovirus is usually acquired by ingestion. Most of the togaviruses are arthropod-borne (hence their earlier name of arboviruses) and enter their human hosts via bites inflicted by their vectors. Other viruses introduced through the skin are those of rabies (via bites from infected animals) and hepatitis B (via transfusions, or injections with contaminated needles). A few viruses are transmitted by direct contact—e.g. those of infectious warts.

Viruses generally invade and replicate in cells around their portal of entry into the host's body. Some do no more than this and produce only local lesions—e.g. in the skin, those of warts; in the upper respiratory tract, those of the common cold. Generally, however, there is lymphatic and blood stream spread from the site of primary infection to other parts of the body. In some cases further replication in some central site and further blood stream dissemination precede the arrival of the viruses at their final target organs. On reaching these final destinations they again have to invade cells and replicate sufficiently to cause local tissue damage before the typical lesions of the disease appear. The incubation periods of virus infections (and of infections of other types) can sometimes be explained in terms of these different cycles of replication which precede development of the final disease-patterns.

As with any other type of infection, the outcome of a virus infection depends on the nature of the virus and on the host's responses. Possible patterns include:

(a) A brief acute episode, ending with the elimination of the virus.

(b) An initial episode followed by low-grade illness that persists for a short or longer period during which new virus particles are being budded off from host cells at a low rate.

(c) An initial episode followed by many years of latent infection, interrupted by occasional reactivation of the virus as a result of some change in the relation between it and host immunity. Recurrent herpes simplex 'cold sores' (p. 185) are well-known example of this pattern.

(d) 'Slow virus' infections, such as the rare human diseases kuru and Creutzfeld–Jacob encephalitis and the much-investigated sheep disease called scrapie, in which no clinical signs appear until many years after the initial symptomless infection.

(e) Total integration of viruses into host genetic material, so that they are no longer detectable as separate entities, but may manifest their presence by causing the development of tumours.

Inclusion Bodies

These are accumulations of virus material up to 30 μm in diameter, which are formed within host cells in some virus infections. Such structures were recognized in association with some diseases long before it was possible to isolate the viruses, and many of them were named after their discoverers—e.g. those found in rabies are called *Negri* bodies and those in smallpox and vaccinia were called *Guarnieri* bodies. Their appearances and situations are often sufficiently characteristic to be of diagnostic value. Those of herpes simplex, poliomyelitis, yellow fever and adenovirus infections are found within the nuclei of the infected cells, whereas others, such as those of poxvirus infections and rabies, are cytoplasmic. Most of them contain active viruses and are intracellular 'colonies', but some intranuclear inclusions seem to be merely deposits of material left over from previous virus synthesis.

RESISTANCE TO VIRUS INFECTIONS

Mechanisms of resistance to virus infections are discussed in numerous places in Chapters 7 and 8. The main differences from resistance to bacterial infections are as follows:

(1) As a defence during the early stages of virus infection, interferon production (pp. 49 and 161) is far more important than phagocytosis, which is the main mechanism for dealing with the early stages of most bacterial infections.

(2) Although antibodies are important in preventing the primary entry of viruses into surface epithelial cells, and can also reach them when they are again released by cells in which they have replicated, viruses are intracellular most of the time. T-cell-mediated immunity is thus of greater importance in virus infections than it is in the majority of bacterial infections.

Immunization against viruses is discussed in Chapter 20.

VIRUS MUTATION

From most animal viruses mutant strains can be readily isolated which differ from their parent strains in antigenic structure, host range, pathogenicity or other properties. Such changes are of great immunological and epidemiological importance.

1 *Changes in antigenic structure.* Type A influenza viruses, and to a lesser extent those of type B, undergo continual changes in antigenic structure, as described on p. 177. These have two important consequences. One is that those who have been attacked by the virus may fail to 'recognize' it when it returns to their community in a second wave; their antibodies may be of only limited relevance to its structure by that time. The other consequence is that prophylactic immunization may be ineffective unless the vaccine used is prepared from a very recent isolate.

2 *Changes in host range and pathogenicity.* These two properties are often interdependent. Thus from a virus which is pathogenic to man it may be possible to select out by animal passage a mutant which becomes adapted to living in an animal host, and which then has little or no pathogenicity for man. At least some strains of vaccinia virus were derived from smallpox viruses in this way. Similarly the 17D strain used in immunization against yellow fever was derived from a virulent strain and has been artificially adapted to grow in hens' eggs. These are two among many possible examples of viruses which are valuable immunizing agents because in the course of host-adaptation they have lost their pathogenicity to man and show no tendency to recover it when reintroduced to him. It is, of course, vitally important to ensure that the attenuation of strains used for such purposes is irreversible (p. 299). Loss of virulence is not necessarily linked with change of host range; for example, some strains of poliovirus used in live vaccines were isolated from human sources but were found to be avirulent, and it is presumed that they were mutants of virulent strains. It is obvious that an avirulent mutant is only of value as an immunizing agent if it is still antigenically much the same as the parent strain.

Not all changes in the heritable characteristics of viruses are to be attributed to mutation. Sometimes infection of a cell by two related viruses results in the production of new viruses having some of the properties of each 'parent'—a process known as *recombination*. This may occur naturally among influenza viruses (for example) and has been used in the laboratory as a means of 'synthesizing' influenza vaccine strains that have the important antigenic components of current epidemic strains but without their virulence.

CHEMOTHERAPY

Most antimicrobial drugs owe their therapeutic usefulness to the fact that they interfere with the metabolic processes of the pathogens but not to any serious extent with those of the host's cells. Clearly there is not much scope for such discrimination in virus infections, though the action of interferons shows that it is possible. Much hard work has gone into the search for antivirus agents, but so far with only limited success. *Methisazone* (a thiosemicarbazone) was of some value in preventing smallpox when given to contacts, and in treating the complications of smallpox vaccination; and *in vitro* it is active against adenoviruses. *Idoxuridine* (IDU), one of a series of halogenated deoxyuridine derivatives that interfere with DNA synthesis, gives good results when applied in aqueous solution to herpetic corneal ulcers. Dissolved in dimethyl sulphoxide, which allows it to penetrate skin, it has been used successfully in treatment of skin lesions due to viruses of the herpes group and even of herpetic whitlows. Although highly toxic and unstable, it has been given intravenously to patients with life-threatening disseminated herpes infections or herpes encephalitis, possibly with some benefit. *Vidarabine* is a purine nucleotide active against DNA viruses. It is used as an ointment for treating herpetic eye lesions, and has been given intravenously with some benefit to immunosuppressed patients suffering from severe varicella-zoster infections. *Acyclovir* is also active against DNA viruses such as herpesviruses, and seems likely to be a useful therapeutic agent. In virus-infected cells it acts as substrate for thymine kinase and so becomes incorporated into the virus DNA; but it is ineffective against some strains for which DNA synthesis does not involve thymine kinase. The value of *amantidine* in prophylaxis against influenza A viruses is still debatable. It is ineffective against other viruses. No antibiotics that can be used against virus infections have been discovered.

SENSITIVITY OF VIRUSES TO OTHER AGENTS

PHYSICAL AGENTS   Viruses differ considerably in their ability to survive outside the body under ordinary atmospheric conditions. Poxviruses can survive in dust for weeks or even months, whereas those of influenza, mumps and measles are extremely labile at room temperatures. Heating to 60°C will inactivate most viruses in 30 minutes, those of poliomyelitis and hepatitis B being important exceptions. Nearly all viruses can be preserved for long periods if they are rapidly frozen to $-70°$C and kept at that temperature. Many, but not all, can be preserved by lyophilization (p. 31). The majority can tolerate pH variations within the range 5–9. Nearly all except the 'slow viruses' (p. 162) are inactivated by ultra-violet light and by other types of irradiation, though there are quite large variations in the dosage required by different viruses.

GLYCEROL   Many viruses, notably those of poliomyelitis, rabies and vaccinia, remain infective for months or years in glycerol concentrations which rapidly kill non-sporing bacteria. Glycerol is therefore used as a preservative in virus vaccines.

DISINFECTANTS   Phenols and cresols are relatively ineffective against viruses. The compounds listed as oxidising agents in Table I (p. 33) are more active against them, but may have to be used in concentrations much higher than those which kill vegetative bacteria; hypochlorite solutions are widely used as disinfectants in virology laboratories. Formaldehyde inactivates viruses, but its action is slow, and glutar-aldehyde is generally preferable.

LABORATORY DIAGNOSIS OF VIRUS INFECTIONS

In many forms of microbial infection the possibility of aiming treatment at the causative agent itself is the main incentive for its rapid identification. In virus infections treatment is mostly symptomatic and seldom directed at the virus. Methods of identifying viruses have in general been slow, and diagnostic virology has tended to be an academic subject, concerned with eventual understanding of virus infections rather than with immediate clinical and therapeutic problems. However, quite apart from the hope of developing antivirus chemotherapy, there are several reasons for wanting to know as soon as possible the identity of a virus that is causing disease. This information may lead to precise diagnosis, more accurate prognosis and the possibility of anticipating a need for special forms of treatment; it may spare the patient an unnecessary exposure to the hazards of antibiotic treatment (p. 305) for an imagined bacterial infection; and it may indicate steps that should be taken to prevent spread of the disease in the community. In an increasing number of virus infections it has become possible to identify the pathogen with reasonable certainty within hours of the specimen reaching a suitably equipped laboratory, instead of having to wait for days or weeks.

Proof that a potential pathogen is present in the body of a patient should never be mistaken for proof that it is causing his illness. In virology as in other forms of microbiology the finding of such an organism has to be interpreted in the light of available information as to how often it can be recovered from healthy people and how likely it is to produce the type of illness from which the patient is suffering. Even a rising level of antibodies, specific for the organism in question, in the patient's blood is evidence only that it has been present, not that it has been acting as a pathogen—though the case against it is stronger if the pattern of antibody rise suggests that it arrived at the right time to initiate the illness.

In the majority of virus infections the organisms are most easily found early in the illness or even in the prodromal period, before the symptoms appear. Decisions about the best times to collect specimens, their nature and the sites from which they should be taken depend on knowledge of individual virus diseases; some of the necessary information is given in later sections of this chapter. Rapid diagnosis depends on microscopic or serological demonstration that virus particles or antigens are present in material from the patient. Isolation of the virus by growing it in tissue culture, in eggs or in animals takes longer but may be more sensitive and more conclusive and may make possible more precise identification. Measurement of the patient's antibody responses may give indirect supporting evidence for the diagnosis or may be the only grounds on which it is based, but such responses take time (pp. 290–1).

Detection of Viruses and Virus Antigens by Microscopy

Only rarely is ordinary *light microscopy* useful in virological diagnosis; examination of stained smears or tissue sections may show characteristic histological changes, or the presence of pathognomic inclusion bodies in rabies, cytomegalic inclusion disease, etc., or even that of individual particles (elementary bodies) in poxvirus infections. *Electron microscopy* can be far more informative, since a much wider range of viruses can be seen and recognized, provided that they are present in adequate numbers and are of distinctive morphology. *Fluorescence microscopy* needs little special apparatus, and immunofluorescence techniques (p. 244) are widely used for the rapid identification of viruses and virus antigens inside host cells. The main technical problem in this field has been the production of antisera of such precise specificity that presence of fluorescence in the microscopic preparation can be confidently interpreted as meaning presence of the appropriate virus antigens in the material.

Immunological Detection of Virus Antigens
Use of specific antisera, raised in animals, to detect antigens is discussed in Chapter 15, and one such procedure—immunofluorescence—has been mentioned in the previous paragraph. CIE (p. 241), passive haemagglutination (p. 242), RIA (p. 244) and ELISA (p. 245) are all used for rapid detection of virus antigens in clinical specimens—e.g. of hepatitis B antigens in blood, of rotaviruses in faeces and of herpesviruses in vesicle fluid.

Virus Isolation
The first essential is to ensure that the viruses survive the period between collection of specimens and setting up of cultures, since it is not usually practicable to set these up at the bedside or in the clinic. Some viruses are relatively robust; for example, poxviruses in material from lesions or polioviruses in faeces require no special precautions during transport so far as their own survival is concerned, though precautions must be taken to prevent infection of those who transport the specimens. Most viruses are unstable at normal room temperatures, and materials containing them should be kept at about $4°C$ (on ice or in a refrigerator) if the delay before culture is likely to be an hour or two, or at lower temperature (e.g. in an insulated flask partly filled with solid CO_2, or in a deep-freeze at $-20°C$ or better still at $-40°C$ or below) if a longer delay is anticipated. However, sub-zero temperatures should be used with discretion, as they are lethal to some viruses—notably respiratory syncytial virus. Repeated freezing and thawing must be avoided. Drying is another hazard to virus survival, especially when the specimens are swabs with only a little material on them; such specimens should be placed in a fluid transport medium (e.g. 0.2% bovine albumin in buffered salt solution).

Most clinical specimens contain bacteria which can interfere with virus isolation, and which therefore must first be killed (usually by incorporation of antibiotics into transport media and the nutrient media of tissue cultures) or removed (e.g. by filtration).

The methods of isolation appropriate to individual viruses are indicated in later sections. If animal inoculation is used, viruses are detected and identified by the diseases and particular lesions which they produce. They may be identified in hens' eggs by the lesions which they produce on the chorio-allantoic membrane, or by the presence of their antigens in fluid from the cavities. However, because of the convenience and low cost of tissue culture, this method of isolation is used in preference to animal inoculation or hen's egg culture whenever the nature of the virus permits it. (The identification of viruses in tissue culture has been discussed on pp. 159–60). The immunofluorescence method mentioned there may make it possible to identify the infecting agent within the first few days of culture, long before it is detectable by most other methods.

Diagnostic Serology

In virology, even more often than in other branches of microbiology, tests with known antigenic preparations are used to detect and measure antibodies in patients' sera. The principles of such diagnostic serology are considered on pp. 245–7. Subject to the qualifications given there, a patient whose serum contains antibodies to a particular virus can be assumed to have encountered that virus, but the encounter was not necessarily recent. Demonstration of *a rising level of specific antibodies* (at least fourfold) in the weeks immediately following onset of an illness, however, indicates recent infection and suggests that the virus in question, or one antigenically related to it, was responsible for the illness—though anamnestic reactions (p. 247) may occur in virus infections. To make a serological diagnosis, therefore, it is always desirable and often essential to examine *paired serum specimens*, one taken at the beginning of the illness and one taken a few weeks later. This is commonly forgotten by those in charge of the patients. There is no difficulty about remembering the acute-stage specimen, when the patient is ill and the doctor is worried; but that specimen is worthless without a second, collected in most cases when all anxiety is passed and the patient may no longer be in hospital or under the doctor's care. A virologist's deep-freeze is often a repository for acute-phase sera which wait in vain for their partners! When no acute-stage specimen has been taken, a single specimen taken later may be of value, either by giving negative results and thus casting doubt on or excluding the suspected diagnosis, or by showing a level of antibodies (notably of IgM—p. 246) high enough to suggest recent infection. In some diseases demonstration of an appropriately timed fall in antibody level may be confirmation of the nature of a recent illness.

The serological methods used in clinical virology include *complement-fixation* tests, *neutralization* tests and *haemagglutination-inhibition* tests (all described below) and all of those mentioned above in connection with immunological detection of virus antigens. The principles of such tests are outlined on pp. 241–5.

COMPLEMENT-FIXATION (CF) TESTS   As antigens, fluids from tissue cultures or from the allantoic cavities of hens' egg cultures of appropriate viruses are commonly used. Tests using such antigens are in general less precise in their specificity than are neutralization and haemagglutination-inhibition tests, and these latter methods are more valuable for distinguishing between related virus types.

NEUTRALIZATION TESTS   The theory of these is simple. The activity of a virus suspension can be demonstrated, according to the nature of the virus, by inoculating it into animals, into hens' eggs or into tissue cultures.

If a serum sample contains adequate amounts of neutralizing antibody for the virus in question, then a dose of virus suspension + serum will fail to produce the effect which is produced by the suspension alone. The amount of antibody can be determined by discovering how much the serum can be diluted before it ceases to neutralize the suspension. Antibodies in the blood of patients or of immunized animals will efficiently neutralize only those viruses that are identical with or closely related to the one that provoked their formation. Conversely, virus isolates can be identified by their susceptibility to neutralization by antisera of known specificity.

HAEMAGGLUTINATION-INHIBITION (HAI) TESTS   These are similar in principle to the neutralization tests, but the activity of the virus which is studied and which is inhibited by specific antibodies is the agglutination of red cells. Such tests can be used for antibodies against any of the assorted viruses which produce one or other of the three kinds of haemagglutination listed on pp. 160–1; and for recognizing particular virus types within groups of haemagglutinating viruses.

NOMENCLATURE AND SUBDIVISION OF VIRUS GROUPS

Attempts to introduce Linnaean binomials for viruses have not been acceptable to many virologists because of the difficulty of applying the concepts of genera and species to these organisms. In the widely accepted system of classification and nomenclature that we are using, virus composition and structure are the chief criteria for primary division into major groups, as we indicated at the beginning of this chapter. Recognition of smaller groups and subgroups relies to a varying extent on similarities of habitat, pathogenicity, mode of transmission, antigenic composition and laboratory behaviour. This diversity of criteria is reflected in the names that have been compounded for the groups and subgroups—e.g. picornaviruses = small RNA viruses; enteroviruses = intestinal viruses; polioviruses = viruses of poliomyelitis. In some cases such names are retained although they are no longer true descriptions of all viruses currently grouped under them, and they should therefore be regarded as convenient labels rather than as statements about the members of the groups (cf. bacterial nomenclature, p. 72). Fine subdivisions into types, designated by letters or numbers, depend on demonstration of antigenic diversity among viruses that are similar in their other properties, including in many cases possession of common group antigens.

Our descriptions of medically important viruses in the next few pages are arranged according to the order in which they are listed in Table VII, p. 156. Many of the groups described include animal viruses with which this book is not concerned.

PICORNAVIRUSES (small RNA viruses)

These are small icosahedral RNA viruses without envelopes. They include two groups that are of considerable importance in medicine—the enteroviruses and the rhinoviruses—and the virus of foot and mouth disease of cattle, which attacks man on rare occasions.

(a) ENTEROVIRUSES (intestinal viruses)

These viruses are primarily inhabitants of the human intestine, though they are also commonly found in the upper respiratory tract. They occur throughout the world, their frequency in temperate climates being higher during the warmer part of the year. They are excreted in faeces, in which they can sometimes survive for many days even in the presence of disinfectants such as cresols. Not much is known about their transmission, but flies can certainly play a part. Infection occurs via the mouth, and the viruses establish themselves in the lymphoid tissue of the upper respiratory and alimentary tracts before travelling via the blood stream to other parts of the body, such as the central nervous system where many of them can produce lesions. Symptomless carriage of enteroviruses is common, and therefore mere isolation of such an organism, unsupported by a rise in appropriate antibody levels, is not evidence of its involvement in the patient's illness. Enteroviruses can be divided into polioviruses (3 types) and coxsackieviruses and echoviruses (about 30 types each).

Polioviruses

Some features of the epidemiology of poliomyelitis have been discussed on p. 51. It is caused by three antigenically distinct types of poliovirus, of which type 1 is responsible for the majority of epidemics. Infection is often *subclinical*, or results only in a mild febrile illness which has no distinctive features and which is due to viraemia following preliminary multiplication of the organism in lymphoid tissue. In a minority of cases this febrile phase may be followed after a few days either by an *aseptic* (i.e. *non-bacterial*) *meningitis* or by true *paralytic poliomyelitis*—a condition due to virus multiplication in cells of the central nervous system and particularly in the anterior horn cells of the spinal cord. Recovery from poliovirus meningitis is rapid and complete, whereas paralytic poliomyelitis may be fatal (particularly if the brain stem is involved) or may leave severe permanent disabilities. Certain types of coxsackie or echoviruses sometimes cause meningitis or encephalitis which may be clinically indistinguishable from illnesses produced by polioviruses.

VIRUS ISOLATION - Polioviruses can be isolated by growing them in human or monkey tissue cultures. They are recoverable from throat swab or washings during the first few days of illness and from the faeces for some weeks longer. They are also to be found in affected parts of the central nervous system in fatal cases, and in the faeces of symptomless carriers. Their isolation from faeces is made easier by treatment of the specimen with penicillin and streptomycin to kill bacteria and with ether to kill viruses of other groups. Polioviruses are pathogenic to monkeys and apes.

DIAGNOSTIC SEROLOGY Neutralizing and complement-fixing antibodies appear in the blood following infection. As a rule they are specific enough in their action to indicate the type of the infecting organism, though there may also be rises of antibodies to other types previously encountered.

IMMUNITY Natural infection results in lasting immunity, but only against the type involved. Active immunization is discussed on pp. 298–9.

Coxsackieviruses (prototype isolated in Coxsackie, USA)
These are distinguished from other enteroviruses by the fact that they are pathogenic to newborn mice. They are divided into two groups, A and B, according to the lesions which they cause in these animals. They are further divided into about thirty types according to their antigenic composition. Group B contains fewer types than group A but they are more often incriminated as pathogens. Diseases caused by coxsackieviruses include *aseptic meningitis* (group A or B); *herpangina*, an acute pharyngitis with vesicle formation (group A); *hand, foot and mouth disease*, characterized by vesicles in all the 3 sites indicated (group A—not the same as foot and mouth disease, p. 170); *epidemic myalgia* or *Bornholm disease*, a febrile illness associated with severe pain in the chest muscles and elsewhere (group B); and *myocarditis* of newborn babies (group B). Also they are among the miscellaneous viruses that cause *colds* (p. 172). Individual types are associated with particular forms of disease. Diagnostic procedures are similar to those used for poliomyelitis, except that inoculation of newborn mice is used as well as tissue culture, and that virus may be recovered from the cerebrospinal fluid in cases of meningitis, whereas such recovery is rare in poliovirus infection.

Echoviruses (= Enteric cytopathic human orphan viruses)
The presence of these viruses in human faeces was first recognized because of their cytopathic effect in tissue cultures; since they did not appear to 'belong' to any disease they were described as orphans. However, it has since then been established that at least some of the thirty or so types can cause *aseptic meningitis, febrile illnesses with or without rashes, diarrhoea* or *mild upper respiratory tract infections*. Isolation procedures are as for polioviruses. Virus may also be recovered from the cerebrospinal fluid in cases of meningitis. Diagnostic serology is seldom practicable until the virus has been isolated, because of the number of viruses in the group, the lack of any common antigen and the impossibility of predicting which type is involved in a particular illness.

Hepatitis A Virus
This is a small (25–28 nm) RNA virus with the morphological features of a picornavirus (p. 170). It has not yet been grown in culture, but has been

transmitted from man to marmosets and chimpanzees. It differs widely from the hepatitis B virus, which is a DNA virus of unusual morphology (p. 191), but the diseases hepatitis A and B are best discussed together; this is done on pp. 190–2.

(b) RHINOVIRUSES and the common cold

The all-too-familiar symptom-complex known as coryza or the common cold was for many years an insoluble problem to virologists. Coxsackie or echoviruses could be incriminated as causing a few cases, and so could some of the myxoviruses (influenza, para-influenza and respiratory syncytial viruses) and some adenoviruses. But most colds remained unexplained until 1960, when the rhinoviruses were discovered as a consequence of growing tissue cultures in a slightly acid culture medium at 33°C (a better approximation to human nose temperature than 37°C). Some rhinoviruses (H strains) grow only in human cells; the rest (M strains) will also grow in monkey cells. Still more rhinoviruses were discovered when organ culture was introduced (p. 160), and over 100 types have now been distinguished. They conform to the description of picornaviruses, and are similar in size and structure to the enteroviruses. Other viruses have also been identified as causing colds, notably the coronaviruses (p. 182), and it is now possible to isolate causative agents from most patients with colds, and indeed quite often to isolate several from one patient. The next obviously desirable step—production of vaccines that will prevent colds—seems to be a long way off. This is because of the embarrassingly large number of different cold-producing viruses (with the further complication that mycoplasmas are also involved—see p. 145). Immunization with a vaccine prepared from one strain may protect the recipient against infection with that strain, but it leaves him still liable to the attacks of some hundreds of other viruses that can give him colds. Immunity resulting from natural infection is equally strain-specific.

REOVIRUSES (= Respiratory Enteric Orphan viruses)

The original members of this group of relatively large icosahedral RNA viruses without envelopes are found in the human respiratory or intestinal tract, often in association with mild inflammatory diseases, but have never been shown to be responsible for these conditions.

Similar viruses, known as *rotaviruses*, are very common causes of infective diarrhoea, especially in children. They can be found in the patients' faeces by electron microscopy, or by an ELISA test, and are divisible into three serotypes.

TOGAVIRUSES (formerly ARBOVIRUSES)

This group consists of icosahedral RNA viruses of variable size (40–70 nm), which differ from the two previous groups in having lipid-containing envelopes. There are more than 300 of them, mostly transmitted by arthropods such as mosquitoes and ticks. They have little resistance to physical or chemical agents, and are unstable outside the bodies of their hosts except at very low temperatures (e.g. $-70°C$) or when lyophilized.

Togavirus diseases are most common where animal hosts and insect vectors are plentiful—e.g. in tropical forests. Individual species show quite sharp geographical localization—e.g. eastern and western equine, Venezuelan, Japanese B and Murray Valley encephalitis viruses are found respectively on the east and west sides of North America, in Central and South America, in East Asia and in Australia. Among the many animals and birds known to act as hosts for togaviruses are monkeys, deer, horses, cattle, sheep, pigs, poultry and pigeons. One virus species may have more than one major host—e.g. birds as well as horses are commonly infected with the equine encephalitis viruses. Only for a few species—e.g. dengue—is man the sole known host. He plays an important part in the cycle of transmission of some others—e.g. yellow fever—but with the majority human infection is incidental, the disease being maintained chiefly in other hosts. One virus species may have more than one cycle of transmission (e.g. in yellow fever, see below). The arthropod vectors are blood-suckers, and their infection depends on the occurrence of viraemia in the vertebrate hosts. The viruses multiply within the bodies of the vectors but cause no disease in them.

Human infection may be subclinical or may produce pictures varying from a mild generalized febrile condition to a severe illness with localization of its main effects—to the brain in the encephalitides and to the liver and kidneys in yellow fever. Such localization is often preceded by a more generalized febrile illness, presumably resulting from virus multiplication at some site other than the point of entry or the final target organs.

Most togaviruses are haemagglutinators. Haemagglutination-inhibition and complement-fixation tests are used to divide them into subgroups containing antigenically-related members. Those that are pathogenic to man are included in the *alphavirus* and *flavivirus* subgroups. Infection-neutralization tests are used in species identification.

Alphaviruses

These include the organisms of *eastern equine*, *western equine*, and *Venezuelan encephalitis* and others which cause dengue-like illnesses (see below). They are mosquito-borne.

Flaviviruses

Some of these are mosquito-borne—e.g. *St. Louis*, *Japanese B* and *Murray Valley encephalitis*; *dengue* and the somewhat similar *West Nile fever*; and *yellow fever*. Ticks are the vectors of *Russian spring-summer* and *Central European encephalitis*, *louping ill* and some haemorrhagic febrile illnesses which occur in Russia and in India.

DENGUE   This disease of tropical and subtropical lands is characterized by fever, severe and widespread pains (hence its other name of 'break-bone fever') and rashes. It is rarely fatal, except in outbreaks of a severe haemorrhagic form of the disease in S.E. Asia. Man is the only known vertebrate host for the virus, and it is transmitted by *Aedes aegypti* (the vector of yellow fever) and related mosquitoes.

YELLOW FEVER   This is a febrile illness causing hepatic and renal necrosis and haemorrhages in various sites. It occurs mainly in equatorial Africa and South America, and caused the death of many early explorers of such regions. Monkeys of many species are susceptible to it, and the 'jungle yellow fever' cycle, maintained by *Haemagogus* mosquitoes in South America and by various *Aedes* species other than *A. aegypti* in Africa, does not include man unless he penetrates into the jungle and allows himself to be bitten. 'Urban yellow fever' has man as its host and *A. aegypti* as its vector. Fortunately this mosquito species, which breeds mainly in small accumulations of water around human habitations, is relatively easy to control, and the urban cycle can therefore be broken. However, the virtually uncontrollable jungle cycle remains as a menace to human beings who enter the jungle, and to nearby communities which allow their *A. aegypti* population to recover.

Vaccination with the egg-adapted 17D strain of yellow fever virus is safe and is effective for 10 years or more following a single injection.

LOUPING ILL   The only arthropod-borne togavirus infection known to occur in Britain is primarily a disease of sheep, causing cerebellar damage and the characteristic ataxic movements from which its name is derived. It is transmitted by a tick, *Ixodes ricinus*, which sometimes bites man, who may then develop a mild encephalitis.

Laboratory Diagnosis of Infections with Arthropod-borne Togaviruses

ISOLATION   Nearly all of these viruses can be detected and isolated by intracerebral inoculation of suckling mice, in which they cause encephalitis. Most of them also grow readily in the yolk-sacs or on the chorio-allantoic membranes of fertile hens' eggs or in tissue culture. Virus isolation may be possible from the blood of patients in the very early days of the illness, especially in yellow fever, but otherwise it may be impossible unless the patient dies and tissue from the brain or other affected organs can be used.

DIAGNOSTIC SEROLOGY   Haemagglutination-inhibition, complement-fixation and neutralization tests are used to detect antibodies in patients' sera. The first two tests are likely to give results which indicate only the subgroup to which the infecting organism belongs, though they can be made more specific by studying the ability of various antigenic suspensions to remove the antibodies. Neutralization tests are more likely to indicate the species of the organism.

Rubella Virus

The virus of rubella (German measles) is classified as a togavirus on morphological grounds, but differs from those already discussed in being purely a parasite of man, with no arthropod or other vector. Rubella infection in childhood may be too mild to attract any attention, or it may be recognizable by the presence of lymphadenopathy and a maculo-papular rash. In adults there may be more constitutional disturbance, and joint pains are a common feature in women, but the illness is still mild, brief and followed by a high level of lasting immunity. However, when a non-immune woman becomes infected during early pregnancy and the infection is transmitted to the foetus, the story is strikingly different. The foetal tissues may become very heavily infected with virus, and this infection is liable to persist throughout pregnancy (if the foetus survives) and for months or years after birth, despite the presence of maternal IgG and foetal IgM antibodies against the virus (p. 65). If the infection occurs early in pregnancy, foetal cells may be damaged at important stages in their differentiation. Some such foetuses die, and others are born with congenital abnormalities, of which cataract, heart abnormalities and deafness are the most important. Probably 50% or more of foetuses infected during the first month of pregnancy have some consequent abnormalities (not necessarily serious), but the risks are less with later infection and by the fourth month are much reduced. Infected babies may be born with large livers and spleens and may be profuse excreters of virus during their early months of life, so constituting a potential danger to other pregnant women and their foetuses.

It is clearly desirable that all women of child-bearing age should be immune to rubella. In Britain at least 80% of them are immune as a result of natural infection, which gives far more solid and lasting immunity than any vaccine at present available. There is thus a strong case for allowing rubella to persist in the community. This is the basis for the current British practice of making rubella immunization available to all girls between the ages of 11 and 13 years and to adult women whose serological tests indicate absence of rubella antibodies. Live attenuated vaccine is used, given subcutaneously. Since it is not certain whether these vaccine strains are themselves hazardous to foetuses, non-immune women should be warned against becoming pregnant within 3 months after immunization, and women who are already pregnant should not be immunized until immediately after delivery.

SEROLOGICAL DIAGNOSIS By no means every illness with clinical features suggesting rubella is due to rubella virus; and rubella infection in a pregnant woman can be subclinical so far as she is concerned but still damage the foetus. The two main reasons for measuring rubella antibodies are (a) to see whether a woman already has an antibody level that indicates that she is immune; and (b) to see whether a rubella-like illness results in a rising titre of rubella antibodies. If a woman who is not known to be immune is exposed to the risk of rubella infection, or develops an illness that might be rubella, during the early months of pregnancy, her blood should be tested for antibodies before there is time for them to rise as a result of the infection—i.e. the blood sample should be collected within 14 days of exposure or within the first day or two of the illness. Such a test is likely to show that she is immune. If it does not, a further sample should be taken 16 days or more after exposure or 7–10 days after the onset of symptoms, and this may show an antibody rise, indicating that she has been infected and that the foetus is at risk. To establish that she has not been infected, it is necessary to obtain negative results from samples taken over the next few weeks. If no sample is taken early enough to allow demonstration of a rising titre, the interpretation of antibody levels found in a late sample may be difficult, but may be made easier by determining whether the antibodies are IgG or IgM (p. 246). The purpose of all these antibody tests is to determine whether there is a risk of foetal infection and consequent malformation, and much anxiety on this score can be avoided by *checking the rubella antibody level as part of the routine early care of a pregnant woman*, rather than waiting until there is a known risk of infection. Indeed, there is no need to wait until the woman is pregnant; there is a strong case for routine screening of women who might become pregnant, especially school-teachers and others particularly at risk of exposure to rubella infection. There is at present nothing that can be done to prevent or treat the infection in an exposed non-immune pregnant woman; passive immunization of the mother with human gammaglobulin has been shown to be of negligible value as a protection to the foetus.

SANDFLY FEVER VIRUS

Sandfly fever is an acute illness with high fever, muscle aches and pains behind the eyes. Recovery is invariable, rapid and complete. The causative agent is an arthropod-borne virus formerly classified with the togaviruses, but now in the bunyavirus group. The disease occurs around the Mediterranean sea and in parts of Africa, India, Russia and China. The vector is the sandfly *Phlebotomus papatasi*. Diagnostic tests are similar to those for arthropod-borne togaviruses (p. 174).

MYXOVIRUSES (ORTHO- AND PARA-)

These two groups of enveloped RNA viruses with helical symmetry derive the shared part of their names from their affinity for mucus. By means of spikes projecting from their envelopes they are able to attach themselves to mucoprotein receptors on the surfaces of host cells (p. 160). The same mechanism is responsible for the phenomena of haemagglutination by virus suspensions and of haemadsorption by virus-infected cells (p. 159). Other more mushroom-shaped projections consist of neuraminidase, which allows the viruses to penetrate through surface mucus to host cell surfaces and also accounts for the reversal of haemagglutination described on p. 160. The envelopes of myxoviruses have high lipid contents and distintegrate when treated with ether, releasing the filamentous nucleocapsids which are then no longer infective. Naturally occurring filamentous forms of the influenza virus, however, are fully infective.

(a) ORTHOMYXOVIRUSES

These are the *influenza* viruses. Human influenza is an acute febrile illness of world-wide distribution, occurring as sporadic cases or in epidemics or sometimes in pandemics. Transmission is mainly by droplets, and the incubation period is only a day or two because the respiratory epithelium is both the portal of entry and the final target organ. The illness itself is also typically of short duration (though recovery of full health may be slow, particularly in the elderly). Though as a rule it is not a serious illness, severe and even fatal pneumonia due to the virus itself can occur; and in some outbreaks there is a high incidence of secondary bacterial infection of the damaged bronchial epithelium and lungs, notably by *Staph. aureus*, which can also be rapidly fatal. Except during epidemics it is often difficult or impossible to make a clinical diagnosis of infection by an influenza virus rather than by one of the other viruses that attack the respiratory tract, and many sporadic cases or small outbreaks of 'flu' are not in fact influenza.

Influenza viruses are relatively stable at room and refrigerator temperatures and can survive for some weeks in dust.

ANTIGENIC STRUCTURE   Viruses that cause influenza in man are divided according to their ribonucleoprotein (S) antigens into three types—A, B and C. Strains belonging to type A can be recovered from various animals and birds as well as from man, and these may well be important sources of new strains causing human outbreaks. Most epidemic strains belong to type A, and the antigenic structure of this type is particularly complex and unstable. Nucleic acid mutation may result in progressive minor antigenic changes ('antigenic drift'), but much bigger changes ('antigenic shifts') also occur as a result of the unusual structure of the virus. Its RNA consists of a 'team' of 8 pieces, each coding for a peptide, which need one another for production of viable virions but are to some extent independent in that each can be replaced by a corresponding member of another team. This can occur when two influenza A viruses meet in one host, and results in changes in the haemagglutinin (H) and neuraminidase (N) proteins—the antigens against which host immunity is directed. So far 16 H and 10 N subtypes are known, though only a few of them have been found in strains isolated from man and by no means all of the 160 possible HN combinations are known to exist. Individual strains are designated according to a complicated code—e.g. A/Hong Kong/1/68(H3N2) was the first influenza A strain isolated in Hong Kong in 1968 and was of H subtype 3 and N subtype 2. Subtyping allows study of the movements of particular strains in epidemics and pandemics. After pandemics particular antigen combinations may disappear from circulation among humans (though it may be that they are maintained in animal or bird reservoirs) for long periods—e.g. H1N1 has reappeared recently after being absent for 30 years, and the pandemic of 1957 was due to a strain with a combination of antigens to which antibodies were found in those who had lived through the 1889 pandemic. Such periods of retirement are probably reflections of herd immunity (p. 51). Antigenic shifts and up-to-date knowledge of prevailing antigenic types are of great importance to the planning of immunization programmes for influenza A. Type B strains undergo some antigenic variation, but type C strains are stable.

VIRUS ISOLATION   The viruses can be found in the throat during the first few days of illness. They can be grown in the amniotic cavities of fertile hens' eggs, where they are detected by their formation of haemagglutinins, or they can be grown in monolayers of human or monkey cells, in which they cause cytopathic changes and endue the cells with the property of haemadsorption.

DIAGNOSTIC SEROLOGY   Haemagglutination-inhibition tests are valuable for precise identification of virus isolates, but they are too highly strain-specific to be suitable for routine diagnostic examination of patients' sera. For this purpose it is better to employ complement-fixation tests, using type-specific antigens each of which will detect antibodies formed in response to infection with any virus strain belonging to its type (A, B or C). Such an antigen is formed when any virus of the appropriate type is grown in hens' eggs, and being soluble it can be separated from the virus particles. Since influenza antibodies are to be found in the blood of healthy people, it is particularly important in this disease to look for a *rising* titre of antibodies, though an unusually high titre in a single specimen may be diagnostic of recent infection.

IMMUNITY   As already indicated, immunity following natural infection with a type A virus is highly strain-specific and therefore of limited value. Similarly, active immunization, using injections of inactivated virus, gives adequate protection only against strains closely related to those contained in the vaccine. However, a vaccine made from current strains is of some use in protecting certain particularly vulnerable groups—e.g. those with existing impairment of respiratory function—for as long as those strains predominate. (The concept of 'original antigenic sin' is discussed on p. 291.)

(b) PARAMYXOVIRUSES

These are larger than orthomyxoviruses, do not undergo recombination, and in some cases are unable to agglutinate red cells.

Parainfluenza Viruses
These include the various myxoviruses formerly called Sendai, croup-

associated or haemadsorption viruses. They cause minor respiratory ailments, and can be distinguished from viruses of sundry other groups found in similar conditions by the haemadsorption phenomenon which they cause in tissue cultures. They are divisible into 4 antigenic types.

Mumps Virus

Mumps occurs mainly in childhood, when it produces acute and painful inflammatory swelling of one or more salivary glands, the parotids being most commonly involved. About 20 % of post-pubertal males who have this disease develop orchitis. Central nervous system involvement is not uncommon, and may occur in the absence of parotitis; it may take the form of an aseptic meningitis or of meningo-encephalitis, but is rarely serious. Transmission of mumps virus is thought to be mainly by droplets. There is no certain explanation for the long incubation period—commonly 18–21 days or more—but it seems probable that generalized dissemination, along the lines indicated on p. 162, precedes localized disease.

In most of its properties the mumps virus has a general resemblance to the influenza virus. It differs in that it rapidly becomes inactive at room temperature, is able to lyse chick red cells, and has a distinct and stable antigenic structure. It can be isolated during the first few days of illness from the mouth, from the salivary ducts or in appropriate cases from the cerebrospinal fluid. It grows in the amniotic cavities of hens' eggs, or in monkey kidney tissue culture; in the latter it induces the formation of syncytia (giant cells). Complement-fixation tests of patients' sera are of greater diagnostic value than haemagglutination-inhibition tests. Antibodies to the S (soluble) antigen of the mumps virus appear in the patient's blood during the acute phase of the illness, but are short-lived; whereas antibodies to the V (virus) antigen appear during convalescence and are more persistent. Active immunization, using either formalin-killed viruses from chick embryo tissue cultures or live attenuated strains of mumps virus, has been reported to give good protection. Passive immunization with human convalescent gammaglobulin is of some value in preventing orchitis. In most cases permanent immunity follows natural infection.

Measles Virus

In most parts of the world measles is a common, usually mild disease of children, characterized by fever, respiratory tract infection and a diffuse macular rash; a small number of deaths occur, either from measles virus encephalitis or from secondary bacterial infection of the respiratory tract. However, isolated communities in which the disease is not endemic are liable to severe outbreaks affecting all age groups and with mortality rates as high as 25 %. Infection is spread by droplets, and the virus multiplies in the respiratory tract epithelium before being spread via the blood stream. In malnourished children or immunodeficient patients an unusual form of measles, characterized by giant-cell pneumonia, may occur (p. 68). Subacute sclerosing panencephalitis (sspe) is a rare fatal disease of children or adolescents who have had measles some years earlier; it is apparently due to reactivation of measles virus latent in the brain.

The measles virus has the general structure of a myxovirus, but its known haemagglutinating activity affects only monkey red cells and it has no neuraminidase. Like many paramyxoviruses it can lyse red cells. It can be grown, with difficulty, in human or monkey tissue cultures, in which it causes the formation of multinucleate cells and syncytia (giant cells). Rising levels of complement-fixing and haemagglutination-inhibiting antibodies may be found in patients' sera, but a single finding of a high level means little because of the likelihood of past infection. These problems are of little practical importance, since laboratory confirmation of the diagnosis is seldom required. Lasting immunity follows natural infection. Passive immunization with human gammaglobulin is indicated when young or delicate infants have been exposed to infection. Active immunization is discussed on pp. 299–300.

Respiratory Syncytial (RS) Virus
Because it survives for only a short time outside the host and cannot tolerate freezing, this common pathogen of the human respiratory tract escaped detection until 1957. It is now known to be widely disseminated in Britain, the USA and many other countries during winter months, presumably by means of droplets, and to be a major cause of respiratory tract infections. In adults these affect only the upper respiratory tract and are not serious; but children may be more severely affected and in particular infants may develop *bronchiolitis* (the syndrome characteristic of this virus) and bronchopneumonia, which may be fatal. The virus can be detected in nasopharyngeal exudate by immunofluorescence. It grows in human or monkey tissue cultures, and as its name implies it shares with mumps and measles viruses the property of causing the infected cells to fuse into syncytia, but it does not cause haemagglutination. Complement-fixing and neutralizing antibodies are formed in response to infection with this virus, even in very young patients.

RHABDOVIRUSES

Rabies Virus
The causative agent of rabies is a helical enveloped RNA virus which differs from the myxoviruses in that its virions are bullet-shaped (typically) or rod-shaped or filamentous.

All mammals are susceptible to this grim disease, which is endemic in many parts of the world, though not in Britain (see p. 257 for further details). It is transmitted chiefly through bites inflicted by its victims upon other animals; vampire bats are exceptional in that they can carry and pass on the virus without themselves having the disease. Human infection is usually the result of a bite from a rabid dog. However, even a lick may be sufficient to transmit the virus, which multiplies in the salivary glands and may be present in large amounts in the saliva. The incubation period of the disease varies from less than 2 weeks to several months. The virus is believed to travel from its point of entry along the nerves or perineural lymphatics to the brain, and the incubation period is to some extent dependent on the length of this journey, being short if the bite is on the face. After multiplying in the brain, where it does extensive damage, the virus travels to the salivary glands and other parts of the body, probably again along the nerves. The outstanding clinical feature of the disease is a violent and painful spasm of the throat on attempting to swallow, with a consequent fear of drinking (*hydrophobia*). Once established, the disease is incurable and invariably fatal.

A bite or an area that has been licked by a possibly rabid animal should at once be thoroughly scrubbed with soap and water and then flooded with 70 % ethyl alcohol or tincture of iodine if available. In hospital it may be thought necessary to carry out more thorough debridement of the wound and other treatment to cover the possibility of bacterial infection from an animal bite—notably with *Cl.tetani* or *Pasteurella multocida*. The other matter for urgent attention is to trace the dog (or other animal), find out whether it has been vaccinated against rabies, and ensure that its subsequent health is carefully observed (see below).

DIAGNOSIS   If the animal causing the bite is available, it is important to determine whether it really has rabies. If it is dead, microscopic examination of its brain tissue is likely to reveal the typical Negri cytoplasmic inclusion bodies in the nerve cells, and the virus can also be demonstrated and identified by immunofluorescence or by electron microscopy. Mice inoculated with infected brain tissue or saliva develop typical nervous system signs in about a week. If the animal is still alive and fails to become paralysed within 10 days, it is not rabid. The diagnosis can be made by mouse-inoculation of specimens from the human patient, but by the time that this is possible it is too late to do anything about treatment. Patients do not live long enough for serological tests to be useful.

IMMUNIZATION   Specific neutralizing antibodies confer protection against rabies. Passive immunization, begun soon after a bite or other exposure and consisting of injection of human rabies-specific immunoglobulin (p. 292) intramuscularly and into tissues around any wound, may prevent development of the disease; but it cannot be relied on to do so on its own. The long incubation period leaves time for the exposed person also to be actively immunized. This was first done by Pasteur. Although he did not know the nature of the rabies organism, he so modified it by drying infected rabbit spinal cords that it was harmless and yet an effective antigen when given by subcutaneous injection. Patients could be given further injections of such cord preparations dried for progressively shorter periods, until they were able to tolerate a preparation containing fully virulent virus. Both Pasteur's live vaccines and inactivated vaccines such as that introduced by Semple had the disadvantage that repeated injections of tissue from the central nervous system were liable to cause allergic encephalitis. The vaccine now used is prepared in human diploid cell culture, and has the advantages that fewer injections are required and that adverse reactions are minimal. It is therefore suitable for routine prophylaxis of those likely to be at risk, as well as for treatment of those who have been exposed.

CONTROL   In countries where there is rabies, stray dogs should be destroyed and all others actively immunized. Quarantine regulations and some other aspects of control of this disease are discussed on p. 257.

CORONAVIRUSES

These pleomorphic enveloped RNA viruses take their name from their crown-like ring of petal-shaped projections. Many distinct types within this group attack the human respiratory tract, usually producing illnesses indistinguishable from common colds produced by rhinoviruses. Coronaviruses were first discovered by inoculating tracheal organ cultures with material from the respiratory tracts of patients with such illnesses, but can now be grown and identified in simple tissue cultures. Infection can also be confirmed by demonstrating rising antibody titres in complement-fixation tests.

ARENAVIRUSES

These are medium-sized enveloped RNA viruses characterized by granularity of appearance in electron micrographs.

Lymphocytic Choriomeningitis Virus
A virus that causes endemic infection in wild mice and is excreted in their urine and faeces is occasionally transmitted to man, by inhalation of contaminated dust or eating of contaminated food. The resultant human illness may be influenza-like, but characteristically it is an aseptic meningitis with a high lymphocyte count (up to 1000 per μl) in the cerebrospinal fluid. The virus may be isolated from the patient's cerebrospinal fluid or blood by tissue culture or by intracerebral inoculation into mice. Antibodies can be detected in patients' sera by complement-fixation tests.

Lassa Fever Virus
A similar virus causes the much more serious human illness first described in Lassa, Nigeria, in 1969, and subsequently seen in outbreaks and as sporadic cases in various parts of West Africa. The illness begins with non-specific symptoms—fever, malaise, muscle pains, headache and sore throat—but after a few days suddenly becomes more severe, with high fever, prostration, diarrhoea and vomiting, chest and abdominal pains,

and a distinctive inflammation and ulceration of the throat. Leucopenia and proteinuria are common. About a quarter of the patients die. The others may remain febrile for a week or two. Serum from those who have recovered from the disease is the only form of specific therapy.

From time to time a patient with what might be Lassa fever arrives in Britain or elsewhere by air from West Africa. Such a patient should immediately be admitted to a hospital with adequate isolation facilities, and virological investigations should be carried out only in a laboratory equipped to handle dangerous pathogens. The virus can be isolated in tissue culture, and can be recognized in the patients' tissues (the usual means of autopsy diagnosis) by electron or immunofluorescence microscopy.

MARBURG AND EBOLA VIRUSES

These as yet unclassified RNA viruses are morphologically similar (resembling elongated rabies viruses), but antigenically distinct. They have caused a number of outbreaks of severe illnesses, with high mortality rates, called *viral haemorrhagic fevers* and characterized by fever, headache, muscle pain, diarrhoea and vomiting, maculopapular rashes and evidence of liver, kidney and central nervous system involvement. The first such outbreak occurred in 1967 and affected laboratory workers in Marburg, West Germany, followed by others in Frankfurt and Belgrade, all of whom had been dealing with tissues and tissue cultures from the same batch of African green monkeys from Uganda. Another outbreak due to the Marburg virus, affecting only 3 people, occurred in South Africa in 1975. Ebola virus disease outbreaks occurred in 1976 in Sudan and Zaire, and again in 1979 in the Sudan. The reservoir for this organism is unknown. Management of a patient arriving from Africa with an illness possibly due to one of these viruses should be as described for Lassa fever. The viruses can be grown in tissue culture, and can be recognized by electron or immunofluorescence microscopy. They form inclusion bodies resembling Negri bodies. Antibodies can be detected in patients' sera by complement-fixation or immunofluorescence tests.

PAPOVAVIRUSES (viruses of PApillomas, POlyomavirus and monkey VAcuolating virus)

These are small icosahedral DNA viruses without envelopes. A virus of this morphology is demonstrable by electron microscopy in common human warts, and since such warts are transmissible to other humans by means of cell-free filtrates they are presumed to be due to the virus. It has not been certainly grown in tissue culture or transmitted to other species. Morphologically similar viruses have been demonstrated by electron microscopy in (but not yet grown from) brain tissue of patients with progressive multifocal leucoencephalopathy, a rare form of encephalitis occurring in the terminal stages of neoplastic diseases or sometimes in association with other diseases in which the reticulo-endothelial system is extensively involved. The other members of this group are all animal viruses. Among those which are found in and are the causative agents of benign papillomas in their various host species, the rabbit papilloma virus is unique in that it can also cause malignant tumours. The polyoma virus, isolated from the tissues of leukaemic mice, produces a wide range of malignant tumours when injected into newborn mice, hamsters and other rodents. The monkey vacuolating virus or simian virus (sv) 40, isolated from monkey kidney tissue cultures, also causes malignant tumours when administered to newborn hamsters; and a 'hybrid' virus, formed when adenovirus type 7 is grown in monkey kidney cells that are infected with sv 40, produces malignant tumours in newborn hamsters more rapidly than does sv 40 itself. These animal viruses are of no direct medical importance, but are mentioned here because their behaviour clearly suggests the possibility that similar DNA viruses may be involved in the aetiology of human malignant diseases. (See also pp. 186 and 187.) Such speculation is not limited to this group of viruses, as some RNA viruses also cause malignant tumours in animals—notably the first two viruses ever shown to do so, the fowl leukaemia virus and the Rous sarcoma virus.

ADENOVIRUSES

These also are icosahedral DNA viruses without envelopes. They are larger than the viruses of the previous group, and nearly all agglutinate red cells of one or more animal species. Those isolated from humans share a group complement-fixing antigen but can be separated into 33 types by haemagglutination-inhibition and neutralization tests. Some types are not known to be pathogenic, but some (notably types 3, 4, 7, 14 and 21) cause *acute febrile illnesses with inflammation of various parts of the respiratory tract*, of which *sore throat* is a frequent component. Epidemics of such infection may occur, and have been particularly noted among large communities of new recruits to the US forces, where they have been sufficiently troublesome to stimulate research into means of active immunization. *Conjunctivitis* is often associated with the respiratory tract infections ('pharyngo-conjunctival fever'). Type 8 has been incriminated in many countries as a cause of *epidemic kerato-conjunctivitis*, notably among shipyard workers and others exposed to abnormal risks of minor corneal abrasions. Outbreaks of this condition have also resulted from cross-infection between patients who were being investigated and treated at the same ophthalmological clinics. There is evidence that enlargement of Peyer's patches as a result of adenovirus infection may lead to *intussusception* in children. The viruses can be recovered from appropriate sites in these infections by growing them in human tissue cultures. Both group and type-specific antibodies appear in the blood following infection; complement-fixation tests for the former are used to provide evidence of adenovirus infection and neutralization tests to indicate the type of virus involved.

HERPESVIRUSES

These are icosahedral DNA viruses which are larger than those of the two previous groups and have envelopes. They multiply inside the nuclei of host cells, producing intranuclear inclusion bodies. The group includes the herpes simplex virus (and their simian equivalent, the monkey B virus, an occasional cause of fatal central nervous system infection in humans who work with monkeys or monkey tissues); the varicella-zoster (chicken-pox and shingles) virus; the cytomegalovirus; and the Epstein–Barr virus of infectious mononucleosis.

Herpes Simplex Viruses
These are probably man's commonest virus parasites. Rarely, infants are infected from their mothers during birth, and severe generalized infection may result. Far more commonly primary infection occurs early in childhood, often without any more specific manifestations than mild fever and malaise, but sometimes in the form of *aphthous stomatitis* (herpetic gingivo-stomatitis), an acute febrile illness with vesiculation and then ulceration of the oral mucous membranes. Primary infection in eczematous children may cause *eczema herpeticum*, in which large numbers of vesicles appear on the eczematous skin. *Herpetic whitlow* is a painful and often destructive finger infection, resulting from direct inoculation of herpes virus into the skin of the finger—sometimes the finger of a doctor, dentist or nurse attending to a patient with herpes. Other possible results of primary infection include mild *aseptic meningitis*, a more severe *encephalitis* and various manifestations of *genital infection*. However, in most cases the primary infection is inapparent, but despite antibody formation by the host the virus establishes itself in a latent state in his tissues. From time to time this host–parasite relationship is disturbed (p. 162) and a crop of vesicles may appear on the skin near the lip margin, near the nose, on the genitalia or elsewhere—commonly recurring many times, possibly as a result of widely different stimuli, and nearly always occupying the same site in a given patient. This is by far the commonest disorder caused by this virus, and is known as *herpes simplex* (or as *herpes labialis* when in its commonest site, or as *herpes genitalis* when on the genitalia, or as *herpes febrilis* on the frequent occasions when the stimulus is a febrile illness). Herpetic lesions, either primary or recurrent, may involve the cornea or conjunctiva or both (*kerato-conjunctivitis*). Treatment of such lesions and of other herpetic infections is discussed on pp. 164–5.

Two types of herpes simplex virus can be distinguished serologically and by some of their cultural features—notably by the pocks that they produce on chorio-allantoic membranes. Type 1 is responsible for virtually all oral and nervous system infections, whereas type 2 is found mainly in the genital tract. Genital herpes is possibly the commonest sexually transmitted disease, and the least treatable. Women with carcinoma or precancerous changes of the cervix uteri have antibodies to the type 2 virus in their blood more commonly than do women from appropriate control groups. It is therefore possible that the virus, though seldom isolated from such lesions, is responsible for inducing neoplastic changes. Alternatively, it may be transmitted in company with a carcinogenic agent.

Herpes simplex virus may be detected in material from lesions by electron microscopy or by immunofluorescence. It can be grown on hens' egg chorio-allantoic membranes or in tissue culture, in which it forms inclusion bodies and is cytopathogenic. Detection of rising levels of neutralizing and complement-fixing antibodies may be of diagnostic value in primary infections, but such antibodies are common in the blood of healthy adults.

Varicella-Zoster (VZ) virus

Chickenpox (varicella) is a highly infectious and usually mild illness, occurring mainly in childhood and characterized by a vesicular eruption. The lesions, unlike those of smallpox, appear in crops on successive days, so that new ones are still appearing when others are well advanced. The trunk is usually affected before the face and limbs. *Shingles* (zoster) is a much less common condition, and almost confined to adults. Its main features are severe pain in the distribution of one or more nerve roots and clusters of vesicles in the same distribution. The pain is due to virus infection of the appropriate posterior horn cells. These two diseases are due to the same virus. An attack of chickenpox commonly confers lifelong immunity against that disease; but the virus may remain latent for years after the attack and then, reactivated by irradiation or a neoplasm or lowering of immunity, it may produce an attack of shingles. It may then go on to produce chickenpox in the susceptible close contacts of the shingles patient—usually, of course, in children.

Despite the clinical resemblance between chickenpox and the poxvirus diseases, the VZ virus is morphologically not a poxvirus but a herpesvirus. Furthermore, characteristic giant cells with intranuclear inclusions (Tzank cells) are seen on microscopic examination of material from the skin lesions that VZ virus produces, and are also found in herpes simplex lesions, but not in those of poxvirus infections. The VZ virus can be differentiated from both poxviruses and herpes simplex virus by electron microscopy and by its failure to produce lesions on the chorio-allantoic membranes of eggs. It can be grown in human-embryo tissue culture, where it produces cytopathic effects and intranuclear inclusions. It has not been transmitted to laboratory animals. Immunofluorescence and immunodiffusion can be used to detect virus antigen. Complement-fixing antibodies for VZ virus antigen can be detected in patients' blood following either chickenpox or shingles, but levels are higher after the latter—a finding which fits in with the concept that shingles is a disease produced by the chickenpox virus in subjects who are already partly immune.

Drugs that can be used in treatment of VZ infections are discussed on pp. 164–5. Local application of idoxuridine accelerates healing of shingles lesions. Human VZ-specific immunoglobulin can be used to prevent or treat severe VZ infections in immunodeficient patients, and vidarabine and acyclovir have each been used with some success to treat them.

Cytomegalovirus

This is another of man's common parasites, and many other animal species have their own equivalent viruses. The names cytomegalovirus and cytomegalic inclusion disease are derived from the characteristic changes found in infected cells, whether in the body or in tissue culture— namely, marked cellular enlargement and the formation of intranuclear inclusions.

Primary infection, which occurs mainly during adolescence and adult life, may be asymptomatic and detectable only by an antibody rise, or may cause a mild fever or occasionally hepatitis, pneumonitis or heterophil-antibody-negative infectious mononucleosis (see below). The virus may also be associated with localized or more generalized disease in debilitated elderly patients or in those with impaired immunological mechanisms, particularly those on immunosuppressive or cytotoxic drugs. A pregnant woman with either a primary or a recurrent infection may transmit it transplacentally, but more often the baby is infected from her genital tract during delivery or postnatally via milk. Intra-uterine infections may result in such manifestations as brain or other neurological damage, liver and spleen enlargement and deranged erythropoiesis; and now that intra-uterine rubella is largely preventable, cytomegalovirus is the more common cause of foetal damage. Perinatal or postnatal infections are usually asymptomatic.

Cytomegalovirus infection can be diagnosed in the laboratory by finding typical infected cells, with 'owl's eye' inclusions, in the patient's saliva or urine or in portions of infected tissue. The virus can be grown in human-embryo tissue culture, and antibodies can be detected by complement-fixation tests or immunofluorescence. It is important to remember that the mere presence of this virus in the human body does not mean that it is causing disease.

No effective drug is available for use against this virus. A vaccine for active immunization to prevent maternal infection is being evaluated.

Epstein–Barr (EB) Virus

In 1962 Burkitt drew attention to the occurrence in certain parts of Africa of an assortment of malignant tumours in children which had many features in common. Their epidemiology was such as to suggest that they are transmitted by insects, and this idea led to a vigorous pursuit of a possible virus agent, both in material from the African tumours and in that from similar conditions since recognized in many parts of the world. As in other attempts to find causative agents for tumours and leukaemias, the results were confusing because too many viruses were found. Presumably some of them at least were innocent 'passengers' in the tissues examined. The most convincing contender for the role of the Burkitt's lymphoma virus is the herpesvirus detected in cell-cultures from lymphoma tissue by Epstein and Barr in 1964. The same virus has been shown to be associated with nasopharyngeal carcinomas in Chinese patients, and its role in the aetiology of these malignant conditions is still a matter for debate and vigorous research. Meanwhile a quite different field of research was opened up when a technician developed infectious mononucleosis after working with the EB virus, and was observed to produce antibodies to that virus during her illness. (Infectious mononucleosis is a disease characterized by prolonged low-grade fever, pharyngitis, abnormal mononuclear cells in the peripheral blood, and lymph-node enlargements. It is alternatively known as glandular fever.) Subsequent studies showed that many patients with infectious mononucleosis produce such antibodies. Those who do so nearly always also give positive Paul Bunnell tests: these depend on the presence of antibodies that are called heterophil because they react with cells from another species (in this case, sheep or horse red cells). It now appears that the EB virus is responsible for most heterophil-antibody-positive and some heterophil-antibody-negative cases of infectious mononucleosis; its role in a particular case can be confirmed by using immunofluorescence to detect virus-specific antibodies. In some (usually heterophil-antibody-negative) cases of this disease rising antibody titres can be demonstrated instead for cytomegalovirus or other viruses. (See also p. 208).

It is now clear that the EB virus resembles other herpesviruses not only in its morphology but in its epidemiology. Natural infection is common in childhood, and indeed almost universal in many communities, but is usually asymptomatic. A substantial minority of those infected have persistent buccal infection with shedding of virus, and are therefore a source of infection to others, particularly by kissing. Persistence of virus can also be demonstrated in some of the circulating B-lymphocytes of some such people. Infectious mononucleosis occurs mainly in those whose primary infection has been delayed to the age-range 15–25 years, but is uncommon in middle age and later. The mononuclear cells in the blood which give the condition its name are T-lymphocytes, proliferating in response to virus–induced 'foreign' antigens on the surfaces of infected B-lymphocytes. Activation or reactivation of latent EB virus infection may follow immunosuppression.

POXVIRUSES

The information necessary for replication of a virus is coded on its nucleic acid. A small virus contains only a small amount of nucleic acid and it is therefore limited to a few structural components and a simple structure. By virus standards the poxviruses are large, and their enveloped particles, which appear brick-shaped on electron microscopy, have a relatively complex structure that is not yet fully elucidated.

Members of this group of DNA viruses cause skin lesions in various bird and animal species. The viruses of greatest interest to us are those of smallpox, cowpox and vaccinia. *Contagious pustular dermatitis* ('orf') is a poxvirus infection occasionally transmitted to man from sheep or goats. *Molluscum contagiosum* is a transmissible human disease which produces multiple warty skin nodules in many parts of the body.

Smallpox (Variola), Cowpox and Vaccinia Viruses

Smallpox, which is said to have killed 60 million people in the 18th century, was still endemic in many countries and liable to appear anywhere in the world until a few years ago. However, a vigorous World Health Organization eradication programme has now eliminated the disease, and the world was officially declared free of it in 1980. The next paragraph is therefore largely of historic interest only.

Smallpox was a febrile illness, with macular skin lesions that became papular, then vesicular, then pustular, and finally crusted after 10 days or so. In severe cases they were confluent and even haemorrhagic, and there was then severe systemic disturbance and many patients died. The lesions differed from those of chickenpox in being more peripherally distributed and in tending to be synchronized rather than appearing in crops.

Cowpox is a disease of cattle. Its lesions resemble those of smallpox, but the infection causes little or no systemic disturbance, either to cattle or to humans who acquire it from them—and were thereby immunized against smallpox, as Jenner discovered (p. 9).

Vaccinia is the condition resulting from infection with the virus used for immunization against smallpox (p. 256). The origins of this virus are uncertain. It may well be that some of the strains used were derived from smallpox viruses and some from cowpox viruses, both types having been so modified by animal passage that they became identical. Although the vast majority of people vaccinated intradermally with live vaccinia virus produced only single local lesions (similar to those of smallpox, as described above), a few developed either a systemic illness with widespread skin lesions (generalized vaccinia) or vaccinial encephalitis, and some of these died. Vaccinia virus should therefore not be used any more, unless smallpox unexpectedly reappears. The possibility of its doing so as an act of microbiological warfare has sadly to be borne in mind, and it may therefore be considered necessary to maintain stocks of vaccinia virus.

Poxviruses can be detected in fluid or crusts from skin lesions by electron microscopy, and although they cannot be distinguished from one another in this way, it does permit their rapid distinction from chickenpox virus, which despite its name is not a poxvirus but a herpesvirus (p. 186).

Poxvirus antigens can be detected in material from lesions by double diffusion (p. 241). Methods for distinguishing between the viruses of this group include growing them on hens' egg chorio-allantoic membranes (where they have different ceiling temperatures for growth and produce different lesions) and DNA analysis using bacterial restriction endo-nucleases.

VIRUS HEPATITIS

Hepatitis due to viruses has a spectrum of severity ranging from subclinial infection through to acute liver necrosis with death of the patient. Intermediate degrees of liver damage may be followed by complete recovery or in hepatitis B (see below) by chronic hepatitis sometimes leading to cirrhosis. Two major epidemiological patterns were recognized in the 1940s—*infective* or *infectious hepatitis*, often occurring in epidemics, spread mainly by the faecal–oral route, and having an incubation period of 2–6 weeks; and *serum hepatitis*, transmitted in blood or blood products, usually occurring as sporadic cases but sometimes in outbreaks associated with receiving particular batches of blood products or with use of one syringe (and sometimes one needle) to inoculate a group of people, and having an incubation period of 2–6 months. Individual cases were often difficult to classify, because of lack of any relevant history. The situation became clearer in the 1960s and 1970s with the discovery of the two principle agents causing virus hepatitis.

Hepatitis A

The RNA virus described on pp. 171–2 is responsible for the pattern of disease formerly called infective hepatitis, but can now be shown also to cause many of the sporadic cases that would previously have been unclassifiable. Patients are mainly children and young people, and outbreaks are common when groups of young people are brought together to live, as in schools, colleges and military camps. Faecal excretion of the virus occurs for 7–10 days before onset of the illness and for a few more days after that, and nearly all transmission takes place during this period—by the faecal–oral route (p. 40), with flies, food, drinking water and other vectors often involved and accounting for the higher incidence of the disease in warm countries with poor standards of hygiene. Transmission in blood is also possible, but there is no persisting viraemia such as occurs in hepatitis B. The diagnosis can be confirmed by demonstrating the appearance of antibodies for hepatitis A virus in the serum, using RIA; IgG antibodies may relate to past infection, but presence of specific IgM antibodies indicates that the current illness is hepatitis A. Active immunization against this infection is not possible yet, but an injection of human normal immunoglobulin (p. 292) provides passive protection for 4–6 months. Such passive immunization is a valuable means of controlling an outbreak in a closed community, such as a school, as it usually prevents the disease even if not given until a few days after exposure; and it is also recommended for travellers visiting countries in which they are at increased risk of acquiring hepatitis A.

Hepatitis B

In 1964 the blood of an Australian aborigine was found to contain an antigen that gave a precipitin reaction with the serum of a much-transfused haemophiliac. This antigen, which became known as *Australia antigen*, was also found in the sera of many patients with hepatitis of the long-incubation type (serum hepatitis, as described above). It is now known to be a capsid antigen of a DNA virus called hepatitis B virus, and it has been renamed hepatitis B surface antigen or HBsAg. The virus has never been grown in culture or transmitted to animals, but it can be seen by electron microscopy of the blood of patients with hepatitis of the long-incubation type (as well as others for whom there is no clue as to the incubation period), and of some other people who are carrying it without symptoms. Three characteristic types of particle are recognized—42 nm double-shelled spheres believed to be the viruses proper, 22 nm spheres and 22 nm diameter filaments. The latter two types consist merely of capsid material. Antigen detection, using RIA or ELISA or a form of passive haemagglutination, is more practicable than electron microscopy as a means of examining numerous blood samples for presence of virus. Presence of any of the particle types is associated with detectable HBsAg. The 42 nm particles contain a core antigen, HBcAg, but this cannot be detected in patients' blood samples; it is found after disruption of the particles in the laboratory. A third antigen, HBeAg, can be found in blood; its presence there correlates with presence of 42 nm particles, with a high level of infectivity and with a propensity to chronic infection. Subgroups of HBsAg and HBeAg have been defined, and are useful in epidemiological studies.

Hepatitis B corresponds roughly to the old definition of serum hepatitis. Before its aetiology was known it was often transmitted by medical procedures—by transfusion of blood or blood products, or by using the same syringe (often with the same needle) for giving injections to a series of people. These routes of transmission can now be closed, by testing blood for presence of hepatitis B antigen before allowing its use for transfusion and by using disposable syringes and needles; but other routes remain open. These including sharing of syringes and needles by drug-addicts, and such procedures as tattooing and acupuncture carried out by non-sterile techniques. Doctors, dentists, nurses, laboratory workers and others may be infected when patients' blood gets on abrasions in their skin, or is splashed in their faces (the conjunctiva being a possible portal of entry for the virus), or when they scratch themselves with needles after inserting them into patients. The virus can also be transmitted during sexual intercourse (particularly among homosexual males), or by sharing a common tooth-brush, and probably in many other ways not yet detected.

HBsAg and HBeAg are detectable in serum during the last few weeks of the long incubation period, before the onset of clinical hepatitis, and as a rule for some weeks afterwards, HBsAg persisting longer than HBeAg and each of them disappearing at about the time that its corresponding antibody becomes detectable. These antibodies are long-lasting, but anti-HBc antibody may be present only in the early stages, and so its presence may indicate recent infection with hepatitis B virus. In some patients, and also in some carriers who have never had clinical hepatitis, the virus persists for years, as indicated by positive tests for HBsAg and HBeAg and by infectivity of their blood to any who may be exposed to it. All potential blood donors must therefore be screened to exclude the possibility of their being carriers of hepatitis B virus. Furthermore, *all* samples of human blood should be regarded and treated as potential sources of hepatitis B infection for medical and nursing staff, laboratory workers and all others exposed to them, until tests for HB antigens have excluded this possibility—though clearly the risk is greater if the samples come from jaundiced patients. The assortment of people among whom persistent carriage of hepatitis B virus is particularly common includes children with Down's syndrome, patients with lepromatous leprosy, patients undergoing haemodialysis and drug addicts. The carriage rate in the community in general is of the order of 1:1000 in Britain, but as high as $5-10\%$ in some countries, notably in the tropics. In S.E. Asia a correlation has been established between HBeAg carriage by young adults and liability to develop hepatoma (a malignant liver tumour).

PROPHYLAXIS   Active immunization, using material derived from the blood of hepatitis B carriers, is now practicable and is undergoing trials in several countries. Passive immunization is also possible, using specific immunoglobulin prepared from plasma samples with high antibody titres for hepatitis B virus. It is used mainly for the protection of those who have been accidentally exposed, as described above, to risk from the blood of proven hepatitis B patients or carriers; if an appropriate type of accident occurs but it is not known whether the patient is a possible source of the virus, his blood should be tested at once, and immunoglobulin given to the exposed person only if the tests show that there was a risk.

Hepatitis Non-A Non-B
Now that it is possible to show which patients with hepatitis are infected with hepatitis A or B viruses or with one of the other viruses (such as cytomegalovirus or EB virus) that can cause hepatitis, there remain some who have similar illnesses for which no agent can be identified. These cases have been called hepatitis C, but it is clear that there are at least two distinct agents, transmissible to chimpanzees but not yet detectable in other ways. Because there is no way of eliminating it by screening blood from donors, non-A non-B hepatitis is still liable to occur following blood transfusion.

BACTERIOPHAGES

Bacterial cultures on solid media sometimes have a 'moth-eaten' appearance, due to the presence of many small areas in which the bacteria have been lysed. This phenomenon was first studied by Twort in 1915. He found that bacterium-free filtrates of a suspension of such a culture of staphylococci could produce similar lysis in other staphylococcal cultures. In 1917 d'Herelle, working with fluid cultures of dysentery bacilli, discovered a similar lytic activity, and concluded that it was due to very small living agents parasitic upon the bacteria. He called them *bacteriophages*, a name which has persisted and is often abbreviated to *phages*.

Bacteriophages are in fact a group of viruses. They have been demonstrated in connection with many bacterial species, but show a high degree of host-specificity, so that any one phage is usually limited not only to a single bacterial species but to certain strains of that species. As we have seen (e.g. pp. 83 and 115), this specificity is of practical value in the subdivision of species for epidemiological purposes.

Bacteriophages can be recovered from such natural sources as faeces, sewage and polluted water. Their presence can be demonstrated by applying bacterium-free filtrates of such materials to cultures of susceptible bacteria, but they are also carried inside bacteria which have only a latent infection and do not undergo lysis (lysogenic bacteria, described more fully later).

Phages differ in size and form, but as a group they have the greatest structural complexity of any viruses. The nucleic acid is DNA in most of those that have been studied, including those that have been the subject of the most intensive investigation, the T phages of *Esch. coli*. Such a phage is tadpole-shaped, its head consisting of a DNA core surrounded by a protein coat that corresponds to the capsid of an animal virus. Taking the T2 phage as an example, the head is about 100 nm long and consists of a short tube, hexagonal in cross-section and about 60 nm across, closed at its ends by caps that are two halves of an icosahedron. From one of these ends emerges a thin hollow tubular tail, with an end-plate and terminal fibres that are the means by which the virus becomes attached and adsorbed to the cell wall of its bacterial host. Such adsorption is possible only if the phage, which is non-motile, happens to come into contact with a bacterium of a strain with the appropriate specific receptors on its surface, and if various other conditions are fulfilled. Once adsorbed, the phage digests a small area of bacterial cell wall and then contracts, injecting its DNA into the bacterial body.

Bacteriolysis

If a large excess of phages is added to a bacterial culture, so that many phages are adsorbed on to each bacterium, the cells may be disrupted because many small areas of their walls are dissolved at once—'lysis from without'. If the infection is not so heavy, the bacteria survive this external assault, but intracellular phage multiplication may then occur, beginning within a few minutes of the injection of the phage DNA. Instead of synthesizing its own DNA, the bacterial cell provides that for new phages, and also supplies them with their protein coats. Within an hour or less, many phages have been formed, which then lyse the cell and are released—'lysis from within'.

As we have already indicated, bacteriolysis by phage can be studied in cultures either on solid or in fluid media. A bacterial 'lawn' can be produced by inoculating the whole surface of an agar plate with the bacterial strain to be studied. Before this culture is incubated, fluid preparations of various phages can be spotted on to it in marked positions. The culture is then incubated overnight, and lytic action of bacteriophages is shown by failure of bacterial growth in the areas on to which the preparations were spotted. If the number of effective phage particles is small, each one produces a separate small defect in the bacterial lawn—*a plaque*—roughly analogous to a single bacterial colony; but a large number of effective phage particles will produce confluent lysis of the whole area covered by the original spot. Bacteriolysis in a fluid culture becomes apparent far more rapidly, a broth culture of a susceptible bacterium becoming crystal clear within 30 to 60 minutes of the addition of a phage preparation; but of course only one phage preparation can be tested for lytic action on any one culture in this way, whereas the lawn procedure on a solid medium allows the testing of many preparations simultaneously on a single plate.

Lysogeny
Infection of a bacterium by phage is not necessarily followed by phage multiplication and bacteriolysis. Sometimes when phage DNA enters a host cell it does not derange its synthetic activities but is integrated into the bacterial chromosome. Such a phage is described as *temperate*, as distinct from *virulent* or *lytic*, and the integrated non-lytic form in which it persists in the cell is called *prophage*. In this form it is reproduced synchronously with the bacterium and handed down to all the progeny of the original cell. This relationship is described as *lysogeny* and the host bacterium as *lysogenic* because in certain circumstances propagation and release of the phage may occur, and it may then cause lysis of other bacterial strains. Such propagation may occur spontaneously, and it can also be induced by using ultra-violet light or various chemicals. A lysogenic bacterial strain is also resistant to lysis by another preparation of the same phage as that which it is carrying.

Transduction and Lysogenic Conversion
The role of temperate phages in the *transduction* of genetic material from one bacterial strain to another has already been mentioned (p. 28). *Lysogenic conversion* is somewhat different, in that the phage does not transfer a property from one strain to another but the phage's own DNA confers new properties upon strains with which it enters into a lysogenic relationship. Thus both erythrogenic toxin production by *Str. pyogenes*

(p. 87) and toxigenicity of *C. diphtheriae* (p. 98) depend on possession of appropriate lysogenic phages.

Suggestions for Further Reading

Virus Hunters by Greer Williams (Hutchinson, London, 1960) for the history of virological research.

Notes on Medical Virology by Morag C. Timbury, 6th edn. (Churchill Livingstone, Edinburgh, New York and London, 1978).

CHAPTER 12

FUNGI

Fungi are eukaryotes (p. 12). The microscopic fungi are a large and varied group, classified mainly according to their methods of sexual reproduction. However, the few species that are pathogenic to man are mostly included in the *fungi imperfecti* because they have no known sexual phase to their life-cycle. The study of fungi is called *mycology*, and diseases caused by fungi are known as *mycoses*.

The fungi with which we are concerned can be divided into four groups:

(1) *Filamentous fungi or moulds* form branching tubular filaments or *hyphae* which are interwoven into a felt-like *mycelium*. Hyphae vary considerably in thickness, but even the finest are much coarser than bacterial filaments. They may be divided by transverse partitions called *septa*. In cultures some of the mycelium is embedded in the medium, some lies on its surface and some is raised into the air, giving to the colonies a fluffy appearance such as is seen also in naturally occurring surface growth of moulds. These fungi produce asexual spores of many kinds, including *arthrospores*, formed by the breaking up of hyphae into short lengths; *chlamydospores*, formed by local hyphal dilatations; and *conidia*. These last may be single-celled microconidia, about 2–6 μm in diameter, or considerably larger macroconidia, containing a number of cells; in either case they are borne on special hyphal structures called *conidiophores*.

(2) *Yeasts* are single round or oval cells which reproduce by forming small lateral buds that enlarge and develop into new cells. Their colonies on culture media resemble those of bacteria.

(3) *Yeast-like fungi*, such as the medically important genus *Candida*, also reproduce by budding. However, the buds tend to elongate into filaments (*pseudohyphae*) which remain linked together in chains that have some resemblance to mould mycelium. They can be differentiated by the facts that pseudohyphae do not form arthrospores or conidia and do not branch, though two or more buds may arise from the same

end of a single filamentous cell and so give an appearance of branching.

(4) *Dimorphic fungi* have a yeast morphology in tissues or when growing in cultures at 37°C, but form mycelium when growing saprophytically in the soil or in cultures at ordinary room temperatures.

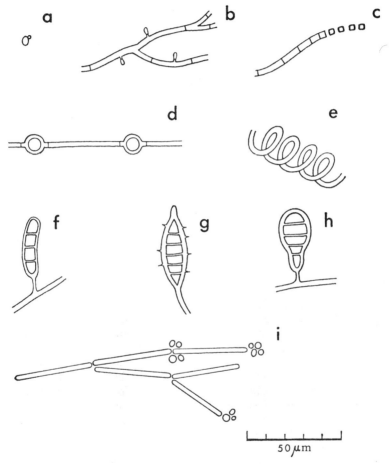

Figure 6 Some morphological features of fungi.

(a) The same yeast as in Fig. 5(q), to emphasize the difference of scale.
(b) Branching septate mycelium with lateral microconidia.
(c) A hypha breaking up to form arthrospores.
(d) A hypha showing chlamydospores.
(e) A spiral hypha.
(f, g and h) Macroconidia of *Trichophyton*, *Microsporum* and *Epidermophyton*.
(i) Pseudohyphae of a yeast-like fungus with yeast forms at junctions.

Although many pathogenic fungi will grow on ordinary bacteriological culture media, they grow better and with less risk of bacterial overgrowth on special mycological media. The commonest of these are *Sabouraud's glucose agar* and *malt extract agar*. Growth of contaminant bacteria and non-pathogenic fungi is suppressed by adding chloramphenicol and cycloheximide to the media. Most of the pathogenic fungi grow as well at room temperatures as they do at 37°C.

The fungi of medical importance are more conveniently discussed according to the diseases that they cause than according to any taxonomic arrangement.

CANDIDIASIS

Candida albicans

This is a yeast-like fungus commonly present in the upper respiratory, alimentary and female genital tracts and on the skins of healthy people. From time to time it becomes pathogenic, often as a sequel to malnutrition, general debility, diabetes, antibiotic suppression of the bacterial flora which normally inhibit proliferation of these and other fungi, use of oral contraceptives, steroid therapy, immunosuppression or other predisposing factors. It can then cause a wide variety of disorders, including the following:

(1) *Thrush*, a superficial infection of the mucous membrane of the mouth, characterized by white adherent patches of pseudomycelium.

(2) *Vulvo-vaginitis*, with white discharge and much irritation, affecting mainly adults and more common during pregnancy.

(3) *Chronic paronychia* of housewives, barmaids, fruit packers and others whose hands are constantly in water.

(4) *Dermatitis*, usually affecting warm moist skin folds (e.g. intra-gluteal or sub-mammary) or obese subjects. The skin becomes red, exudative and irritant.

(5) *Bronchial candidiasis*, a rare condition in Britain, in which the fungus invades the bronchial walls and lungs and may go on to produce a generalized infection. This must be clearly distinguished from the multiplication of *C. albicans* in the bronchi which often follows vigorous antibiotic treatment of bacterial infections, and which usually ceases spontaneously when treatment is stopped, though on rare occasions it may develop into a true bronchial candidiasis.

(6) *Candida enteritis*, almost always a consequence of suppression of the normal bowel flora by broad-spectrum antibiotics.

(7) *Candida endocarditis*, formerly a disease mainly of drug addicts (who presumably introduce the organism into their blood when giving themselves injections) and of diabetics, but more recently a serious and all-too-common complication of heart-valve replacement.

(8) *Candida septicaemia*, with abscess formation in kidneys and other organs, and sometimes endocarditis. Common predisposing factors are immunosuppression, malignant disease, broad-spectrum antibacterial treatment and parenteral feeding.

(9) *Chronic muco-cutaneous candidiasis*—a rare condition, consisting of persistent and disfiguring infection of skin, mucous membrane and nails. There may be underlying defective cell-mediated immunity and endocrine hypofunction.

LABORATORY INVESTIGATION   The oval yeast cells, $2-5\,\mu m$ in diameter, and the larger pseudohyphae are strongly Gram-positive and are easily recognized in stained films. Alternatively they may be demonstrated in skin and nail scrapings by the methods described below for the dermatophytes. Their mere presence in clinical specimens means little, and even their presence in abundance is significant only if the specimen is fresh, as they multiply rapidly at room temperatures. They give visible growth on blood agar after overnight incubation at $37°C$, but are more easily recognized on Sabouraud's medium, on which they form moist creamy colonies. *Candida* species show characteristic submerged growth with budding (*blastospore* formation) when inoculated into the depths of a plate of corn-meal agar, and *Candida albicans* can be differentiated from other species of the genus by its formation of chlamydospores in such circumstances, by its carbohydrate fermentation reactions, and by its formation of germ-tubes within a few hours of inoculation into neat human serum. *C. tropicalis* and other species of this genus are also sometimes pathogenic to man.

TREATMENT   The first step is to remove the predisposing cause, if possible—in particular, to stop or change antibacterial therapy if candidiasis threatens to be troublesome. Local application of 1 % gentian violet is effective in the treatment of thrush. The antibiotic *nystatin* is valuable for treatment of accessible candida infections on the skin or mucous surfaces (including intestinal candidiasis) but is poorly absorbed when given by mouth and cannot be given by injection. Another antibiotic, *amphotericin B*, is an alternative for topical use and can also be given intravenously for systemic candidiasis (and other systemic mycoses—see below). However, when given in this way it is liable to be toxic, particularly to the kidneys. This problem can be overcome in part by giving it in the lower dosage, which is possible if the synthetic drug *flucytosine* is also given, by mouth or intravenously. Flucytosine is less toxic than amphotericin B, and can be used for treatment of systemic candidiasis, provided that the *Candida* strain is fully sensitive to it; partial or more complete resistance is fairly common. The *imidazole* group of drugs (clotrimazole, miconazole, econazole and others) give good results when used topically for candida infections; their value in treating systemic candidiasis is still being assessed.

RINGWORM (THE DERMATOMYCOSES)

Fungi of the genera *Trichophyton, Epidermophyton* and *Microsporum*, collectively known as the *dermatophytes*, cause superficial infections of the keratinized layers of the skin, hair and nails (*ringworm* or *tinea*) but never attack deeper tissues. There is considerable overlap in the clinical syndromes which they produce, but *Epidermophyton floccosum* (the only species in its genus) does not attack hair and *Microsporum* species do not attack nails. Infection is commonly from man to man. For example, *tinea pedis* (athlete's foot), usually due to *T. rubrum* or *T. mentagrophytes*, is frequently transmitted via wet floors around swimming pools and bathrooms; and *tinea capitis* (scalp ringworm) due to *M. audouini* or *T. tonsurans*, can be transmitted by direct contact or via infected combs and brushes. Other species are acquired from animals—e.g. *M. canis*, which affects dogs, cats and other animals, may be transmitted to humans, particularly children, in close contact with them; and *T. verrucosum*, a common cause of cattle ring-worm, is also transmissible to man. Human infections with such animal pathogens tend to provoke vigorous local reactions and to be self-limiting.

LABORATORY INVESTIGATION   Scales are collected from skin lesions by scraping with a blunt scalpel; swabbing the skin first with 70 % alcohol may help to reduce bacterial contamination. The scales should be placed in a folded piece of paper (preferably black) for transmission to the laboratory. Infected hairs are carefully extracted from their follicles, using forceps; dull, broken hairs should be taken, and recognition of hairs infected with *Microsporum* species is helped by the fact that they fluoresce in UV (Wood's) light. Full thickness clippings of affected nails are taken for examination, together with debris from under the nails.

Portions of these specimens are placed on slides in drops of 20–30 % KOH, covered with coverslips and warmed gently. This treatment dissolves the host cells, and the highly refractile fungal elements can then be seen, using a microscope with a dry objective. Nail clippings usually need preliminary softening in KOH in a test tube before they can be made into microscopic preparations. In skin or nails all of the dermatophytes form branching hyphae and arthrospores, and are indistinguishable from one another. Hyphae also abound in and around the roots of hairs, but spores predominate further up the hairs. In those infected with *Microsporum* and some *Trichophyton* species, the spores are closely applied to the outside of the hairs (ectothrix), whereas those of other *Trichophyton* species are within the hairs (endothrix).

Material that has not been treated with KOH is inoculated on to Sabouraud's or other suitable media and incubated at 30 °C. Colonies take 1 to 3 weeks to appear, and species recognition depends on the fluffiness, texture and colour of the colonies and on the liberation of pigment into the medium, and also on the microscopic appearances of the growth. Among the most important distinctive features are the macroconidia, which may be cylindrical (*Trichophyton*), spindle- or boat-shaped (*Microsporum*) or pear-shaped (*Epidermophyton*). The number, shape and distribution of the macroconidia and the presence or absence of other structures such as chlamydospores and spiral hyphae help in species identification (Fig. 6, p. 197).

TREATMENT In some dermatophyte infections, notably athlete's foot, secondary bacterial infection may have to be dealt with before the fungal infection can be controlled. Ointments of benzoic, salicylic or undecylinic acid or combinations of these, for many years the best treatments for skin ringworm, still have a place in topical treatment of localized skin infections, as have the imidazoles (p. 199). The antibiotic *griseofulvin*, which is valueless in treatment of bacterial or monilial infections, cures most forms of ringworm. Taken by mouth for a number of weeks, it is incorporated in newly formed cells of the skin and its appendages, and makes them unsuitable media for the growth of most dermatophytes. These cells then gradually replace the existing keratinized epithelial layers, hair and nails, causing the dermatophyte infection to die out. Nail infection is the form of ringworm that most commonly fails to respond to such treatment. Surgical removal may then be necessary.

Pityriasis versicolor
This common and benign form of skin ringworm produces red, scaling patches on the body and limbs. It is caused by *Malassezia furfur*, a yeast-like fungus which is readily recognized in KOH preparations of scales by its characteristic mixture of round budding cells and short irregular lengths of mycelium. If confirmatory culture is required, olive oil or other suitable lipid must be added to the medium. Pityriasis versicolor usually responds well to treatment with a sulphur ointment or with any of the topical antifungal agents.

ASPERGILLOSIS

Members of the genus *Aspergillus* are common saprophytic moulds, such as grow on stored foods. They are recognized by their conidiophores. These are swollen ends of hyphae from which radiate large numbers of sterigmata (short lengths of narrower hyphae) ending in short chains of spores. As aspergilli are common saprophytes and multiply at room temperature, their presence in clinical specimens needs cautious interpretation, particularly if the specimens are not freshly collected. However, species of this genus can cause disease in man, including:

1 *Otomycosis.* A chronic condition in which fungal growth fills the external auditory meatus. Imidazoles are useful in its treatment.

2 *Allergic aspergillosis.* Some of those exposed to repeated inhalation of aspergilli—e.g. from dust of farm buildings or from air-conditioning systems in which these organisms have established themselves—become hypersensitive to them. The consequences of this are discussed on pp. 203–4.

3 *Invasive aspergillosis.* In some immunocompromised patients aspergilli (usually *A. fumigatus*) invade lung parenchyma and other tissues, with serious and commonly fatal results. Temporary withdrawal of immunosuppressive drugs and intravenous administration of high doses of amphotericin B may eliminate the infection in some cases.

4 *Aspergilloma.* This name is given to a spherical mycelial mass or giant colony of an aspergillus—usually *A. fumigatus*—that is sometimes formed in a lung cavity left by an abscess or an old tuberculous lesion or an infarct. There is no lung invasion; radiography shows that the ball moves freely in the cavity so that there is always a crescent of air above it on the picture, regardless of the position of the patient. Detection of serum antibodies (multiple precipitin lines) gives further confirmation of the diagnosis. Treatment is by surgical removal of the affected portion of the lung.

THE DEEP MYCOSES

Apart from candidiasis, fungus infections that involve deep structures are rare in Britain. In the absence of suitable treatment they are commonly fatal, but good results have been obtained with amphotericin B in each of the conditions described below, and other effective treatments for some of them are indicated in the appropriate paragraphs.

Cryptococcus neoformans (*Torula histolytica*)
This is a true yeast found in soil throughout the world. It is an occasional cause of disease in man and animals. Human infection begins as a local cutaneous or pulmonary lesion but usually becomes generalized, its commonest feature being a form of subacute or chronic meningitis which is liable to be mistaken for a brain abscess or tumour. Immuno-compromised patients, especially those with Hodgkin's disease, are particularly liable to develop this disease. The yeasts can be seen by microscopic examination of the cerebrospinal fluid, and their characteristic large capsules are well demonstrated if india ink is first added to the fluid to provide a dark background. They grow well on Sabouraud's glucose agar, forming creamy colonies and differing from other saprophytic yeasts in that they grow rapidly at 37°C. Cryptococcosis is best treated with both amphotericin B and flucytosine.

Blastomyces dermatitidis
Blastomycosis, the disease caused by this dimorphic fungus which is thought to have its main habitat in soil, was formerly believed to be restricted to eastern parts of the USA and Canada and was known as N. American blastomycosis. However, there is increasing evidence of its occurrence in S. America and in many parts of Africa. The fungus probably enters the human body via the respiratory tract. It may then cause chronic lesions of skin, bones, viscera and meninges. The organisms can be seen in their yeast state in the lesions, and can be grown on

ordinary mycological media. Amphotericin B is the most effective form of treatment, with hydroxystilbamidine as a less toxic and often successful alternative.

Paracoccidioides brasiliensis

Paracoccidioidomycosis (formerly known as S. American blastomycosis, and indeed apparently restricted to S. America, with its highest reported incidence in Brazil) is due to another dimorphic fungus, of which the natural habitat is not known. Initial ulcerative lesions of the oral or nasal mucous membranes may be followed by systemic spread, mainly to lymphatic tissues. Surprisingly for a fungus infection, sulphonamides are of some value in controlling (though not usually curing) the disease, and can be used to enhance the rather unreliable activity of amphotericin B. Successes with imidazoles have been reported.

Histoplasma capsulatum

This is another dimorphic fungus found in soil, notably in parts of the USA. In endemic areas symptomless human infection is common, as judged by the frequency of skin hypersensitivity to an extract of the organism called histoplasmin. Miliary lung lesions, similar to those of tuberculosis but healing spontaneously, are often found in such people. In a few subjects the infection progresses to involve lymph nodes and other organs, causing a febrile and often fatal illness, for which amphotericin B is once again the treatment of choice.

Coccidioides immitis

This is also a dimorphic fungus found in the soil. It is largely restricted to certain areas of the south-west of the USA. Almost all of the inhabitants of those areas are infected, most of them without symptoms but with the development of a coccidioidin hypersensitivity. A very few of those infected develop a generalized tuberculosis-like illness with a bad prognosis, for which the treatment is either amphotericin B or miconazole.

IMMUNOLOGY OF THE MYCOSES

IMMUNITY All except the most superficial of fungus infections (e.g. hair ringworm) elicit immune responses. T-cell-mediated immunity is of predominant importance in resistance to fungi, and patients with T-cell defects are particularly susceptible to opportunist fungus infections.

RESPIRATORY ALLERGIES Many fungi produce numerous spores less than $5\,\mu m$ in diameter, which can penetrate to the lung alveoli (p. 46). Many of the deep mycoses are initiated in this way; but it is also the basis of various respiratory allergies to fungi. Some allergic individuals form IgE antibodies to aspergilli, and then develop Type I hypersensitivity reactions (p. 63), with asthma and rhinitis, when they again inhale aspergillus spores. In *allergic bronchopulmonary aspergillosis* precipitating antibodies are formed as well, skin tests show both Type I and Type III responses, and there is pulmonary eosinophilia and consolidation as well as asthma. The hypersensitivity mechanisms underlying the various forms of extrinsic allergic alveolitis (hypersensitivity pneumonitis) have been discussed on p. 64; the prototype of this group of diseases, 'farmer's lung' is due to inhalation of spores of thermophilic actinomycetes such as *Micromonospora faeni* or *Thermoactinomyces vulgaris* which have grown in mouldy hay. Acute episodes of allergic alveolitis commonly present as fever, dyspnoea and cough, starting a few hours after exposure; but repeated exposure over a long period may lead to progressive pulmonary fibrosis and incapacitating limitation of respiratory function.

IMMUNODIAGNOSIS   Detection of fungal *antigens* in body fluids may be helpful in the diagnosis of deep mycoses. For example, in a case of cryptococcal meningitis it may be possible to detect the capsular polysaccharide of *C. neoformans* in cerebrospinal fluid, using a latex agglutination method, before antibodies have been formed—and indeed, antibody responses may never be detectable in patients with this condition because of immunosuppression (p. 202). Tests for serum *antibodies* may also be of value in diagnosing systemic fungus infections, including candida endocarditis, provided that due allowance is made for the frequency of such antibodies in the sera of healthy people. For example, *Candida albicans* is part of the normal flora of the human body, and many people have some antibodies to it, whereas this is not true of aspergilli. *Skin tests* similar to the tuberculin test (p. 253) can be used to demonstrate delayed-type hypersensitivity to antigenic extracts of fungi responsible for various mycoses, but like most such tests they indicate only whether the patient has at some time been exposed to the relevant antigen. Thus the histoplasmin skin test is of no diagnostic value in those parts of Kentucky where it is positive in about 95 % of people!

Suggestions for Further Reading
Medical Mycology by C. W. Emmons and others, 3rd edn. (Lea and Febiger, Philadelphia, 1977).
Also Section V of *Bacteriology Illustrated*—see p. 145.

CHAPTER 13

PROTOZOA

Protozoa are unicellular eukaryotes (p. 12), in most cases considerably larger than bacteria but still of microscopic dimensions. They all have nuclei clearly differentiated from their cytoplasm. They vary greatly in shape, structure and habitat. The phylum is divided into *Sporozoa, Mastigophora, Sarcodina* and *Ciliophora.*

All four of these subphyla are represented among man's parasites. Only a few of them are pathogenic, but since they include the causative organisms of malaria, trypanosomiasis and amoebic dysentery they make a formidable contribution to human illness and mortality.

SPOROZOA

THE GENUS PLASMODIUM

Malaria was formerly endemic in Britain and other temperate countries but is now mainly restricted to the tropics and subtropics. The four plasmodial species that are pathogenic to man—*P. vivax, P. falciparum, P. malariae* and *P. ovale*—respectively cause *benign tertian, malignant tertian, quartan* and *ovale* malaria. The terms tertian and quartan refer to the periodicity of the bouts of fever associated with the disease, with the days counted according to the Roman convention so that tertian fever recurs every 48 hours and quartan every 72 hours. Malaria seen in Britain today has invariably been acquired abroad, and most such imported cases are due to *P. vivax*; but it is important that those due to *P. falciparum* should be recognized promptly, as delay in their treatment may be fatal.

Man becomes infected when he is bitten by a female *Anopheles* mosquito in which the parasites have completed the sexual cycle to be described below. Entering the human blood stream as minute spindle-shaped *sporozoites*, the plasmodia pass to the liver where they develop into larger multicellular *schizonts*. Usually about 5 to 10 days after infection (depending upon the plasmodial species) the schizonts disrupt into many *merozoites*. This completes the *pre-erythrocytic* cycle. Some of the merozoites re-enter the liver and the same cycle, now called the *exo-erythrocytic cycle*, is repeated over and over, except in *P. falciparum* infections. Meanwhile, other merozoites have entered the red cells of the blood and initiated a similar but shorter *erythrocytic cycle*, which ends with the rupture of the infected red cells and the release of further batches of merozoites. The length of the erythrocytic cycle determines the periodicity of the fever, though the patient does not experience symptoms during the first few cycles, which involve relatively small numbers of red cells. *P. falciparum* causes infected red cells to agglutinate, with consequent capillary obstruction and the high incidence of severe cerebral and other complications which have earned for this form of malaria the name 'malignant'.

Instead of developing into schizonts, some of the merozoites which invade red cells become either male or female *gametocytes*. It is on these sexual forms that transmission of malaria depends, for when sucked up by a female *Anopheles* they fuse to form zygotes, which develop into *oöcysts* in the mosquito's stomach wall. Mature oöcysts rupture and release *sporozoites*, which make their way to the insect's salivary glands and are then ready to initiate a fresh human infection.

LABORATORY INVESTIGATION   Plasmodia can be recognized in blood films stained with haematological stains, and this is the definitive procedure for diagnosis of malaria. Since parasites may be few, thick films are used for their detection, but their morphology is more easily studied in thinner films. Species recognition depends upon the appearances of the *trophozoites* (ring-shaped precursors of schizonts), of the schizonts and of the gametocytes, and also upon the presence and colour of pigment granules in infected red cells. *P. ovale* takes its name from the fact that the infected red cells tend to be of oval shape.

TREATMENT AND CONTROL   Antimalarial drugs can be used for any of three purposes:

1 *Prophylaxis*.   Drugs cannot prevent malarial infection, but they can suppress the erythrocytic cycle, and so the clinical manifestations, until the infection has died out. Chloroquine or proguanil are suitable for this purpose, except in areas—notably in S.E. Asia and S. America—where there are chloroquine-resistant strains of *P. falciparum*, which necessitate the use of pyrimethamine (p. 325) with either a sulphonamide or dapsone (p. 136). Even a brief stop in a malarial region—e.g. for aircraft refuelling—may be long enough to become infected. Taking of prophylactic drugs should begin a week before entering a malarial region (to allow development of adequate blood levels) and *must be continued for four weeks after leaving the area*. This is because the drugs mentioned so far do not kill the exo-erythrocytic stages of the parasite, and cessation of prophylaxis soon after leaving the malarial area may therefore be

followed by clinical malaria a few weeks later—though not malignant tertian malaria, since *P. falciparum* has no exo-erythrocytic cycle.

2 *Treatment of an attack.* For this purpose chloroquine is usually the best drug, except for treatment of the chloroquine-resistant *P. falciparum* strains. Against these, the time-honoured drug quinine can be used, preferably together with pyrimethamine and a sulphonamide; but some strains in Thailand are resistant to pyrimethamine as well as to chloroquine, and for them a combination of quinine and tetracycline seems to be the best available treatment.

3 *Eradication of infection.* Primaquine kills the exo-erythrocytic stages, and so can be used with one of the other drugs to eradicate infection by species other than *P. falciparum*.

Elimination of malaria from a community depends upon a two-pronged attack—treatment of infected human beings so that there is no source of gametocytes, and control of the mosquito vectors. The methods used in achieving the latter vary considerably from place to place because of the varied habits of different *Anopheles* species. They include swamp drainage and other measures to eliminate suitable breeding grounds, oiling the surface of exposed waters to asphyxiate larvae, and spraying houses with long-acting insecticides. Although *P. falciparum* can now be grown *in vitro* and the possibility of making a vaccine for immunization against this species is being actively explored, the problems involved in doing so are formidable and there is no immediate prospect of success.

THE GENUS TOXOPLASMA

Toxoplasma gondi

First described in 1908, and named after one of its earliest known hosts, an African rodent called the gondi, this species has a world-wide distribution in animals and birds, but its pathogenicity to man was unrecognized until 1939. The probable major source of human infection is the domestic cat; it becomes infected by eating rodents, a sexual phase of the life-cycle of *T. gondi* then takes place in the cat's intestine, and oocysts excreted in its faeces are ingested by humans. Humans can also acquire the infection by eating inadequately cooked meat from infected animals; and infants can be infected from their mothers as described below. The majority of human infections are sub-clinical. Of the various clinical manifestations, all of them rare, the most important are:

(1) Transplacental transmission of *T. gondi* from a mother who acquired her primary infection during the pregnancy may result in stillbirth, neonatal death or congenital deformities. Hydrocephalus, microcephaly, intracerebral calcification, chorio-retinitis and psycho-motor retardation are common features of congenital toxoplasmosis.

(2) Infection acquired in early childhood may cause fatal encephalitis.

(3) Infection during later childhood or adult life may cause a benign febrile illness with the clinical and haematological features of infectious mononucleosis; heterophil antibodies are not formed (p. 188).

(4) Chorio-retinitis and other eye lesions may occur as part of one of the above pictures or separately.

LABORATORY INVESTIGATION   The crescent-shaped nucleate protozoa, about 6 μm by 3 μm, can be demonstrated inside and between the cells of affected tissues by staining smears with haematological stains. They may also be found in blood or other body fluids. They can be grown in tissue cultures or in eggs, but intracerebral and intraperitoneal injection into young mice are generally employed for their identification and maintenance.

Antibodies can be detected in the blood of patients, and of many healthy adults who have presumably had subclinical infections. The methods in current use include a fluorescent-antibody procedure similar to the FTA test (p. 251), indirect haemagglutination and complement-fixation procedures and the Sabin–Feldman dye test, which depends upon the fact that after exposure to specific antibodies the parasites resist staining with alkaline methylene blue.

Combined therapy with a sulphonamide and pyrimethamine (p. 325) has given good results in this previously untreatable disease.

PNEUMOCYSTIS CARINI

Although this protozoon has been recognized as a pathogen of animals since 1912 and of man since 1928, its *in vitro* culture (in chick embryo cells) was not reported until 1977, and its classification as a Sporozoon is still provisional. Serological surveys suggest that subclinical (possibly persistent latent) infection is common from early life. Overt disease, however, is restricted to those with immunodeficiencies (p. 67), and takes the form of a diffuse interstitial pneumonia. Epidemics of such infection were reported among debilitated infants in central Europe during and after World War II; but nearly all of the patients reported in recent years have been adults on immunosuppressive drugs or with leukaemias or other malignant diseases. The diagnosis is made by microscopy of lung tissue (obtained by biopsy or at autopsy) or of tracheal aspirates (sometimes positive) or of sputum (seldom positive). The organism's various cystic and extracystic forms can be recognized in smears or sections stained by any of a number of histological procedures, but immunofluorescence microscopy allows the most certain identification. The mortality of untreated *P. carini* pneumonia is very high; but treatment with co-trimoxazole (trimethoprim + sulphamethoxazole, p. 324) or with the relatively toxic pentamidine isethionate is successful in about 75% of cases.

MASTIGOPHORA (FLAGELLATES)

THE GENUS TRICHOMONAS

Trichomonas vaginalis
This is a pear-shaped organism, usually 15–20 μm long, with four flagella arising from its blunt end and an undulating membrane down one side. It is found throughout the world, in the genito-urinary tracts of both sexes. In the male, infection is commonly symptomless but there may be a white urethral discharge. In the female *T. vaginalis* may cause vulvo-vaginitis, with a characteristic frothy, yellow or cream-coloured alkaline discharge. It cannot survive at the pH level of the healthy adult vagina, and probably depends upon disturbance of the normal flora for its establishment there. Transmission is commonly but not exclusively by sexual intercourse.

LABORATORY INVESTIGATION   In wet microscopic preparations made as soon as the specimen of discharge is collected, *T. vaginalis* is easily recognized by its shape, its ungainly movements and the undulations of its membrane. Identification is considerably more difficult in older specimens or in stained films. In most cases it is possible to grow the organism in artificial culture media.

TREATMENT   Metronidazole (p. 325), which is given by mouth and reaches all relevant sites, is usually highly effective in treatment; it should be given also to any sexual consort, to prevent reinfection.

T. hominis and T. tenax
These flagellates, similar to *T. vaginalis* but smaller, appear to be harmless commensals of the intestine and the mouth respectively.

GIARDIA INTESTINALIS (*G. lamblia*)

The *vegetative form* of this species is similar in size to *T. vaginalis*, and is also pear-shaped if seen 'full-face', though flattened in 'profile'. It has in fact quite a striking resemblance to a human face, with its two symmetrically placed nuclei as 'eyes'. It has eight flagella. The *cyst form* is a thick-walled ellipsoid, 10–15 μm long. Structural features similar to those of the vegetative form can be recognized inside it.

G. intestinalis infection, known as *giardiasis*, occurs world-wide. Chronic infection of the upper intestinal tract is common; it may cause chronic malabsorption, but it may be virtually or totally asymptomatic and is therefore often unrecognized. The presentations of acute infection best known in Britain are:

(a) Outbreaks of diarrhoea, with foul-smelling bulky stools typical of impaired fat absorption, among children attending day or residential nurseries. Faecal-oral transmission is the important means of spread in such situations.

(b) Sudden onset of diarrhoea, as described above, with abdominal cramps in many cases, affecting people who have recently been on holidays abroad—notably in the USSR, but there have also been outbreaks associated with cruise ships. Water supplies are the usual sources of such infections, and the 8–14 day incubation period allows many of the patients to reach home before becoming ill.

Vegetative forms and cysts are easily found in the faeces in acute infection, but duodenal aspiration and biopsy are more sensitive means of diagnosing chronic giardiasis. Metronidazole is effective in treatment of most cases. Some advantages are claimed for the related drug tinidazole. Mepacrine has been widely used, but is less effective than metronidazole and has more side-effects.

THE GENUS TRYPANOSOMA

There are many trypanosomes that are pathogenic to vertebrate animals. Most of them are restricted to Africa or S. America, and all are transmitted by biting insects, in which parts of their life-cycles take place. Only three of them are pathogenic to man. Of these, *T. gambiense*, transmitted by the tsetse fly *Glossina palpalis*, and *T. rhodesiense*, transmitted by *G. morsitans*, cause *African sleeping sickness*, whereas *T. cruzi*, transmitted by reduviid bugs, causes *S. American trypanosomiasis* or *Chagas' disease*. Insects become infected by biting human beings or animals (e.g. cattle and antelopes in Africa, opossums and armadillos in S. America). After appropriate intervals for the completion of the insect stages of their life-cycles, the trypanosomes are to be found in the saliva of the flies and in the faeces of the bugs, and enter the human body through bites contaminated with these materials. In each case an indurated local lesion develops over the course of a few weeks, accompanied by regional lymphadenitis, blood stream spread to other parts of the body, and intermittent fever. The African forms multiply while free in the blood, whereas *T. cruzi* does so in the tissues. Meningo-encephalitis with the characteristic lethargy of sleeping sickness takes a month or so to develop in infections with *T. rhodesiense* and longer with *T. gambiense*. Myocarditis and smooth muscle damage are usually more prominent than nervous system involvement in Chagas' disease. Involvement and enlargement of the liver and spleen may occur in any of the three forms, but are most common in Chagas' disease.

When in the human blood stream parasites are long sinuous structures, 15–30 μm wide. Each organism has a longitudinal undulating membrane and a single anterior flagellum. In smears stained with haematological stains it can be seen that each has a central macronucleus and a posterior micronucleus. In wet preparations of fresh blood the trypanosomes are actively motile.

LABORATORY INVESTIGATION   Diagnosis of African trypanosomiasis is based upon microscopy of blood, lymph node aspirates and cerebrospinal fluid and upon inoculation of such materials into laboratory animals. In Chagas' disease, *xenodiagnosis* is more likely to be positive: this consists of allowing uninfected reduviid bugs to bite the patient and examining their faeces for trypanosomes 7 to 10 days later.

TREATMENT AND CONTROL Intravenous suramin has various toxic side-effects but is highly effective in African trypanosomiasis if given early enough. Pentamidine, given intramuscularly, is less toxic and is highly effective, against *T. gambiense* only, for early treatment or for prophylaxis. For treatment of late cases the arsenical melarsoprol is required, as the other drugs do not penetrate into the brain. There is no effective treatment for Chagas' disease. Prevention of trypanosomiasis depends upon control of animal reservoirs, destruction of insect vectors and protection of human beings against the risk of being bitten.

THE GENUS LEISHMANIA

The three closely similar species of this genus resemble certain stages in the trypanosome life-cycle. All three are pathogenic to man and also have animal hosts, and all three are transmitted by sandflies of the genus *Phlebotomus*. *L. donovani* causes *kala-azar* or *visceral leishmaniasis*, a disease which is patchily distributed throughout the tropical and subtropical zones. The infection spreads from the site of the sandfly bite to involve the liver, spleen, lymph nodes and bone marrow, with resultant fever and emaciation. In the absence of treatment the mortality is high. *L. tropica* causes *cutaneous leishmaniasis*, otherwise known as *oriental sore*, *Baghdad button* and *Delhi boil*. It is predominantly an Asiatic disease, but also occurs around the Mediterranean Sea and in N. Africa. Local ulcerative lesions occur at the sites of sandfly bites, but there is no spread from the skin to internal organs, and no risk to life. *L. braziliensis* causes *muco-cutaneous leishmaniasis* or *espundia*, which differs from oriental sore in that it occurs in S. America and that it commonly affects the mucous membranes of the nose and pharynx. It is readily transmitted from patient to patient by direct contact as well as by sandflies.

The flagellate stages of leishmaniae occur in the sandfly or in artificial culture, which is possible in a medium consisting largely of defibrinated horse or rabbit blood. (This is also suitable for the culture of trypanosomes.) In human tissues small oval non-flagellate forms called Leishman—Donovan bodies are found. They are of the order of 2–6 μm in diameter, have macronuclei and micronuclei as do the trypanosomes, and are found inside endothelial cells. One such cell often contains a tightly packed mass of parasites as a result of their multiplication within it.

LABORATORY INVESTIGATION The organisms can be recognized in smears or sections of scrapings or of biopsy specimens from superficial lesions or of aspirates from lymph nodes or the liver or spleen. Blood or bone marrow smears are also likely to show them in kala-azar. Culture of such materials or inoculation into hamsters or monkeys may also be helpful in diagnosis. So may estimations of the serum proteins, since very high serum globulin levels are common in this disease.

TREATMENT AND CONTROL   Pentavalent antimony compounds, given intravenously, are usually effective in the treatment of kala-azar. They may also be valuable in the superficial conditions when these have failed to respond to simple measures, such as curetting, protective dressings and control of secondary infection by antibiotics. Sandflies are difficult to control. Animal reservoirs can be reduced, dogs and rodents being particularly important in relation to kala-azar and oriental sore respectively. Artificial immunization is of some value in preventing oriental sore.

SARCODINA

THE GENUS ENTAMOEBA

Entamoeba histolytica
This is a common cause of dysentery in the warmer parts of the world. However, in such areas it is also commonly found in the faeces of people who have never had any symptoms, and we do not know whether all of the strains assigned to this species are pathogens.

Infection occurs through taking water or food contaminated with cysts, which usually come from a symptomless excreter. Poor sanitation and food hygiene, assisted by flies, make such contamination possible. In the intestine of the new host the cysts turn into vegetative forms. They may then multiply vigorously in the large intestine and invade its mucosa, producing multiple ulcers. The onset of diarrhoea is less rapid than in bacillary dysentery due to shigellae, and amoebic dysentery is more likely to become chronic. Passage of non-purulent blood-streaked mucus is characteristic of the early stages, but secondary bacterial invasion of the ulcers may cause formation of pus later. In addition to attacking the intestine, amoebae may reach the liver, causing amoebic hepatitis or liver abscesses. The latter may be difficult to diagnose, and may first call attention to themselves by rupturing through the diaphragm into the lung, with consequent expectoration of brown material consisting of altered blood and necrotic liver tissue.

The characteristics of the parasite itself are discussed in the next section.

LABORATORY INVESTIGATION   The vegetative forms of *Ent. histolytica* are present in fresh faeces from patients with active dysentery, and are most easily seen by examining a specimen as soon as it is passed, using a warm slide so that the amoebae remain active. A small portion of blood-stained mucus should be mixed with saline on the slide and examined under a cover-slip. It is not sufficient to detect the presence of irregularly shaped organisms, 15–30 μm in diameter, moving by projecting pseudopodia; these may be the common non-pathogenic *Ent. coli* or other commensal amoebae. Full discussion of this differentiation is beyond the scope of this book. It is sufficient to note here that in suitable preparations *Ent. histolytica* moves more rapidly than *Ent. coli* and that its cytoplasm often contains ingested red cells, whereas that of *Ent. coli* contains bacteria and other small particles. If examination of the specimen is delayed, the vegetative *Ent. hystolytica* will have encysted (see below).

The faeces of patients with chronic amoebic dysentery and of symptomless carriers contain *Ent. histolytica* cysts rather than vegetative forms. These are round structures, 10–20 μm in diameter (or down to 5 μm in the case of small-cyst variants). Their recognition is made easier by using iodine solution (which stains their internal structures) rather than saline when making a wet preparation of faeces for microscopy. Since cysts are non-motile, the freshness of the specimen is less important than when looking for vegetative forms. Once again the chief problem is to distinguish *Ent. histolytica* from *Ent. coli*. Cysts of the latter tend to be larger and to have eight nuclei (well shown in the iodine preparation), whereas those of *Ent. histolytica* have four or less. We would stress the point that the finding of cysts in a patient's faeces and their identification as *Ent. histolytica* do not mean that the patient is suffering from amoebiasis.

The detection of specific antibodies, by immunofluorescence, indirect haemagglutination, gel-diffusion or complement-fixation procedures, may be helpful in the recognition of active amoebic infection, especially when it is in the liver.

TREATMENT Metronidazole has now largely replaced the assortment of drugs that have been used in this disease. However, in the high dosage required it may cause vomiting—a problem which can be reduced by giving it in lower dosage together with diloxanide furoate. There are good reports of tinidazole as a possible alternative to metronidazole. Emetine hydrochloride, first used for amoebiasis in 1912, has to be given by injection and is potentially toxic; but it can be valuable in the rapid control of severe acute amoebic dysentery, or in treatment of amoebic liver abscesses that have not responded satisfactorily to treatment with metronidazole. (Surgical drainage of such abscesses may also be necessary.)

THE GENERA NAEGLERIA AND HARTMANNELLA

Since 1965 *Naegleria fowleri*, an amoeba found living free in fresh water and soil, has been reported from many countries as causing a rare acute and usually fatal disease, *primary amoebic meningo-encephalitis*. Most of the patients have been adolescents or children who had recently swum or played in fresh water lakes, pools or puddles. Infection is thought to be by inhalation. Amoebae of the genus *Hartmannella* have been shown to cause a more chronic but otherwise similar disease in older patients, not associated with recent swimming or playing in water.

CILIOPHORA (CILIATES)

Balantidium coli

Man's only ciliate pathogen is also his largest intestinal protozoon, its vegetative form being an oval structure 50 μm or more in length. It is motile by means of short cilia distributed all over its surface. At its anterior end it has a mouth-like recess, the cytostome, and its cytoplasm contains a single large kidney-shaped nucleus, two contractile vacuoles and various ingested particles. The thick-walled cysts are somewhat smaller than the vegetative forms.

This organism is commonly carried by pigs. In man it is a rare cause of severe dysentery which closely resembles that caused by *Ent. histolytica*. It is probable, but not certain, that man usually acquires his infection from pigs. Metronidazole is again the drug of choice, with arsenicals and (surprisingly) tetracyclines (p. 332) as possible alternatives.

IMMUNITY TO PROTOZOAL INFECTIONS

Immune responses to protozoa depend on their situation in the patient.

(1) Plasmodia and trypanosomes are blood parasites. In each case the important immune response is antibody formation (thymus-dependent—see p. 62). Maintenance of immunity to malaria requires continuing exposure. In areas where this disease is endemic, babies are protected by maternal antibodies for the first few months of life (p. 58), and the period of highest incidence and mortality is between 6 months and 5 years old. Trypanosomiasis resembles relapsing fever (p. 143) in that emergence of a succession of new antigenic variants allows the pathogen repeatedly to evade the existing host defences. Antibodies are formed to each new variant, and many other antibodies result from non-specific activation of B-lymphocytes. The patient's lymphoid tissues are heavily infiltrated with plasma cells, and the blood and cerebrospinal fluid contain high levels not only of specific antibodies but also of total IgM—a useful pointer to the diagnosis.

(2) *Toxoplasma gondi* and the leishmaniae are intracellular parasites, able to survive and multiply in host macrophages (p. 48). *T. gondi* prevents fusion of the vacuole with the cytoplasmic granules, but loses this ability when coated with antibody. One attack of toxoplasmosis confers solid resistance; T-cells activate macrophages to suppress intracellular multiplication of the parasites. In immunosuppressed patients disseminated infection may occur. Leishmaniasis resembles tuberculosis and leprosy (pp. 131–5) in that the clinical manifestations of the diseases depend on the state of the host's resistance, which is T-cell mediated. If T-cell immunity is weak or absent, primary lesions fail to heal and after a time metatstatic lesions appear—diffuse cutaneous leishmaniasis (*L. tropica*) or kala-azar (*L. donovani*). Parasitized macrophages are abundant in the lesions, but lymphocytes

are few. At the other end of the spectrum of immunity (recidiva leishmaniasis) there is a destructive local lesion at the primary site due to a T-cell-mediated (Type IV) hypersensitivity reaction which can also be elicited elsewhere on the patient's skin by injecting leishmanin (the Montenegro test—cf. the tuberculin test, p. 253). There are few parasites in the healing lesions, local infiltration with lymphocytes is heavy and there are no metastatic lesions.

Both groups of protozoa discussed so far can induce secondary immunodeficiency by suppressing host immune responses.

(3) *Trich. vaginalis, G. intestinalis* and *Ent. histolytica* are mucous membrane parasites, and immunity to them depends largely on locally produced secretory antibody. Some patients with giardiasis, particularly those with malabsorption, have specific antibodies in their blood, suggesting some mucosal penetration. There is an increased incidence of giardiasis in patients with hypogammaglobulinaemia , especially if they lack secretory IgA. Antibodies are found in the blood of patients with invasive amoebiasis, but not as a rule of those who are asymptomatic cyst-excreters. However, invasion is limited not by these antibodies but by cell-mediated immunity.

Suggestion for Further Reading
Section IV of *Bacteriology Illustrated*—see p. 145.

PART V

PART V

LABORATORY DIAGNOSIS
OF MICROBIAL DISEASES

CHAPTER 14

COLLECTION AND EXAMINATION OF
SPECIMENS FOR MICROSCOPY
AND CULTURE

We have already dealt quite extensively with diagnostic procedures when discussing particular organisms or groups of organisms. In practice, however, diagnostic microbiology begins not with a known organism but with a patient who is ill, from an unknown cause. We need, therefore, to rearrange our knowledge so as to provide a coherent scheme for the investigation of patients. While we cannot here give a comprehensive account of what specimens are appropriate to each clinical problem that the reader is likely to meet, we can indicate how specimens are commonly collected from different parts of the body, how they should be transmitted to the laboratory, and the results that they are likely to give in health and disease.

The amount of help that a microbiological laboratory can give to a clinician depends largely on what it receives. As has been said of computers: 'Garbage in, garbage out'. The laboratory needs:

(1) Careful and well-informed selection of the right specimens to send to the laboratory. If in doubt about this, it is wise to ask the laboratory staff; this often saves time and money, and avoids the tragedy of discovering too late what should have been done.

(2) Proper collection of such specimens. (*Whenever possible, this should be done before antibacterial treatment is given.*) Even the best of specimens may be useless without a label showing what it is and the patient's name.

(3) Rapid transmission of the specimens to the laboratory.

(4) Completion of an appropriate laboratory request form, giving the name, whereabouts, age, sex and (when relevant) occupation of the patient; a legible indication of the name of the doctor concerned (often not the same as a signature); and clear concise indications of the diagnostic problem, relevant treatment already given (particularly antimicrobial drugs) and the reason for sending the specimen.

The importance of these points is illustrated by the following all-too-common situations:

(1) A vaginal swab is often the only specimen sent to the laboratory from a woman with suspected gonorrhoea. Because of the acidity of the adult vagina (p. 24), gonococci do not thrive there and are better sought in the cervix uteri or in urethral discharge.

(2) In the absence of supervision or clear instructions, a patient who has difficulty in producing sputum will often spit out saliva instead. This is, of course, useless as a source of information about his lower respiratory tract. Indeed, if it is examined and reported upon as though it were sputum, the clinician may be totally misled.

(3) Urine is quite a good bacterial culture medium. If it is left to stand at room temperature for some hours after collection, its bacterial content may increase considerably, and subsequent culture may give a highly inaccurate picture of what was in the specimen when it left the patient. This problem is compounded by the fact that the common urinary tract pathogens are particularly good at growing in urine, and therefore on standing a lightly contaminated urine can come to resemble a heavily infected urine.

(4) The more delicate pathogenic species—e.g. the gonococcus and many anaerobes—are liable to die before reaching the laboratory if the specimen is allowed to become dry or is excessively delayed in transit. Their failure to grow in cultures may then give a misleading impression.

(5) The presence of a large number of *Esch. coli* or related organisms in the upper respiratory tract can be interpreted in various ways. In infants it is a common finding, probably a result of regurgitation, and is of no importance. It is also common in patients of all ages who have received antibiotic treatment sufficient to derange their normal flora; in such circumstances the most that is usually called for is modification or cessation of the antibiotic treatment. But in the absence of either of these explanations such a finding requires further investigation, and the enterobacteria may require specific treatment. The bacteriologist who has not been told anything about the patient's age or treatment is in no position to give intelligent co-operation.

Having received a satisfactory specimen in good condition and with adequate accompanying information, the laboratory staff have to decide what to do with it. Routine procedures in busy laboratories are planned to extract the maximum of useful information from each specimen and yet keep the amount of work within bounds. When the specimen comes from a part of the body that is normally sterile, any organism found is abnormal—though it may have entered the specimen as a contaminant during or after collection. However, it is clearly impossible to apply to each such specimen a routine calculated to detect any known micro-organism; the best that can be done is to look for those which are not excessively rare in such situations and are likely to be relevant to the patient's condition. This is one reason why it is important that the laboratory should be told if any unusual infection is suspected. With specimens from sites that have a normal microbial population it is essential to have clearly defined aims—one of which is usually the discouragement of organisms normally present, in order to increase the chances of detecting those that are abnormal. There can be few hospital bacteriologists who have not at some time received a faecal specimen 'For organisms please'. Isolation and identification of all bacteria, viruses, fungi and protozoa in a single faecal specimen might well take years, whereas the question 'Does this specimen contain known intestinal pathogens?' can usually be answered by a few minutes' work spread over 2 or 3 days.

The presence of a normal microbial population creates problems of reporting. Clearly the report should include the names of any known pathogens found which might be responsible for the patient's illness or which it is undesirable that he should continue to carry. As a rule it will also include information about the sensitivity of such pathogens to appropriate antimicrobial agents. Organisms which are common commensals but also potential pathogens—e.g. pneumococci in the respiratory tract—need to be assessed in the light of circumstances. An unexplained and unusual predominance of one of the normal commensals may be of some significance—e.g. an almost pure growth of viridans streptococci is sometimes obtained from a swab of an inflamed tonsil, and possibly indicates that this organism is in fact causing the tonsillitis. The correct wording of 'negative' reports is a subject of controversy. 'No pathogens isolated' gives the clinician a minimum of information, though it is probably the best formula for some specimens for which the range of normal findings is very wide. A list of pathogens which have been sought but not found is sometimes appropriate but is liable to be cumbrous. A report of the predominant organisms in the cultures—e.g. 'viridans streptococci and commensal neisseriae' from a throat swab—does not convey much useful information, and obscures the fact that this predominance was probably determined by the methods of culture. 'Normal flora' is defensible provided that it is taken to mean: 'The varieties and proportions of organisms identified appear to be within normal limits for such specimens when examined by the procedures in routine use in this laboratory.' The last point is important; an abnormality will be detected only if the procedures used are appropriate to its detection.

With these points in mind we will now consider methods of collecting and examining specimens from human beings, first in general terms and then in relation to different parts of the body.

METHODS

Infection Hazards

Nearly every specimen sent to a diagnostic microbiology laboratory may contain pathogenic micro-organisms and is therefore potentially hazardous to the one who collects it, to those who carry it to the laboratory and to the laboratory staff. The degree of hazard varies greatly. A number of reports issued in Britain in recent years have high-lighted the danger from blood and other fluids from hepatitis B carriers (p. 191), and the special precautions indicated below should be taken when collecting these and specimens from other patients who are likely sources of readily transmissible and highly virulent pathogens. However, specimens from patients who are *unsuspected* sources of such organisms are equally dangerous, and so all microbiological specimens must be treated with due care. Furthermore, it is important to remember that a blood sample is no less dangerous when sent to a biochemical, haematological or other laboratory than when microbiological investigation is requested! The following guide-lines should be observed:

(*a*) When collecting specimens from 'high risk' patients, disposable gloves should be worn and other special precautions may be appropriate.

(*b*) Specimens should be securely enclosed in protective containers, and fluid specimens should be in properly closed leak-proof bottles or tubes.

(*c*) Care must be taken to prevent contamination of the outside of the container.

(*d*) Ideally in all cases, and certainly when there is any special hazard, the container should be enclosed in a sealed plastic bag for transmission. The request form should *never* be wrapped round the container or enclosed in the same plastic bag; bags with 2 compartments, one for the specimen and one for the form, are best.

(*e*) Any known special hazard—e.g. of hepatitis B—should be indicated by agreed coloured markings on the specimen and the request form.

Collection of Specimens

Most clinical specimens are collected in one of the following ways:

(1) Materials such as saliva, sputum, faeces, urine, crusts, and scabs and freely discharging pus can be collected *directly into suitable sterile containers.* (Special containers for faeces are described on p. 231.) Because of the labour involved in efficient cleaning and resterilization of screw-capped glass bottles and jars after they have been used for such purposes, they are increasingly being replaced by plastic bottles and

jars with watertight caps and by disposable waxed cardboard or plastic cartons with tightly fitting lids.

(2) Sometimes it is convenient to collect small quantities of fluid—e.g. vesicle contents for examination for poxviruses, or exudate from a suspected syphilitic chancre for dark-ground microscopy—into *capillary tubes*, which can then be sealed by heating their ends, so that the fluid does not dry up.

(3) For collection of material from skin and mucous surfaces, and also of exudates and discharges which are too small in amount for direct collection as in (1), a *swab* can be used. This usually consists of a wooden or wire rod about 6 inches long, with a small quantity of cotton wool tightly twisted around one end and the other end inserted into the cork or stopper of the tube in which it is supplied. The swab and the inside of its container are sterile. For use, the swab is withdrawn from the tube, applied to the patient and then replaced in the tube for transmission to the laboratory, or else placed in a suitable *transport medium* (see below). Modifications of swab design for special purposes are discussed under appropriate headings later in this chapter. Collection of organisms from dry skin is more efficient if the swab is moistened with sterile broth immediately beforehand. Use of serum- or albumin-coated cotton wool swabs may increase the chances that relatively delicate bacteria, such as *Str. pyogenes*, will reach the laboratory alive. The efficiency of transfer of organisms from the patient to the culture media by means of a swab is low, particularly if the amount of material on the swab is small, for some of it becomes entangled in the cotton wool. For certain purposes this difficulty can be overcome by using alginate wool; this is soluble in sodium hexametaphosphate solution, so that all of the trapped material is released into the solution and can be concentrated by centrifugation.

It needs to be emphasized that *swabbing is not a satisfactory substitute for the direct collection of such materials as pus or other exudates* when these could have been collected in a bottle or syringe; it should be used only when inadequacy of materials or other factors make direct collection impossible.

(4) *Washings* from cavities are used in certain circumstances. Throat washings, sometimes preferred to throat swabs for virus investigations, are obtained by asking the patient to gargle with physiological saline and then expectorate it. Gastric washings for examination for tubercle bacilli, from patients who cannot produce sputum, are obtained by running saline into the empty stomach and then withdrawing it through a Ryle's gastric tube. Washing out the maxillary antrum is a therapeutic procedure, but the washings may be sent for bacteriological examination.

(5) *Aspiration*, usually through a needle and often with the assistance of suction from a syringe, is used to collect materials confined within the patient's body, such as blood, cerebrospinal fluid, effusions into

body cavities and joints, and closed abscesses. Organ biopsies can be carried out in the same way. Care must be taken to avoid contamination of the specimens, either from the apparatus used or by collecting organisms in the needle as it passes through the skin. (See p. 268.) Aspirated materials are either placed in a sterile container or added to suitable media directly from the syringe.

Transmission

Correct choice and collection of a specimen is of little use if the pathogens die on the way to the laboratory. The best way to prevent this is to take it there, or see that it is taken, without delay. (Inoculation of media at the bedside or in the clinic, while necessary in some cases, is unsuitable for general use because of administrative difficulties and the risks of contaminating the cultures.) If delay is inevitable, virtually all specimens other than blood cultures are better kept in a refrigerator than at room temperature; but it is usually better still to use suitable *transport media*, which are designed to keep the pathogens alive. This can be achieved in a general-purpose bacterial transport medium by incorporating reducing substances to protect the anaerobes from oxygen, and charcoal to neutralize components of the specimen that might be toxic to bacteria, and by excluding any nutrients to prevent overgrowth of fast-growing bacterial contaminants. Most virus transport media contain antibacterial drugs, and are therefore inappropriate for transport of bacteriological specimens.

Special regulations govern postal transmission of microbiological specimens and other pathological materials. Those operative in the UK are given in *Medical Microbiology* (Churchill Livingstone, Edinburgh, J. P. Duguid and others, 13th edn., vol. 1, 1978) p. 645.

Microscopy

WET PREPARATIONS   These are used for counting leucocytes and other cellular elements in such specimens as urine, cerebrospinal fluid and effusions, and are usually more satisfactory than stained smears for the identification of such structures. Wet preparations are also used for the examination of skin scrapings and hairs for fungi and of faeces, vaginal swabs, etc. for protozoa.

GRAM-STAINED SMEARS   These are made from a large proportion of specimens sent for bacteriological examination, and often give valuable leads as to the most appropriate culture procedures. Such smears are of limited value, however, in the study of specimens from the alimentary tract and many of those from the respiratory tract, since even those from healthy subjects are likely to contain commensal bacteria of many different morphological types.

ZIEHL–NEELSEN-STAINED SMEARS   These are made from specimens sent specifically for investigation for tubercle bacilli. Whether they are also made routinely from sputa and other specimens sent for general bacteriological investigation depends on the local prevalence of tuberculosis.

Appropriately stained smears are made from specimens that may contain virus inclusion bodies or elementary bodies (p. 166).

Cultures

Many of man's parasitic bacterial species grow on *blood agar incubated aerobically* at 37°C, and therefore this medium is used for most clinical specimens. *Anaerobic cultures on blood agar* are also put up routinely from most specimens taken from situations to which there is not free access of air; and incorporation of the antibiotic kanamycin in the blood agar is often a help in the isolation of anaerobes from specimens giving mixed growths, as it suppresses many facultative organisms. (Anaerobic culture techniques are described below.) *MacConkey's agar* (p. 76) is valuable for specimens likely to contain enterobacteria—including, among others, faeces, urine, most pus samples and wound swabs and many ulcerative skin lesions, especially those on the lower half of the body. *Cooked meat medium* (boiled minced lean meat in peptone water—p. 109) supports the growth of most aerobic and anaerobic bacteria, and is commonly used in addition to the solid media for primary culture of pus and of swabs from many sites. Particularly when there has been delay in transport of the specimen or when the patient has been on antibiotic treatment, growth may occur in the cooked meat medium when there is none on the primary plate cultures; the cooked meat medium is then subcultured to further blood agar plates for aerobic and anaerobic incubation. Organisms from a patient receiving a β-lactam (penicillin or cephalosporin) will sometimes grow in *broth containing β-lactamase* when they fail to grow in or on other primary culture media. They too can then be subcultured to blood agar. Less straightforward and in general less effective means are available for neutralizing antibiotics of other groups, but *p*-aminobenzoic acid successfully antagonizes sulphonamides (p. 33).

The few media mentioned so far are sufficient for the examination of most clinical specimens except faeces, for which a highly selective approach is necessary (pp. 218 and 232). Specially nutritious media—notably *chocolate agar* (p. 93)—must be provided for unusually exacting bacteria. Various media containing selective inhibitors for the isolation of particular groups of bacteria have already been mentioned in discussing the relevant organism, as have those for the growth of viruses and fungi; some of them will be referred to again at appropriate points in the next section of this chapter.

ANAEROBIC CULTURE This is commonly carried out in metal or polycarbonate *anaerobic jars*, which are large enough to hold piles of plate cultures; they can also be used for cultures in tubes or bottles, provided that these have cotton-wool stoppers or loose caps rather than air-tight closures. The lid of the loaded jar is clamped down onto an air-tight seal, and the air is then evacuated and replaced by a mixture of 90 % hydrogen and 10 % carbon dioxide (or 80 % nitrogen, 10 % hydrogen and 10 % carbon dioxide, which is safer and probably as suitable). The remaining traces of oxygen are removed by combination with some of the hydrogen, a reaction which is catalysed by palladium in a capsule fixed to the under surface of the lid. When its preparation has been completed, the whole jar can be placed inside an incubator.

There are other ways in which anaerobes can be grown—e.g. reducing agents such as *glucose* and *sodium thioglycollate* can be added to the medium; and *cooked meat medium* is suitable for growing anaerobes because of the reducing activity of the pieces of meat at the bottom of the bottle. However, none of these methods is as reliable, or as suitable for the stricter anaerobes, as the use of anaerobic jars. Special anaerobic cabinets, in which all plating of specimens and all subculturing can be carried out as well as incubation, are a help to those doing a lot of anaerobic culture work but are not essential for good routine anaerobic bacteriology.

CULTURE IN 10 % CO_2 A simple and inexpensive way of achieving approximately the right atmosphere for isolation of CO_2-requiring bacteria, such as the meningococcus and *Br. abortus*, is to place the cultures and a lighted candle in any suitable container which can then be closed with an air-tight lid. The candle goes out when the CO_2 level is of the desired order. An anaerobe jar containing 10 % CO_2 in air instead of the anaerobic culture mixture is rather more reliable; but these simple methods are increasingly being replaced by use of special incubators in which the proportion of CO_2 in the atmosphere can be precisely controlled.

SPECIMENS FROM DIFFERENT PARTS OF THE BODY

This section has the following aims:

(1) To indicate the *commensal organisms most commonly found* and the *pathogens of greatest importance* in specimens from various situations. The lists are deliberately brief and far from comprehensive, and little reference has been made to pathogens that are rare in Britain.

(2) To indicate *reasonable basic routines* for the collection and initial investigation of specimens. These are by no means the *only* reasonable routines, and they would often need to be supplemented by further investigations. Laboratories differ widely in their choices of methods, and are influenced by many local factors. We indicate appropriate specimens to collect for investigation of virus infections, but say nothing here about laboratory procedures for examining them, which are considered in Chapter 11. Nor do we include in this chapter any mention of serological investigation, which is often more important and informative than microscopy and culture, especially in virus infections, but is discussed in Chapter 15.

Except where otherwise indicated, examination of bacteriological specimens is generally completed within one or two days of receiving them, with the addition of a further day if antibiotic sensitivity determinations are carried out after the organisms have been isolated. A minority of specimens require a few more days for the sorting out of mixed cultures or the identification of unusual organisms, and on rare occasions the latter causes further delay. Culture for tubercle bacilli takes 2 to 6 weeks. Mycological cultures for dermatophytes and some other slow-growing fungi may also take several weeks.

The Skin

COMMON COMMENSALS

Staphylococci (mainly *Staph. epidermidis*) and diphtheroid bacilli. Many other bacteria and some fungi are often present on the skin, but only transiently.

IMPORTANT PATHOGENS

Staph. aureus—pustules, boils, carbuncles, paronychial infections, impetigo, and secondary infections of blisters, bites, burns, ulcers, dermatitis and many other lesions.

Str. pyogenes—much the same, but not pustules, boils or carbuncles.

Esch. coli, *Proteus* species, *Ps. aeruginosa*, enterococci—secondary infection (but sometimes only harmless colonization) of various lesions, especially on the lower part of the trunk and the lower limbs.

Bacteroides—ulcers and gangrenous areas.

Candida albicans—exudative dermatitis of the skin folds (intertrigo) and chronic paronychia.

Dermatophyte fungi—ringworm.

Pox and herpesviruses—appropriate vesicular lesions.

CHOICE AND COLLECTION OF SPECIMENS

Rubbing a dry swab over a dry area of skin is unlikely to provide the laboratory with a useful specimen, but the operation is usually more productive if the lesion is exudative or if the swab is moistened in sterile broth or saline before use. Crusts or scabs, in a sterile bottle, may be even more valuable, especially from suspected virus lesions, from which vesicle fluid in capillaries (p. 220) should also be collected if possible. From possible dermatomycoses, skin scrapings, hairs and nails should be collected as appropriate (p. 200).

ROUTINE INITIAL INVESTIGATIONS

For bacteria—Gram-stained smear and aerobic culture on blood agar; also on MacConkey's medium if enterobacteria are suspected or if Gram-negative bacilli are seen in the smear; and anaerobic culture from necrotic lesions. For *C. albicans*, if suspected clinically or seen in the smear—cultures on mycological media.

For dermatophytes—wet preparation of scrapings, etc., in KOH (p. 200) and cultures on mycological media.

Wounds, Abscesses, Sinuses etc.

COMMON COMMENSALS

Such lesions have no 'normal flora' of their own, but the organisms isolated from them commonly include commensals from any surfaces with which they are in communication.

IMPORTANT PATHOGENS

Staph. aureus—the commonest pathogen in skin wounds and abscesses.

Esch. coli, Proteus species, *Ps. aeruginosa*—abdominal wounds, intra-abdominal abscesses.

Cl. perfringens and other clostridia—abdominal wounds, contaminated accidental wounds.

Bacteroides species—wounds and abscesses, especially in association with the alimentary and female genital tracts; also lung abscesses, brain abscesses, gangrenous lesions.

Myco. tuberculosis—'cold' abscesses (i.e. chronic abscesses without the warmth and other features associated with acute inflammation) derived from breakdown of infected lymph-nodes, occurring in many sites but notably in the neck.

Actinomyces israeli—abscesses around the jaw and elsewhere, usually discharging to the surface through multiple sinuses.

CHOICE AND COLLECTION OF SPECIMENS

All too frequently a bacteriology laboratory receives a minute amount of pus on the end of a swab, accompanied by a form that refers to incision and drainage of a large abscess. *Whenever pus is present in sufficient amount, it should be collected in a bottle*—a syringe and needle being usually the best means of getting it there. A small portion of the wall of an abscess or sinus may also be a good bacteriological specimen. When a sinus suspected of being actinomycotic has discharged into a dressing, the dressing should be sent to the laboratory, as 'sulphur granules' (p. 138) may be found on its contaminated surface.

ROUTINE INITIAL INVESTIGATIONS

Gram-stained smear; culture on blood agar (aerobic and anaerobic) and MacConkey's agar and in cooked meat medium. Anaerobic cultures need to be incubated for at least 2 days for some *Bacteroides* and 5 days for *A. israeli*. Gas-liquid chromatography (p. 3) may give rapid information about the presence of anaerobes in pus.

For *Myco. tuberculosis*—see under Lower Respiratory Tract.

The Conjunctivae and Lid Margins

COMMON COMMENSALS

Bacteria are usually scanty, but they may include staphylococci, diphtheroid bacilli, viridans streptococci, non-pathogenic neisseriae and many others.

IMPORTANT PATHOGENS

N. gonorrhoeae, *Staph. aureus*, *Str. pneumoniae*—neonatal conjunctivitis.

Staph. aureus—styes and blepharitis.

H. influenzae—conjunctivitis.

Chlamydia trachomatis—inclusion conjunctivitis (investigations, p. 152).

Adenoviruses and herpesviruses—conjunctivitis, kerato-conjunctivitis.

CHOICE AND COLLECTION OF SPECIMENS

A conjunctival swab is seldom an adequate specimen for bacteriology, except when there is visible purulent discharge; even then, the swab should be delivered to the laboratory immediately or sent in a bacteriological transport medium. In most cases it is better to have microscope slides and culture plates to hand in the clinic or ward, or to send the patient to the laboratory, so that smears can be made and cultures inoculated with material taken straight from the conjunctival surface by means of a sterile bacteriological loop (made of platinum, not of nichrome wire, because the latter is liable to abrade the conjunctiva). Material for chlamydia culture should be sent in an appropriate transport medium. Conjunctival swabs for virology should be sent in virus transport medium (p. 167), together with a throat swab if adenovirus infection is suspected.

ROUTINE INITIAL INVESTIGATIONS

Gram-stained smear; culture on blood agar and chocolate agar, aerobically and in 10% CO_2.

The Ears

COMMON COMMENSALS

External ear: as for skin. Middle ear: normally sterile.

IMPORTANT PATHOGENS

Staph. aureus, *Str. pyogenes*, *Ps. aeruginosa*—otitis externa.

Str. pneumoniae, *H. influenzae*, *Str. pyogenes*, *Staph. aureus*—otitis media.

Bacteroides—chronic otitis.

CHOICE AND COLLECTION OF SPECIMENS

A swab can be used to collect material from the external ear—i.e. from an otitis externa or from an otitis media that is discharging through a perforated ear-drum. In the absence of perforation, it is usually possible to aspirate fluid from an infected middle ear by passing a needle through the drum, but this is rarely justified, as treatment can be based on probabilities. Despite the communication between the healthy middle ear and the nasopharynx via the Eustachian tube, swabbing of the nasopharynx is not useful as a means of determining the probable pathogens in otitis media.

ROUTINE INITIAL INVESTIGATIONS

Gram-stained smear and aerobic culture on blood agar and MacConkey's agar and, in the case of otitis media in a child, chocolate agar for the possible *H. influenzae*. Anaerobic culture and fungal culture in chronic otitis.

The Upper Respiratory Tract (including the mouth)

COMMON COMMENSALS

Staph. epidermidis and *Staph. aureus* (particularly in the anterior nares), viridans and non-haemolytic streptococci, diphtheroid bacilli, lactobacilli, non-pathogenic neisseriae, haemophili, bacteroides group, various spirochaetes; also in young children, *Esch. coli* and related organisms, probably regurgitated from the alimentary tract.

IMPORTANT PATHOGENS

In the mouth:

C. albicans—thrush.

Vincent's organisms (p. 130).

Herpes simplex virus type 1—herpes labialis, aphthous stomatitis.

In the throat and nasopharynx:

Str. pyogenes and *Staph. aureus*—tonsillitis.

C. diphtheriae.

H. influenzae (type b)—acute epiglottitis.

Vincent's organisms.

The many viruses that cause respiratory tract infections.

Other pathogens are sometimes to be found in these sites although they produce their main ill effects elsewhere—e.g. *N. meningitidis, Bord. pertussis*, polioviruses and the causative organisms of pneumonia (see below).

In the paranasal sinuses:

Staph. aureus, Str. pyogenes, Str. pneumoniae, H. influenzae, Bacteroides (chronic infections).

CHOICE AND COLLECTION OF SPECIMENS

Swabbing a mouth lesion is usually a straightforward procedure. So is swabbing of the anterior nares, except that when there is no nasal discharge (e.g. when the purpose is to detect nasal carriage of *Staph. aureus*) the swab should be moistened as for skin swabbing (p. 224). Throat swabbing is carried out with the patient's mouth wide open and his tongue depressed, and care must be taken not to touch the swab against anything other than the pharyngeal mucosa. (The results of culture may be vitiated if antiseptics or antibiotics have been applied to the throat in the previous 12 hours or so—a statement which is, of course, equally true about specimens from other sites, but is most commonly forgotten in relation to throat swabs.) The nasopharynx can best be swabbed by passing a *pernasal swab*, made with fine and fairly flexible wire, along the floor of one nostril; this is the recommended procedure for isolation of *Bord. pertussis.*

Swabbing the epiglottis or even the throat of a child with haemophilus epiglottitis may provoke a fatal supraglottic spasm, and should therefore not be attempted unless steps to maintain the airway have been taken or can be taken immediately. Blood culture, while it does not provide information soon enough to help in the management of this fulminating condition, is usually positive for *H. influenzae* type b and should be carried out, as the best means of confirming the diagnosis.

Pernasal aspiration of nasopharyngeal fluid through a fine plastic tube provides the best sample for rapid diagnosis of respiratory syncytial and other respiratory virus infections by immunofluorescence. Nose and throat swabs for culture of viruses should be sent in virus transport medium (p. 167).

Investigation of infections in the paranasal sinuses is difficult because of their inaccessibility. If there is a purulent discharge it may contain relevant bacteria. The surgical procedure of washing out the affected sinus provides the best information about what is happening inside it, but clearly is indicated only when the infection has failed to respond to simpler measures.

ROUTINE INITIAL INVESTIGATIONS

Gram-stained smears; smears stained with dilute carbol fuchsin for Vincent's organisms; aerobic cultures on blood agar and on the following media as indicated—Loeffler's serum and a tellurite medium for *C. diphtheriae*, chocolate agar for *H. influenzae* and for *N. meningitidis*, special media (p. 126) for *Bord. pertussis* and mycological media for *C. albicans*. Anaerobic cultures when appropriate.

Information about the diagnosis of diphtheria is available at the following times:

(1) *No information* is available *immediately* after receipt of the specimen; this diagnosis cannot be confirmed or refuted by examination of direct smears made from the specimen. (Exception: some laboratories undertake rapid diagnosis from smears by immunofluorescence.)

(2) *Provisional identification* of *C. diphtheriae* may be possible 18 hours or less after receipt of the specimen, on the basis of its characteristic appearances in films made from Loeffler's serum culture at this stage and stained with methylene blue or by Albert's or Neisser's method.

(3) *More definite identification* may be possible 48 hours or more after receipt of the specimen, by examination of colonies on a tellurite medium.

(4) *Confirmation that the strain isolated is C. diphtheriae* usually

takes a further day, during which the fermentation reactions of the organisms are tested.

(5) *Confirmation that the strain is toxigenic* takes a few more days. Further details of all these procedures are to be found on pp. 97–9.

Bord. pertussis may take 4 days to form visible colonies. (As with diphtheria, immunofluorescence may permit more rapid diagnosis.)

The Lower Respiratory Tract

COMMON COMMENSALS

In the larynx and trachea, much the same as in the nasopharynx. The bronchi are sterile when healthy.

IMPORTANT PATHOGENS

Str. pneumoniae, Staph. aureus, Mycoplasma pneumoniae—pneumonia.

H. influenzae, Str. pneumoniae—chronic bronchitis and bronchiectasis.

Legionella pneumophila—pneumonia.

Bacteroides, Fusobacterium species—lung abscess.

Myco. tuberculosis.

Viruses, notably influenza and (from children) parainfluenza and respiratory syncytial virus.

(Also *C. diphtheriae* in the larynx and *Bord. pertussis* in the trachea and bronchi, but these organisms are more commonly *isolated* from the upper respiratory tract.)

CHOICE AND COLLECTION OF SPECIMENS

The commonest specimen obtained from the lower respiratory tract is sputum. Ideally this is coughed up from far down the bronchial tree, expectorated immediately with minimal contamination from the throat and mouth, and delivered to the laboratory without delay, since such contaminant bacteria and fungi as have been picked up are likely to multiply in the specimen at room temperature far more rapidly than the pathogens. Even such an ideal specimen (which is rare) may not give straightforward information about the infection that is being investigated. For example, in the early stages of lobar pneumonia (as well as in various other lung infections) the sputum— if there is any—may merely reflect conditions in a bronchus at some distance from the lung lesion; better information may come from blood culture, or from looking for pneumococcal polysaccharide or other relevant bacterial products in the patient's blood. In acute bronchopneumonia the sputum may well come straight from the 'battlefield' and be highly relevant. Especially in chronic bronchial disease, any one sputum is likely to consist of somewhat diverse contributions from different sources which have stuck together but not mixed, and consecutive sputa may represent different parts of the bronchial tree and give markedly divergent bacteriological results. The problem of contamination from the upper respiratory tract can be minimized by aspirating material direct from the bronchi through a bronchoscope, or from the lumen of the trachea by passing a needle through the skin and anterior wall of the trachea, but such procedures are not suitable for routine use. In children too young to expectorate, the causative organisms of broncho-pulmonary infections can sometimes be found in the nasopharynx; and from patients with pulmonary tuberculosis but no sputum, tubercle bacilli may be found by swabbing the larynx (using a long curved *laryngeal swab*) or by obtaining gastric washings. These two procedures both depend upon the fact that ciliary currents carry mucus from the bronchi up the trachea and larynx, after which it is swallowed if its quantity is insufficient to provoke coughing.

For investigation of virus infections of the lower respiratory tract the specimens indicated for upper respiratory tract infections are appropriate.

ROUTINE INITIAL INVESTIGATIONS

Important information may be given by the naked-eye appearance of the sputum—mucoid, mucopurulent, purulent, blood-stained, etc. (In sputum from asthmatics, apparent pus may in fact consist of eosinophils, as can be shown by staining a smear with a suitable haematological stain.) Sometimes the specimen obviously consists mainly or entirely of saliva. Frequently its non-homogeneity is evident. A sample for microscopy or culture which is taken by dipping a loop into an untreated sputum is likely to contain a disproportionately large contribution from the irrelevant surface coating of throat and mouth contamination, together with material taken from only one part (not necessarily a representative part) of the underlying sputum. A better procedure is first to shake up the specimen with a homogenizing agent; any sample from it should then contain a fair representation of all parts of the specimen, and any organism that was present in very large numbers in some part of the original sputum should also be plentiful in the sample. The homogenate can be used for all of the investigations listed below:

Gram-stained smear (which gives further information about purulence, shows the extent of upper respiratory tract and mouth contamination and may give useful indications as to the predominant organisms). Aerobic culture on blood agar and chocolate agar; culture of the homogenate in 1:1000 saline dilution as well as neat helps to show which organisms are present in very large numbers and therefore probably important. Anaerobic culture on blood agar when there is a possibility of lung abscess or of bronchial obstruction leading to failure of aeration of part of a lung.

For *Myco. tuberculosis*—Ziehl–Neelsen-stained smear (which must be carefully searched, as the bacilli may be scanty), and aerobic culture on Löwenstein–Jensen or other suitable medium after concentration of the specimen as described on p. 133. (Ziehl–

Neelsen-stained smears of concentrate may reveal tubercle bacilli when these were not seen in smears of untreated sputum.) Processing of laryngeal swabs is easier and more effective if they are made with alginate wool (p. 220). Gastric washings must be examined and cultured without delay, as the tubercle bacilli may not long survive the action of gastric juice.

The Alimentary Tract

COMMON COMMENSALS

Bacteria of very many varieties are to be found in the alimentary tract, especially in its lower parts, and make a large contribution to the bulk of faeces. The culture procedures used by medical laboratories are selective and give a false impression that enterobacteria are overwhelmingly predominant, but other groups usually present in large numbers and in considerable diversity include lactobacilli, anaerobes of the *Bacteroides* and *Bifidobacterium* groups, clostridia and streptococci. Commensal protozoa are also common, as are viruses, though the latter are not usually regarded as commensals.

IMPORTANT PATHOGENS

Salmonellae—enteric fever and gastro-enteritis (food-poisoning).
Campylobacters—diarrhoea
Certain serotypes of *Esch. coli*—gastro-enteritis, mainly of young children; 'traveller's diarrhoea'.
Clostridium difficile—pseudomembranous colitis.
Shigellae—bacillary dysentery.
Ent. histolytica—amoebic dysentery.
V. cholerae—cholera.
Staph. aureus—staphylococcal enteritis (rare).
C. albicans—enteritis.
Rotaviruses.

CHOICE AND COLLECTION OF SPECIMENS

In cases of food poisoning it may be possible and desirable to send vomit to the laboratory, in a suitable water-tight container and with care not to contaminate the outside of the container. The same precaution is essential on the many occasions when it is appropriate to send faeces. All too often a laboratory receives faeces, in unnecessarily large amount, filling and overflowing from an unsuitable container, the outside of which was contaminated during collection and during transport; the hazards of this to nurses, porters, laboratory staff and others are easy to conceive (p. 219). It is far better to use a screw-capped, watertight container with, inside it and attached to its cap for convenience of handling, a small plastic spoon that can be used to transfer safely into the container the small amount of material which is all that the laboratory needs. From young children and other patients from whom there is difficulty in obtaining a faecal specimen uncontaminated with urine, a swab inserted into the rectum may be adequate.

ROUTINE INITIAL INVESTIGATION

Naked-eye inspection for consistency and the presence of blood, pus and mucus. Aerobic culture on blood agar (when appropriate) for pathogenic serotypes of *Esch. coli* (since these give their most satisfactory slide-agglutination reactions when grown on this medium) and for *Staph. aureus*; on primary selective media for salmonellae and shigellae (p. 114); and in selenite F or other enrichment broth, to be subcultured next day, for salmonellae. Selective culture for campylobacters (p. 122). Gram-stained smears should be made if either staphylococcal or candida enteritis is suspected, and in either condition usually show the respective pathogens in large numbers. Mycological cultures should be set up when candida enteritis is suspected. Wet microscopic preparations, usually in iodine solutions, are used for the detection of *Ent. histolytica* and other protozoa (as well as worm ova and larvae, which are outside the range of this book). Investigations for suspected pseudomembranous colitis or cholera are described on pp. 108 and 122 respectively.

The Urinary Tract

Apart from skin commensals and transient organisms in the female and the anterior part of the male urethra, the tract is normally sterile.

IMPORTANT PATHOGENS

Esch. coli, Proteus species, enterococci, *Myco. tuberculosis*—cystitis, pyelitis, pyelonephritis.

Staph. saprophyticus—acute cystitis in young women.

Typhoid and paratyphoid bacilli, while not primarily pathogens of the urinary tract, may be found in the urine (pp. 114 and 115).

CHOICE AND COLLECTION OF SPECIMENS

For non-tuberculous infections—a mid-stream specimen of urine whenever possible, collected as follows. The foreskin of a male should be retracted and the glans penis carefully cleaned with gauze soaked in sterile saline (not disinfectant, because of the risk of some getting into the specimen). The vulval area of a female should be cleaned similarly (or in a bath, if convenient) and dried, the vagina occluded with a tampon, and the labia should be held apart while the specimen is passed. After some urine has been voided to flush out urethral bacteria, the specimen is collected in a suitably wide-mouthed sterile receptacle. Ideally this should be a glass or plastic jar with a water-tight lid, which can be sent directly to the laboratory without the specimen having to be transferred to another container and so incurring an additional risk of contamination. Even the best of mid-stream specimens is likely to be contaminated with some of the patient's surface organisms (especially if it comes from a female), and therefore needs to reach the laboratory without undue delay, as explained on p. 217. Special procedures for use when delay is inevitable are discussed below, in relation to the routine investigations. A cleaner specimen can usually be obtained by passing a catheter into the bladder; but since this procedure may itself initiate infection of a previously sterile urinary tract, specimens should be collected in this way only when it is in any case necessary to pass an instrument into the bladder, or when the patient is unable to co-operate. In the latter circumstance, particularly with young children, it is often better to collect a specimen by supra-pubic aspiration—i.e. by using a syringe and needle to withdraw urine from the full bladder through the abdominal wall. Sometimes, especially when it is important to find out whether urinary tract infection is limited to one kidney, specimens are collected direct from the ureters, by means of fine catheters inserted via the bladder with the aid of a cystoscope. For *Myco. tuberculosis*—repeated early morning urine specimens, since these are likely to be the most concentrated and so to offer the best chance of finding the scanty bacilli. If the investigation is solely for tuberculosis, there is no need to take special precautions to avoid contamination of such specimens during collection.

ROUTINE INITIAL INVESTIGATIONS

Microscopy of a wet preparation of urine (preferably concentrated about 10-fold by centrifugation) to assess its cell content. Precise counting of the cells in a random urine specimen is pointless, since their number depends on the patient's level of hydration and other factors. (Counting of pus cell excretion per hour is sometimes more informative.) Presence of more than a few pus cells suggests infection, but their absence does not exclude it; non-purulent *bacteriuria* is not uncommon, especially in pregnant women, and may progress to frankly purulent infection. Presence of vaginal or vulval epithelial cells indicates contamination of the specimen, and so casts doubt on the origins of any pus cells or bacteria.

Semi-quantitative aerobic culture using a standard wire loop or a specially designed strip of filter paper to transfer a measured amount of urine to the surface of a suitable culture medium—usually MacConkey agar or CLED (cysteine lactose electrolyte-deficient agar, devised to meet the particular requirements of urine bacteriology). The heaviness of the resulting growth allows an estimate of the number of bacteria per ml of urine. *If a carefully collected specimen is cultured within 3 hours, contaminant bacteria picked up during collection are unlikely to exceed 1000 per ml* and these are usually a mixture, including staphylococci and diphtheroid bacilli. On the other hand, *a specimen from a patient with a non-tuberculous urinary tract infection is likely to contain 100 000 or more organisms per ml* and these are usually of a single bacterial species which grows well on both the media used and in most cases are Gram-negative bacilli. Delay in examination of the specimen is likely to confuse the distinction between contaminants and pathogens (p. 217). One way of overcoming this problem is to collect the urine into a container in which is enough boric acid powder to give a final concentration of about 2 %. This inhibits bacterial growth (as well as preserving the pus cells, which otherwise gradually disintegrate) but also substantially reduces the numbers of a few enterobacterial strains. Another approach is to adapt the semiquantitative culture method for use at the time of collection of the specimen. 'Dip-slides' (plastic slides, about the size of microscope slides, coated with culture media) can be dipped into freshly passed urine and then returned to their screw-capped air-tight containers for transmission and incubation (or even incubation in a doctor's surgery). As with the plate method, the heaviness of the growth indicates the number of bacteria in the urine—but this time in the urine as passed, not after transmission. However, interpretation is not always easy, heavy contamination is difficult to tell from infection, and the additional information provided by microscopy is not available. A similar semi-quantitative culture, rather more convenient for subsequent laboratory manipulations, can be achieved by using a wide-mouthed pot that has a layer of culture medium over its base; this is easier and as a rule cheaper to produce than a dip-slide. Freshly passed urine is added to the pot for about half a minute and then poured off, and the pot is left for a short while inverted over its lid, which contains absorbent paper to remove any surplus urine. The rest of the procedure is as for a dip-slide.

All that we have said about the importance of heavy growths is inapplicable to chronic renal parenchymatous infection, in which the pathogen may be excreted in the urine intermittently and in small numbers—a difficult condition to detect.

For *Myco. tuberculosis*—Ziehl–Neelsen-stained smear, and aerobic culture on Löwenstein–Jensen or other suitable medium, of concentrated deposit from a large volume of urine which has been allowed to stand in a refrigerator for a day or two. The possibility of tuberculosis should be considered whenever other pathogens are absent from a purulent urine, unless this situation is due to antibacterial treatment.

The Female Genital Tract

COMMON COMMENSALS

A bacterial population similar to that of skin is found in the vulva and lower vagina, and also in the vaginal vault before puberty, late in pregnancy and after the menopause. During the child-bearing period, lactobacilli, micro-aerophilic or anaerobic streptococci and some *Bacteroides* species usually predominate in the vaginal vault. The cervical canal, uterus and Fallopian tubes are normally sterile.

IMPORTANT PATHOGENS

T. pallidum—syphilitic chancres and condylomata.

N. gonorrhoeae—urethritis, cervicitis, endometritis and salpingitis of adults, vulvo-vaginitis of children.

Trich. vaginalis, C. albicans—vaginitis.

Str. pyogenes, Staph. aureus—puerperal sepsis.

Cl. perfringens, Esch. coli, Proteus species etc.—septic abortion.

Bacteroides species, CO_2-dependent streptococci, anaerobic cocci—puerperal sepsis, septic abortion, chronic vaginitis and endometritis, bartholinitis.

Myco. tuberculosis—endometritis, salpingitis.

Chlamydia trachomatis—urethritis, cervicitis, salpingitis, lymphogranuloma.

Herpes simplex virus—genital ulcers.

CHOICE AND COLLECTION OF SPECIMENS

For *T. pallidum*—exudate collected in capillary tubes from the surfaces of lesions which have first been thoroughly cleaned with gauze and sterile saline.

For *N. gonorrhoeae*—swabs of urethral discharge and of cervical mucopus (*not* a high vaginal swab) placed in transport medium; or preferably, when possible, material collected with a sterile wire loop and used at once to inoculate suitable media; and in either case, smears of discharge suitable for Gram-staining (and, if the technique is available, immunofluorescence for *N. gonorrhoeae*) in the laboratory. When there is no evident discharge but chronic gonococcal infection is suspected, it is important also to send a rectal swab for culture for *N. gonorrhoeae*.

For *Trich. vaginalis*—if immediate microscopic examination of a wet preparation of the discharge is not possible in the ward or clinic, a swab of discharge sent immediately to the laboratory in a suitable transport or culture medium.

For *Myco. tuberculosis* or other causes of chronic endometritis—uterine curettings or other surgical specimens.

For *C. trachomatis*—cervical swab, in appropriate transport medium.

For other organisms—swabs of the vaginal vault ('high vaginal' swabs) or of discharges of lesions.

ROUTINE INITIAL INVESTIGATIONS

For *T. pallidum*—immediate dark-ground microscopy of the exudate. The laboratory should be warned in advance, so that the specimen can be given prompt attention.

For *N. gonorrhoeae*—Gram-stained smears (and immunofluorescence); culture on suitable selective medium in $5-10\%$ CO_2.

For *Trich. vaginalis*—immediate microscopy of wet preparation.

For *Myco. tuberculosis*—Ziehl–Neelsen-stained smears or sections, aerobic culture on Löwenstein–Jensen or other suitable medium, and guinea-pig inoculation when considered appropriate.

For *C. trachomatis*—tissue culture.

For other organisms—Gram-stained smears. Culture on blood agar aerobically and anaerobically and on mycological media if *C. albicans* was suspected clinically or seen in the smears.

The Male Genitalia

Exudate from syphilitic chancres and discharge from gonococcal and chlamydial urethritis are collected and examined in the same way as similar specimens from female patients. *Bacteroides* species and other anaerobes may cause balanitis, genital ulceration and scrotal abscesses.

The Central Nervous System

When healthy this system is free from micro-organisms.

IMPORTANT PATHOGENS

N. meningitidis, Str. pneumoniae, Myco. tuberculosis—meningitis at all ages.

H. influenzae (type b)—meningitis, mainly in children aged 2 months to 3 years.

Staph. aureus—abscesses with secondary meningitis at all ages.

Haemolytic streptococci group B, *Esch. coli, Listeria monocytogenes*—meningitis in new-born infants.

Bacteroides species, *Str. milleri*—brain abscesses.

Coagulase-negative staphylococci—infections of shunt prostheses.

T. pallidum—the various forms of neurosyphilis (p. 140).

Many viruses, notably: polioviruses—poliomyelitis; mumps coxsackie and echoviruses—meningitis; herpes simplex virus and togaviruses—encephalitis.

(*Cryptococcus neoformans*, p. 202, and *Naegleria fowleri* and *Hartmannella* species, p. 213, are rare causes of meningitis that need to be borne in mind.)

CHOICE AND COLLECTION OF SPECIMENS

Cerebrospinal fluid, by far the commonest microbiological specimen from the central nervous system, is sometimes collected from the ventricles of the brain or elsewhere inside the skull, particularly by neurosurgeons; but far more often by the procedure known as lumbar puncture. In outline, a wide-bored sterile needle is passed between the spines of two lumbar vertebrae and through the dura, and cerebrospinal fluid is allowed to drip from it into a sterile container. From the bacteriological point of view, the most important technical problem is to avoid introducing contaminant organisms either into the subdural space or into the specimen. This calls for rigorous aseptic technique and for antimicrobial treatment of the skin—e.g. by applying povidone-iodine or chlorhexidine in 70% alcohol (p. 268).

When a virus infection of the central nervous system is suspected, other specimens besides cerebrospinal fluid should be sent to the laboratory—nose and throat swabs in virus transport medium, and also faeces if an enterovirus infection is a possibility. Brain biopsy may be appropriate when virus encephalitis is suspected.

ROUTINE INITIAL INVESTIGATIONS

The cerebrospinal fluid specimen should be sent to the laboratory and examined without delay. Normal cerebrospinal fluid is crystal clear and colourless; any turbidity indicates either infection or the presence of blood (possibly as a result of trauma during collection of the specimen). In tuberculous meningitis a 'spider web' clot often forms in the fluid shortly after collection. Investigations of a turbid fluid should include a total and differential cell count and estimations of its glucose and protein contents. If, as commonly occurs, these are to be carried out elsewhere than in the bacteriological laboratory, two specimens should be collected so that there is no risk of the specimen for culture being contaminated during the removal of material for other purposes. In most cases of acute bacterial meningitis there are thousands of cells per μl, virtually all polymorphonuclear leucocytes (in contrast to the very small number of lymphocytes normally present), glucose is absent or present in much smaller amounts than normal and the protein level is raised. Later, there is commonly a lower total cell count with a larger proportion of lymphocytes, a picture which is also common in tuberculous meningitis. In virus meningitis, predominance of polymorphonuclear cells, if present at all in the early stages, is usually short-lived and there is little or no alteration of the glucose level.

Unless it is very turbid the fluid is centrifuged for bacteriological examination and the deposit is used for making smears and for inoculating cultures.

For *Myco. tuberculosis*—Ziehl–Neelsen-stained smears of deposit, or if a spider web clot is present, part of it should be spread out on a slide, dried, fixed by gentle heating, and stained by the Ziehl–Neelsen method; culture on Löwenstein–Jensen or other suitable medium; and guinea-pig inoculation when considered appropriate.

For other bacteria—Gram-stained smear; aerobic culture on blood agar and chocolate agar. Because the identity of the pathogen may have an important bearing upon the treatment of acute bacterial meningitis, initial investigations applied directly to the cerebrospinal fluid may include such procedures as attempted identification of the organism itself by capsule-swelling or immunofluorescence, or of its products by cross-over immuno-electrophoresis or co-agglutination.

The Blood Stream

Although many oral, intestinal and other bacteria enter the blood in small numbers from time to time, it has no normal microbial flora.

IMPORTANT PATHOGENS

Staph. aureus, Str. pyogenes, Esch. coli and many other bacteria— acute septicaemia.

N. meningitidis—septicaemia (acute or chronic).

Viridans streptococci, enterococci—subacute bacterial endocarditis.

Coagulase-negative staphylococci—infections of prosthetic heart valves and other prostheses.

Salmonellae—enteric fever.

Brucellae—undulant fever.

Plasmodia—malaria (see p. 206 for investigation).

COLLECTION OF SPECIMENS

Venepuncture should be carried out with the same scrupulous care to avoid contamination as is required for lumbar puncture, using a sterile needle attached to a sterile syringe (or to a sterile evacuated ampoule specially designed for the purpose). The veins in the antecubital fossa or on the forearm are commonly used, and are distended by means of a tourniquet. It may be best to take blood at a time when the patient's temperature is rising, as this is the time at which the number of bacteria in the blood is likely to be greatest. The blood should be transferred as soon as it is taken (before it has time to clot) into two or more bottles containing appropriate broth culture media, as a general rule adding about 3–5 ml of blood to 50 ml of broth. (Laboratories differ in their choice of general-purpose blood culture broths, and may issue special broths for some species.) In addition to the direct inoculation of broth cultures, blood can be added in a ratio of about 2:1 or 3:1 to broth containing 0.05% Liquoid (sodium polyanethol sulphonate), which both prevents it from clotting and inhibits its bactericidal mechanisms. In the laboratory some of this treated blood can be mixed in a 1:20 ratio with melted nutrient agar, poured into Petri dishes and allowed to set. All cultures are usually incubated at 37°C. The poured plate technique may provide colonies of bacteria on or beneath the surface of the medium within 18 hours or so of setting up the cultures, in which case identification of the organism is possible sooner than if it is merely growing in broth; and it gives a quantitative estimate of the number of bacteria in the blood—heavy growth indicates that there were many organisms, and contamination during collection is most unlikely to account for more than a very few colonies. Broth culture, on the other hand, is a far more sensitive means of detecting small numbers of bacteria, especially of organisms like brucellae and some of the streptococci that cause endocarditis; but it is also a good means of producing heavy growths from a small number of contaminant organisms. Opinions differ as to whether a broth culture should be subcultured to solid media every few days (thus hastening the detection of any organisms present, but at the risk of introducing contaminants into the bottle and thus confusing the interpretation of subsequent subcultures) or should be left alone until colour change of the blood layer at the bottom of the bottle or turbidity of the supernatant indicates that bacterial growth has occurred. One solution to this dilemma now available is to use broths that include bacterial nutrients containing radio-active carbon; and a machine that can sample the atmosphere in the tops of culture bottles daily (or more often) and can detect the arrival there of radio-active CO_2 released by the metabolic processes of multiplying bacteria. As soon as the machine records a positive finding, the bottle can be subcultured. The need for very great care to avoid contamination of the cultures arises from the difficulty of deciding that any organism grown from blood is not a pathogen; bacteria of almost every group have at some time or other been at least suspected, if not convicted, of causing subacute endocarditis or low-grade chronic septicaemia.

Pleural and Peritoneal Cavities, Joints etc.

When fluid from one of these sites is required for microbiological investigation, aspiration should be carried out with the same care to avoid contamination as is required for cerebrospinal fluid or blood. The investigations appropriate to the specimen are determined by clinical indications as to the likely pathogens and by its own nature— e.g. it may be thick pus as from an abscess, it may be a relatively clear fluid on which cell counts and protein determination could be helpful, or it may be virtually pure blood.

Suggestions for Further Reading

Manual of Clinical Microbiology by E. H. Lennette and others, 3rd edn. (American Society for Microbiology, Washington, D.C., 1980).

Clinical Bacteriology by E. J. Stokes and G. L. Ridgway, 5th edn. (Edward Arnold, London, 1980).

Also Section III of *Bacteriology Illustrated* by R. R. Gillies and T. C. Dodds, 4th edn. (Churchill Livingstone, Edinburgh, London and New York, 1976).

CHAPTER 15

IMMUNODIAGNOSIS OF INFECTION

ANTIGEN–ANTIBODY INTERACTIONS IN THE LABORATORY

Many experimental and diagnostic microbiological procedures make use of the fact that antibodies 'recognize' antigenic groupings with a precision that is often much finer than that of the most discerning chemical tests. This specificity of antigen–antibody interactions has a number of important practical applications, including the following:

(1) Two substances can be shown to be identical or closely similar by the fact that each reacts with antibodies produced in response to the other, and to some extent it is possible to estimate degrees of dissimilarity between substances by differences of reaction with the same antibodies.

(2) Consequently the identity of a micro-organism in culture can be established and its antigenic composition analysed by testing its reactions with antisera of known specificity—that is, sera containing antibodies against known antigens.

(3) Current infection with a particular micro-organism can some-times be detected by demonstrating that the patient's body fluids contain antigens which react with antisera specific for products of such organisms—e.g. toxins, capsular polysaccharides, hepatitis B virus antigens.

(4) The presence, in human or animal serum, of antibodies specific for components or products of a particular micro-organism is pre-sumptive evidence of infection at some time with that organism or with one that is antigenically related; and if the amount of such antibodies is still increasing, the infection was a recent one.

Some of the techniques for demonstrating these and other interactions are outlined in this section. Many examples of their application to the problems of medical microbiology are to be found in earlier chapters and in later sections of this chapter.

PRECIPITATION   A soluble antigen may combine with an appropriate antibody to form a precipitate. This happens maximally when the two meet in approximately *optimal proportions* and are both used up in the formation of large lattice complexes with alternating antigen and antibody layers. In the presence of substantial excess of either, there is a tendency to form much smaller complexes, each possibly consisting of just a single molecule of the scarcer component and enough molecules of the other to use up all of its binding sites; in antigen excess in particular such complexes are still soluble.

A precipitation reaction may be demonstrable by drawing up a small volume of antigen followed by a similar volume of antiserum into a capillary tube; the reaction then manifests itself as a layer of white precipitate near to the interface between the two fluids. This is one of the methods commonly used for Lancefield grouping of streptococci (p. 87).

Alternatively, a *double-diffusion* procedure may be used. Antigen solution and antiserum are placed in two suitably spaced holes cut in a layer of agar gel on a flat glass or plastic surface. Antigen and antibody diffuse out into the gel, and where they meet in optimal proportions a white line of precipitate is formed. Since the position of the line can be brought nearer to one hole by putting less of the relevant reactant into the hole in the first place, this procedure can be made quantitative. Multiple lines may appear if the two fluids contain several sets of antigens and corresponding antibodies. By using 3 holes it is possible to compare the reactions of, say, one serum and two antigen solutions, and so to arrange things that the lines formed by the two interacting systems meet at an angle. If the two antigens are the same, the two lines will merge into a curve—*the reaction of identity*; if the two are different, the lines will 'ignore' one another and cross. The Elek method for detecting toxin production by *C. diphtheriae* (p. 99) is another form of the double-diffusion procedure.

In *immuno-electrophoresis* an electric current is used to separate out the components of an antigen mixture (or an antibody mixture) so that they are located at different points along a line in agar gel on a microscope slide or other suitable surface. Antiserum (or antigen solution) is then placed in a trough cut in the gel parallel to and at an appropriate distance from the electrophoresis line. Diffusion is then allowed to take place, and since the electrophoresed components set out from point sources on their line and meet a linear front of the reactant from the trough, precipitate lines are arc-shaped.

Cross-over or *countercurrent immuno-electrophoresis* (CIE) is a rapid and very sensitive variant of double–diffusion, in which an electric field is used to hasten the diffusion of the reactants towards one another. This technique is widely used for detecting antibodies—e.g. specific fungal precipitins in the sera of patients with fungal infections or allergies—and also for detecting microbial antigens—e.g. pneumococcal polysaccharide in the blood of a patient with pneumonia or in the cerebrospinal fluid of one with meningitis. Detection of specific antigens can be particularly helpful when bacterial cultures are negative because antibiotics have already been given.

AGGLUTINATION   Bacteria are commonly identified by preparing aqueous suspensions of them on glass slides or in tubes and seeing whether these are agglutinated into visible clumps on the addition of antisera specific for known bacterial surface antigens. Conversely, suspensions of known bacteria can be used to detect and quantitate antibodies in sera. Quantitation is achieved by testing a series of dilutions of the serum against a standard bacterial suspension and determining the highest dilution of the serum which still gives definite agglutination (the *titre* of the serum, more fully defined on p. 246).

For many purposes agglutination tests are easier and more satisfactory than precipitation tests. For *indirect* or *passive agglutination tests* soluble antigens are made particulate and therefore agglutinable. This is done by allowing or persuading the soluble antigens to adhere to the surfaces of particles that are themselves immunologically inert, at least so far as the test system is concerned. For example, many polysaccharides adhere readily and firmly to the surfaces of washed red blood cells; many protein antigens adhere similarly to red cells that have been treated with tannic acid or various other agents, or to particles of polystyrene latex; and antigens of many kinds adhere to particles of the mineral bentonite.

CAPSULE SWELLING   This phenomenon, alternatively known by its German name 'quellung', consists of a change in appearance of the bacterial capsule when it is exposed to a serum containing antibodies specific for the capsular polysaccharide. The change in appearance is probably due in part to actual swelling of the capsule and in part to an increase in its refractility. The phenomenon is highly type-specific—i.e. it occurs only if the organism being tested shares a polysaccharide antigen with that against which the antibodies were formed. Accordingly, capsulate strains of *Str. pneumoniae* can be divided into a number of types, differing in their capsular antigens; and a similar process can be applied to the typing of other capsulate species, such as *Haemophilus influenzae* and *Klebsiella pneumoniae*.

COMPLEMENT FIXATION   It has been known since the end of the last century that certain antigen–antibody interactions which produce no visible result (such as a precipitate, agglutination or changes in the appearance of organisms) can be detected by the fact that they use up or 'fix' complement (see p. 60 for a comment on the use of the word *complement* as though it referred to a single substance) so that it is no longer available to take part in other interactions. To demonstrate that such fixation has occurred in a tube which originally contained only a small known amount of complement, another antigen–antibody mixture can be added which will undergo a visible change only if complement is still present in adequate amounts. This is the basis of the *complement-fixation test* (CFT), which is most easily understood if considered in stages.

(i) Into a test tube are placed known amounts of antigen and of the serum to be tested for the presence of an antibody that will combine with the antigen and fix complement. This serum has previously been heated to inactivate the unknown amount of complement that it contained.

(ii) A known amount of complement is added to the mixture, usually in the form of guinea-pig serum. The amount is related to the known amount of antigen present, so that if the serum contains enough antibody all of the complement will be fixed.

(iii) After the antigen–serum–complement mixture has been given an adequate opportunity to combine, an indicator system is added. This commonly consists of sheep red cells and rabbit serum containing lytic antibodies for such cells. The serum must of course be heated to inactivate its own complement before it is added to the mixture in the test tube. If the original guinea-pig complement is still present in adequate amounts, the red cells will be lysed:

(i) Antigen + serum containing no antibody→ No COMPLEMENT FIXATION

(ii) Complement —————————————→ ⎫
(iii) Red cells + haemolytic serum ————→ ⎬ LYSIS

whereas if the complement has been fixed in the first reaction, no lysis will occur:

(i) Antigen + serum containing antibody —→ ⎫ COMPLEMENT
(ii) Complement —————————————→ ⎬ FIXATION
(iii) Red cells + haemolytic serum ————→ No LYSIS

The result is described as 'positive' if lysis fails to occur (indicating that antibody was present in the serum being tested) and as 'negative' if lysis does occur.

COOMBS' TEST The presence of non-agglutinating antibodies on the surfaces of particles can be demonstrated by the technique developed by Coombs and his associates. This depends upon the fact that the antibody is of necessity a globulin of a type peculiar to the animal species in question. Particles coated with it are therefore agglutinated by serum of an animal of another species which has received repeated injections of globulin derived from the first species. Thus, for example, the presence of human globulin on particles can be shown by exposing them to the action of the serum of a rabbit which has been stimulated to produce anti-human globulin (AHG) antibodies. Furthermore, if the AHG has been prepared by using purified immunoglobulin of one class only (e.g. IgM or IgG), it will agglutinate the particles only if they are carrying antibody molecules of that class. Originally devised for detection of blood-group antibodies, this technique has found various applications in microbiology—e.g. the exposure of a suspension of brucellae to the serum of a patient with possible brucellosis and then to AHG to see whether they have acquired non-agglutinating antibodies.

NEUTRALIZATION, BLOCKING, INHIBITION   Many antibodies can be detected and quantitated by means of their ability to interfere with the actions of micro-organisms or their products. Neutralization of toxin, as tested by comparing the action on susceptible animals of untreated toxin and of toxin mixed with the serum being investigated, is a simple example. Similarly, virus neutralization tests measure the ability of a serum to protect animals or tissue cultures against viruses. Other examples of this interference approach are metabolic inhibition tests, haemagglutination-inhibition tests and immobilization tests, which respectively test the ability of sera to prevent measurable metabolic activities of micro-organisms, to prevent the agglutination of red blood cells of various animal species which normally follows their exposure to certain viruses (p. 169) and to stop the spontaneous movement of flagellate or other motile organisms. Since such interference by antibodies is confined to particular species of organisms or even types within species, similar tests using antisera of known specificity can be used in identification of organisms.

LABELLING   Attachment of recognizable labels—radio-isotopes, fluorescent dyes or enzymes—to antigen or antibody molecules is the basis of an increasing number of methods for immunodiagnosis of infection.

1 *Radio-immunoassay* (*RIA*)   The amount of radio-labelled antigen bound by a known amount of antibody is decreased in the presence of unlabelled antigen, which competes for binding sites. Quantitation of this competitive inhibition allows precise measurement of the amount of an unlabelled antigen—e.g. hepatitis B surface (Australia) antigen—in a sample of serum or other fluid. A similar system can be used to measure antibodies.

2 *Immunofluorescence.*   When antibodies labelled with a fluorescent dye combine with antigens in a tissue section or otherwise fixed on a microscope slide, the complex is visible by ultraviolet microscopy (p. 16). Variations of this technique include:

The *direct test*, in which labelled antibody specific for the antigen in question is applied directly to the specimen.
The *indirect test*, in which the specific antibody is unlabelled but is itself the target for labelled antibodies specific for immunoglobulins of the animal species in which it was produced. For example, rabbit antibodies are allowed to attach themselves to their specific antigens and are then located by means of labelled guinea-pig anti-rabbit-

immunoglobulin antibodies. Use of this procedure for detection of antibodies (and particular immunoglobulin classes) in human serum is illustrated by the account of the FTA test on p. 251.

The sandwich test, in which antibody is detected in a specimen by first treating the specimen with a solution of its corresponding antigen, then washing off any unbound antigen and finally locating the bound antigen as in the direct test.

3 *Enzyme-linked immunosorbent assay (ELISA).* Antigens or antibodies carrying enzyme labels can be located, after they have attached themselves to fixed antibodies or antigens of appropriate specificity, by adding a substrate that undergoes a visible change when exposed to the enzyme. At microscopic level this technique permits detection and localization of antigens in tissues, but on a larger scale changes visible to the naked eye may be used. The ELISA procedure for detecting and measuring antibodies in serum uses antigen firmly attached to a solid phase, such as the inner surface of a tube or a well in a plastic tray. The serum to be tested is given an opportunity to react with this fixed antigen and is then washed off. Enzyme-labelled anti-immunoglobulin of appropriate specificity (as in the indirect immunofluorescence test described above) is then given a chance to attach itself to any antibody bound by the original antigen. Finally, after a further wash, retention of labelled anti-immunoglobulin by bound antibody is detected by adding enzyme substrate to the tube or well and looking for the visible change (usually of colour). By starting with specific antibody (instead of antigen) fixed to the solid phase, the ELISA procedure can be used to detect and measure antigen in serum or other fluids.

DIAGNOSTIC SEROLOGY

Since microbial infection commonly provokes the host to make specific antibodies, the demonstration of such antibodies in a patient's serum is often of considerable diagnostic value—particularly in conditions in which isolation of the causative organism takes a long time or is difficult or even impossible. However, important points to be borne in mind when interpreting the results of antibody determinations include the following:

(1) Sometimes antibodies are found which react with a particular organism or its products although they were formed in response to infection with a different organism. For example, antibodies that agglutinate various *Proteus* strains are formed as a result of infections with some of the rickettsiae (p. 148, the Weil–Felix test).

(2) The duration of detectable antibody responses to different organisms varies. After infection with some species, antibodies may be detectable for many years, and in such circumstances their presence is evidence only of infection *at some time*, not necessarily of *recent* infection. For example, the finding of rubella antibodies in the serum of

a woman a few weeks after she had been exposed to rubella during early pregnancy may mean either that she became infected at that time, with the possibility that her foetus was severely damaged, or that she had her infection some years earlier and was immune at the time of exposure, and so the foetus was not at risk. Two lines of evidence in favour of an infection being recent are the demonstration of a rising titre (see below) and the identification of some of the antibody molecules as IgM, since in many infections—notably rubella and brucellosis—antibodies of this class are the first to appear in the serum after a primary antigenic stimulus but may persist for only a few weeks. In other infections IgM antibodies may persist much longer but their presence can be taken to indicate that the disease is still active. (However, IgM antibodies to some bacterial antigens may persist long after the infection is extinct, so far as we can tell by any other means.)

(3) As a corollary of the preceding points about cross-reaction and persistence of antibodies, the significance of a given level of the antibody measured by a particular test cannot be assessed without knowing the levels to be expected in the blood of normal healthy individuals of the same age, habitat and social background as the patient.

(4) In general, antibody responses are not detectable for at least a week, and often not for several weeks, after the onset of an infection with an organism of which the host has no previous experience. Thus examination of a serum sample collected during the first few days of an illness cannot be expected to give useful direct information about the cause of the illness. However, in virtually all acute infections for which specific serological tests are available, *it is desirable to collect a serum sample in the acute stage*. This is because demonstration of *a rising level of specific antibodies* is often the best way of identifying a recent infection. If antibodies are found in a serum sample collected 3 weeks or so after the onset of an illness, it may be impossible to say whether they have any connection with that illness and it may be too late to demonstrate a further rise (however, see p. 168). But the situation is much clearer if an acute-stage specimen is available to be tested at the same time as the later specimen, and contains a significantly smaller amount of the antibodies in question. It is generally accepted that a 4-fold rise in titre is beyond the range of experimental error of most routine procedures, provided that the two specimens are tested at the same time, and is therefore indicative of a true increase in the amount of antibody in the patient's blood. (The *titre* of a serum is the highest dilution of that serum which gives a positive reaction in a given test for antibodies of a given specificity.)

(5) Even a rising titre of specific antibody is not unequivocal evidence that the organism in question was responsible for the illness that is being investigated. Contact with the organism may have occurred coincidentally at about the time of onset of the patient's

illness—though this possibility can reasonably be ignored if the patient's condition is strongly suggestive of that which the organism commonly produces. The position may also be obscured by an *anamnestic reaction*—i.e. a rise in the level of a previously formed antibody in response to the non-specific stimulus of some quite different infection. This is particularly well recognized in connection with salmonella H agglutinins, which may increase in amount following a wide variety of unrelated febrile illnesses.

(6) When a patient is suspected of suffering from an illness in which detectable antibodies are usually formed, but no appropriate antibodies are found in his blood several weeks after the onset of his illness, considerable doubt is thrown upon the diagnosis—unless there is some derangement of his antibody-forming mechanism.

(7) Detectable antibodies are not necessarily protective antibodies, and therefore the results of serological tests may have nothing to do with the patient's immunity or lack of it.

Tests used to detect infection with particular organisms have been indicated in Chapters 9 to 13, in relation to the following conditions:

> *Str. pyogenes* infections—pp. 87–8
> *Enteric fever—p. 115 and below (the Widal test).
> *Yersinia* infections—p. 118
> *Brucellosis—p. 128 and below.
> Legionellosis—p. 129.
> *Syphilis—p. 141 and below.
> Leptospirosis—p. 143.
> *Mycoplasma* infections—p. 144.
> Rickettsial infections—p. 148.
> Q fever—p. 151.
> Chlamydial infections—p. 152.
> Most virus infections—pp. 168–9.
> Candidiasis, aspergillosis and deep mycoses—p. 204.
> Toxoplasmosis—p. 208.
> Amoebiasis—p. 213.

There are many other infections in which diagnostic serological tests can be used, at any rate by workers with special interest and expertise, and no doubt in some of them such tests will in due course be widely adopted. The serological approach to diagnosis is used far more generally in virology than in bacteriology, but the techniques are more standardized and have been described adequately for our purposes in Chapter 11. In this chapter we shall deal with serological tests for the bacterial infections marked * in the list above, since between them these account for the great majority of the serological workload of most diagnostic bacteriology laboratories and since the tests used illustrate many general principles and involve certain theoretical complexities that need to be explained.

The Widal Test

In many cases of fever it is necessary to investigate the possibility of enteric fever or other salmonella infection. The serological part of such an investigation is measurement of the ability of the patient's serum to agglutinate various salmonella suspensions.

THE TEST   The nature of the three types of salmonella antigen—H, O and Vi—has been discussed on pp. 112 and 115. Standard bacterial suspensions can be so prepared that each is of known agglutinability by antibodies to one of these antigen types only. In Britain, H and O suspensions of *S. typhi* and of *S. paratyphi* B are routinely used in the test, usually accompanied by a 'non-specific salmonella H' suspension that is made from a salmonella with phase 2 antigens shared by a wide range of salmonellae. Use of *S. typhi* Vi suspension as a means of detecting typhoid carriers has a long but unimpressive history, but purified Vi antigen preparations now available may provide the basis for a more reliable test for this purpose. When a salmonella other than *S. typhi* or *S. paratyphi* is suspected of causing a generalized infection, H and O suspensions of that organism may be used in the Widal test.

Serial dilutions of the patient's serum in saline are pipetted into special small tubes, one complete set of dilutions being prepared for each bacterial suspension that is to be used in the test. An equal volume of the appropriate bacterial suspension is then added to each tube. Control tubes are also set up, containing suspensions mixed with saline instead of serum, to ensure that the bacteria do not agglutinate spontaneously.

H and O agglutination tests are incubated in a water-bath at 37°C (or at 50–55°C). Floccular agglutination of the H suspensions becomes apparent within 2 hours or so, whereas the more granular agglutination of O suspensions takes from 4 to 24 hours. The results of the tests are expressed as antibody titres, as defined above.

INTERPRETATION   Low levels of antibodies that agglutinate salmonella suspensions are common in the blood of patients with no history of relevant illness or of immunization. The picture is greatly confused by previous immunization, especially when TAB (killed bacilli of *S. typhi* and *S. paratyphi* *A* and *B*) or TABC (the same + *S. paratyphi* *C*) have been used (p. 296), and it is important that all relevant information on this matter should accompany any request for a Widal test. Following such immunization, high levels of H agglutinins for the species used may be present for many years, and rising H agglutinin titres are of doubtful significance because they may represent anamnestic reactions (p. 247). Similarly, after natural infection the H agglutinin level may be high and variable for many years, but in this case it is only the H suspension belonging to the appropriate species which is agglutinated or those which are antigenically related to it. O agglutinin levels, on the other hand, remain high for only a few months after immunization or natural infection, and are less liable to anamnestic rises. Furthermore, O agglutinins are formed more rapidly and more constantly than H agglutinins following typhoid or other salmonella infections, usually being detectable in the serum by about the tenth day of the illness. For these reasons the most reliable serological evidence of a salmonella infection is a 4-fold or greater increase in the O agglutinin level between the first week and the second or later weeks of the illness. However, because there is considerable sharing of O antigens between salmonellae, a rise in the H agglutinin level may give more precise information as to the particular organism causing the patient's illness. Absence of agglutinin response does not exclude the possibility of typhoid, as occasionally patients fail to produce detectable levels of antibodies.

Serological Tests for Brucellosis

Since brucellosis is a possible cause of persistent pyrexia, agglutination tests using suspensions of the appropriate brucella species (in Britain, *Br. abortus* and sometimes *Br. melitensis*) are commonly carried out in conjunction with the Widal test. The technique is essentially that of the Widal test for O agglutinins, and, since the organisms are not flagellate, only a single suspension of each species is required. Neither agglutination tests nor any of the other tests mentioned below can be relied upon to establish firmly the diagnosis of brucellosis, since antibody levels found in the blood of some apparently healthy people, notably of farm workers and others who have long been exposed to risks of brucella infection, may exceed those found in some patients with undoubted brucellosis. If the patient is seen early in the illness, it may be possible to demonstrate that his blood contains IgM antibodies, and such a finding strongly supports the diagnosis of brucellosis. Demonstration of a rising antibody titre may also be possible at this stage, and is a help to diagnosis. But because the onset of this disease is often insidious, the IgM antibodies may have disappeared and the initial IgG antibody rise may be over before the patient presents for investigation.

Serological Tests in Pyrexia of Unknown Origin (PUO)

The patient with persistent pyrexia and no clear indication as to its cause is a common diagnostic problem. Serological tests may provide vital clues. Tests which it is reasonable to carry out in such circumstances in Britain include the Widal and brucella-antibody tests already described in this chapter and those which we have mentioned in earlier chapters in connection with leptospirosis, toxoplasmosis and Q fever; with the addition, in influenza-like illnesses, of tests for influenza and other viruses capable of producing such illnesses, and for psittacosis and mycoplasma infection. Special circumstances or features of the illness may suggest other possibilities.

Serological Tests for Syphilis

NON-SPECIFIC OR REAGIN TESTS For over half a century the Wassermann reaction (WR) test was the mainstay of the laboratory diagnosis of syphilis. It is a complement-fixation test and therefore conforms to the outline given on p. 243. Wassermann's problem was to find a source of a suitable antigen, since the causative organism of syphilis could not be grown in artificial culture. He thought that he had solved the problem by using an aqueous extract of the liver of a dead human syphilitic foetus, since the organ was teeming with syphilitic spirochaetes. The resulting test was highly successful, but it was soon discovered that the liver of a non-syphilitic foetus was equally good, and that alcoholic extracts of various other organs worked even better. Cardiolipin from ox heart was adopted as the standard antigen. It reacts with an IgG serum component which is called *reagin* (though it is not related to the similarly named IgE antibodies mentioned on p. 63). Many other cardiolipin-based serological tests for syphilis have been devised, in which the reaction between the cardiolipin and a positive serum is manifested by formation of a visible floccular precipitate rather than by complement-fixation. These too are known as reagin tests, though the serum component is IgM rather than IgG. Most of them are now obsolete, but the *Venereal Disease Research Laboratory* (VDRL) test and its variant the *Rapid Plasma Reagin* (RPR) test are widely used, as they are simple and easy to perform and give consistent results. They become positive within 2–3 weeks of syphilitic infection, before some of the more specific tests mentioned below, and they are valuable screening tests for determining which specimens for syphilis serology need further investigation. However, in view of the basis of the reagin tests it is not surprising that they give positive reactions in conditions other than syphilis—'biological false positives'. These may occur in many infections, notably in malaria, leprosy, tuberculosis, leptospirosis and infective hepatitis, after smallpox and other vaccinations, and also (by far their commonest cause in Britain) in pregnancy. Such false positives are usually transitory, except in certain chronic diseases such as rheumatoid arthritis and disseminated lupus erythematosus.

SPECIFIC TESTS USING TREPONEMA PALLIDUM ANTIGENS   These more specific tests use genuine *T. pallidum* antigens. The organism can be propagated by serial intratesticular passage in rabbits—though this is a procedure for a specialized reference laboratory only. Where such a preparation of live *T. pallidum* is available, it can be kept alive for several days in a special fluid medium under carefully controlled environmental conditions, and shows itself to be alive by continual flexuous movements that can be observed by dark-ground microscopy. If serum from a syphilitic patient, together with guinea-pig serum, is added to such a suspension of *T. pallidum*, the organisms cease to move. This is the basis of the *Treponema pallidum immobilization* (TPI) test, a highly specific and useful confirmatory test but one which is necessarily limited to reference laboratories. It fails to detect very early infections, but apart from that it is the most sensitive and most specific serological test for syphilis, with the possible exception of the TPHA test (see below). It cannot, however, be carried out on sera that contain antibiotics or other substances which themselves would be toxic to, and immobilize, the treponemes. The *fluorescent treponemal antibody* (FTA) indirect immunofluorescence test depends on the same source of *T. pallidum,* but they do not have to be alive, and so it can be carried out in a routine laboratory. It is performed by applying dilute serum from a patient to a fixed smear of dead *T. pallidum* on a microscope slide, so that any anti-treponemal antibodies present attach themselves to the treponemes during a period of incubation; the serum is then washed off and antibody-coated treponemes are detected by means of rabbit serum containing fluorescent anti-human-gammaglobulin antibodies (p. 244). The version of this test now in general use is the FTA-Abs, in which antibodies that react with treponemes in general and not specifically related to *T. pallidum* are absorbed out of the serum before it is tested. This test has the advantages that it becomes positive early in the disease, at about the same time as the reagin tests and before the other treponemal tests, and that, by use of rabbit serum specific for particular human immunoglobulin classes it is possible to detect IgG and IgM antibodies separately. In an adult, presence of IgM antibodies suggests continued active infection; in an infant, it indicates infection of the infant itself, since maternal IgM (unlike IgG) cannot cross the placenta. The *Treponema pallidum haemagglutination* (TPHA) test is a passive haemagglutination procedure (p. 242) in which red blood cells (from animals or birds) are coated with a *T. pallidum* extract and are then agglutinable by sera containing appropriate anti-*T. pallidum* antibodies.

CHOICE OF TESTS FOR ROUTINE USE A system of serological tests for syphilis should ensure diagnosis early in the disease, allow monitoring of the effects of treatment so far as possible (see the next paragraph), be able to detect evidence of old syphilitic infection that might be still active or in other ways relevant to the patient's condition, and be readily applicable to large numbers of sera without undue cost in materials or time. Most of these criteria are fulfilled by combining either the VDRL or the RPR test with the TPHA test. The reagin test permits early diagnosis, and in a quantitative form reflects progress in response to treatment; and the TPHA test aids recognition of false positive results in the reagin test and has a much longer 'memory' for past infection. The FTA test requires careful examination of slides under a microscope, and so is not suitable as a screening test; but it is a valuable confirmatory test within the competence of a routine bacteriological laboratory, and can also be applied to selected sera from patients who might have very early syphilis.

Effective treatment very soon after syphilitic infection may prevent development of any serological responses. Treatment some weeks later, during the secondary stage, usually results in disappearance of detectable reagins some 6 months to a year later, but specific tests are likely to remain positive for years. If treatment is still further delayed, all tests may remain positive for many years, those using *T. pallidum* being the more persistent. This happens despite eradication of the infection by treatment, and subsequent attempts to reverse the positive findings by further antibiotic treatment are of no avail.

The serological tests for syphilis can be applied to cerebrospinal fluid, with positive results in most cases of active neurosyphilis.

The serological responses to T. pallidum infection cannot be distinguished from those to any of the other treponematoses—yaws, pinta etc. (p. 141). Clearly this is most important in parts of the world in which these conditions are endemic, but it needs to be remembered elsewhere. For example, a bacteriologist in Britain is frequently confronted with a set of results which would undoubtedly indicate a past *T. pallidum* infection if they came from the blood of someone who had always lived in this country, and could therefore be used to support a diagnosis of vascular, neurological or other late syphilitic disease; but in fact they come from the blood of an immigrant from the West Indies or some other appropriate area who had had untreated yaws in childhood and had been left with permanent serological memorials of it.

SKIN TESTING

Skin tests used in microbiological diagnosis mostly fall into one of two categories—those for detecting immunity and those for detecting hypersensitivity.

Tests for Immunity

THE SCHICK TEST   If a small amount of diphtheria toxin is injected into the skin of a human being who is not immune to it, local damage results. In such a subject, the minute standard amount used in the Schick test causes a reaction that begins to appear one or two days after injection, reaches a maximum after about four days and persists for a week or two. Its chief component is erythema of the skin in an area a few cm in diameter around the injection site, though there may also be some swelling. However, if the same dose is injected into a subject whose level of diphtheria antitoxin is sufficient to protect him against an attack of the disease, the toxin is neutralized and produces no reaction. The picture is complicated by the fact that diphtheria toxin is prepared from cultures of diphtheria bacilli, and the material used for the test therefore contains other products of the bacilli as well as the toxin. Some patients, probably only those with previous experience of diphtheria bacilli, produce a local erythematous reaction to these other components. However, this 'pseudo-reaction' begins within about 12 hours of injection and lasts only a few days; furthermore, it is produced equally well by an injection of toxin preparation in which the toxin itself has been inactivated by heating.

In a community in which there is very little diphtheria, such as Britain at present, there is no need to carry out routine Schick tests on small children coming to be immunized for the first time, but they should always be done as a preliminary to immunizing older children or adults, in order to exclude both those who do not need immunization and those in whom it might cause severe reactions.

The Dick test, used in the past to determine the need for immunization against scarlet fever, was essentially similar to the Schick test except that the test material was a preparation of streptococcal erythrogenic toxin and the skin reaction produced was more rapid and transitory.

Tests for Hypersensitivity

THE TUBERCULIN TEST   The theoretical basis of tuberculin testing has been discussed on p. 65. It depends on a Type IV hypersensitivity reaction. (delayed type)

It is important to appreciate certain features in which the tuberculin test is fundamentally different from the Schick test:

(*a*) The test material—old tuberculin (OT) or its Purified Protein Derivative (PPD)—is not itself toxic. Any reaction that follows its injection is due to the host's acquired hypersensitivity, not to the properties of tuberculin itself.

(*b*) Whereas a positive Schick reaction indicates lack of immunity and a negative reaction indicates immunity, it is the positive tuberculin reaction which is associated with immunity. This association is only an indirect one, however, for there is no clear evidence that tuberculin hypersensitivity is itself part of the mechanism of immunity. All that can be said is that those who have had and overcome tuberculous infections (natural or resulting from BCG vaccination) generally have some degree of immunity to further infection; and, therefore, since tuberculin hypersensitivity indicates past tuberculous infection, it also indicates probable immunity.

(*c*) The important component of a positive tuberculin reaction is palpable induration, which is maximal two or three days after injection of the tuberculin. Erythema also occurs but is in part non-specific and is difficult to interpret.

Tuberculin testing of human patients can be carried out in various ways. In the *Mantoux* test 0.1 ml of OT or PPD solution is injected intradermally by means of a syringe and needle. Since some patients, especially those with active tuberculosis, may give very strong reactions, it is necessary to start with a dilute solution and to repeat the test using stronger solutions if indicated. The inconvenience of the Mantoux test for screening large numbers of people led to the introduction of speedier multiple-puncture techniques. The *Heaf* test employs a number of very short needles mounted on a spring-loaded device which drives them into the skin through a drop of tuberculin solution placed on the skin in the appropriate site. Although this procedure sounds formidable when described, it is in fact more acceptable to children than is the Mantoux test, and is less liable to produce excessive reactions. Positive reactions range from multiple small papules at the sites of individual punctures to a zone of induration including all of the puncture sites and the surrounding skin. The *Tine test* is a variant of the Heaf test that uses a disposable multiple-puncture instrument with a coating of dried tuberculin on its tines (prongs). It is simpler to use than the Heaf gun, and eliminates any risk of transmitting hepatitis viruses from person to person; but is liable to give false negative results because of inadequate tuberculin coating of the tines. Use of a disposable instrument and liquid tuberculin may be the best answer to this problem.

Purposes for which tuberculin testing of human subjects is useful include:

(*a*) *Diagnosis* of individual patients. The test is positive in all cases of active tuberculous infection except those which are very early or of overwhelming severity. However, its diagnostic value is limited by the fact that it is also positive in a high proportion of older children and adults who are not suffering from active tuberculosis, these being people with healed primary infections (natural or from BCG vaccination). A negative reaction, contraindicating the diagnosis of tuberculosis, is often helpful to the clinician; and a very strong reaction suggests an active tuberculosis infection.

(*b*) *Detection* of foci of infection. In the absence of widespread vaccination, a high incidence of positive reactions in the children of any social unit—e.g. a family or a school—suggests the presence of an active disseminator of the disease.

(*c*) *Surveys* of population groups to determine the frequency of tuberculosis in the communities which they represent. This use also depends upon the situation not having been obscured by widespread vaccination.

(*d*) *Selection* of subjects for BCG vaccination. In the absence of any better criterion of immunity, a negative tuberculin reaction is taken as indicating that vaccination is required.

(*e*) *Assessment* of a patient's capacity for cell-mediated immunity.

Use of tuberculin testing in follow-up of BCG vaccination is discussed on pp. 294–5.

Tuberculin testing of cattle, with elimination of those giving positive reactions, is the basis of the creation of tuberculosis-free herds, which has played an important part in eliminating the risk of human infection with tubercle bacilli of the bovine type.

OTHER TESTS   There are many other microbial antigens that can be used in skin tests with the aim of providing evidence of past or present infection. The usefulness of any such test depends upon the frequency with which positive reactions, due to subclinical infections, are found in healthy members of the community. For example, a positive histoplasmin test is a most unusual and potentially important finding in a patient normally resident in Britain, but far less interesting if the patient comes from an area of the USA in which histoplasmosis is endemic.

PART VI

PART VI

PREVENTION AND TREATMENT OF MICROBIAL DISEASES

CHAPTER 16

PRINCIPLES OF PREVENTION

Everyone knows, and most victims of infectious diseases would heartily agree, that 'prevention is better than cure'; but medical teaching and practice have traditionally been preoccupied with treatment of sick individuals. Today we have therapeutic capabilities, both medical and surgical, far beyond the dreams of only a few years ago; but even so, when prevention of a disease is practicable it is usually 'better than cure' because it does more to reduce suffering and costs less money.

Microbial disease can be prevented by:

(*a*) eliminating sources of the responsible organisms;
(*b*) preventing transmission of the responsible organisms; or
(*c*) raising the resistance of potential hosts so that they are not susceptible to the attacks of the organisms.

The extent to which each of these lines can be followed varies greatly from one disease to another. In many cases it is possible and necessary to advance along two or all three of them at the same time.

ELIMINATION OF SOURCES

The great majority of human microbial infections are acquired from other human beings or from animals. Whether their sources can be eliminated depends upon the ease with which cases and carriers can be found and then treated or destroyed.

That the sources of a disease can be totally eliminated is illustrated by the recent history of smallpox. In 1967 this disease was still a major problem, endemic in 38 countries; but by 1980 the World Health Organization could declare the whole world free of it. Rapid eradication, despite the lack of any drug effective in treatment, was possible because this was a disease of humans only, with no animal carriers, and because patients either died or overcame the disease completely—they did not become carriers. Success was achieved by identifying and isolating all cases (the only sources of infection, though viruses shed by them into dust could remain infective for many weeks), and by immunization of all possible contacts, for their own protection and to break the chain of transmission. Provided that laboratory cultures of the virus are all destroyed or properly controlled, and that the organism does not prove to be capable of survival outside the body for longer than is currently believed, smallpox should never occur again.

Tuberculosis provides a somewhat more complicated illustration of the possibility of eradication, since man may be infected from cattle as well as from humans—and indeed cattle may acquire their infections from badgers and other wild animals. In a highly developed community all cattle can be located, and those with latent or active tuberculous infection can be identified by tuberculin testing. If those giving positive reactions are destroyed the human population is freed from any risk of tuberculosis of bovine origin. Finding human sources of tuberculous infection is a bigger problem, in that human beings are more numerous than cattle and less easy to round up for regular testing. Furthermore, the value of the tuberculin test as a means of detecting latent or active tuberculosis has been considerably reduced by widespread BCG vaccination, which also causes positive tuberculin reactions. However, since infection with the human type of tubercle bacillus usually involves the lungs, it can often be detected on chest X-ray films. Mass-radiography campaigns, involving the collection of such films of as many members of a community as possible, have been widely and effectively used in the search for infected human beings, but as the incidence of tuberculosis decreases as a result of such measures, further routine screening of the apparently healthy population ceases to be cost-effective. As for the active cases that are discovered by one means or another, treatment (with temporary isolation of those that are 'open'—i.e. discharging tubercle bacilli in their sputum or by any other route), must be followed by prolonged surveillance, since it is never safe to regard any tuberculous infection as permanently cured. The contacts of all active cases must also be carefully followed up.

Brucellosis presents a simpler control problem than tuberculosis because domestic animals (cattle in Britain) are the only sources of human infection and elimination of infected farm stock puts an end to the disease (p. 128).

Anthrax is predominantly a disease of domestic animals. As Pasteur demonstrated, the most dangerous source of this disease, at any rate for other animals, is the dead body of one of its victims. Here the problem is not to find the source but to deal with it, since the bacillus is a spore-former and hard to eradicate. Bodies of animals that die from anthrax should either be destroyed by burning or be buried deep in the ground. These are simple procedures when small animals are involved but less simple, when, as in an English zoo some years ago, the victims are elephants! The main sources of anthrax in countries such as Britain are hides, hair and bone-meal imported from countries where anthrax is endemic and where skin and bone are the marketable components of sick or dead animals. The hazards from such materials are reduced by hypochlorite or other appropriate treatment, preferably before shipment but, failing that, on arrival in the receiving country.

It may be difficult or impossible to eliminate the sources of diseases carried by wild animals. A thickly populated island such as Britain has great advantages in this respect, for there are no large tracts of uncontrollable waste land, and land animals cannot enter the country without human help. The rabies virus is not carried by any native wild animals, and has not been endemic among domestic animals since the beginning of the century, although there have been a few localized outbreaks following importation of infected pets. The strict quarantine regulation governing importation of dogs or other potential carriers have been of great value to the country, but are defied—usually for sentimental or commercial reasons—with a frequency which is particularly disturbing at a time when rabies among the fox population has been spreading westward across Europe. Control is far more difficult on a continent than on an island, and particularly in a country such as Canada, where various wild animal species suffer from rabies—some of them roaming over vast uninhabited areas and others, such as squirrels, coming into close contact with man and his domestic animals.

Persistent hunting for cases and carriers, which is so valuable in controlling chronic widespread diseases such as tuberculosis, is less well rewarded in connection with more acute and less common infections. With some of these the best way to locate sources of infection is to co-ordinate information about new cases. This is the purpose of legislation which makes certain diseases notifiable. To search Britain for carriers of typhoid, for example, would be an enormous undertaking with little likelihood of reasonable reward; but as soon as a new case is reported, public health authorities can institute an intensive local detective operation. This may be made easier if there are several new cases due to the same phage-type of typhoid bacillus, since the search for a carrier can then be concentrated in spheres of contact that are common to the people involved. However, finding a typhoid carrier is only part of the problem; eradication of his infection may be a much slower process (p. 114).

There is no possibility of eliminating the sources of some of man's commonest and most important pathogens—e.g. *Staph. aureus* and *Str. pyogenes*—since these are normally carried by a high proportion of healthy people. However, all possible steps must be taken to ensure that people in certain types of employment—e.g. operating theatre staff and food-handlers—are not disseminating strains of such organisms with known propensities for causing trouble (pp. 274 and 289).

PREVENTION OF TRANSMISSION

Control of Migration and Local Movement
We have already touched upon the importance of quarantine regulations in preventing transmission of disease on the international scale. Such regulations require animals or human beings, entering a country in circumstances in which they might be incubating one of certain specified diseases, to be kept in isolation for a period which exceeds the incubation period of that disease. Such an approach is of no use in excluding carriers or those with diseases that have long and unpredictable latent periods. There are other ways of dealing with these, such as insisting that intending immigrants undergo appropriate investigations—e.g. chest radiographs, examinations of their faeces for pathogens, or serological tests for syphilis—before leaving their countries of origin, or that they are effectively immunized against diseases for which this is possible.

Unwanted and undocumented animal immigrants can be a serious problem. Hence ships in port have shields on their hawsers which prevent 'hitch-hiking' by plague-carrying rats, and aeroplanes which pass through yellow fever zones are sprayed with insecticides in case they pick up infected mosquitoes.

Quarantine regulations can be imposed on a local basis. It is no longer generally regarded as necessary to restrict the movements of children during the incubation stages of the common infectious fevers of childhood, but similar restrictions can be applied to members of small units, such as families or schools or military camps, who are possibly incubating more serious diseases.

Isolation of infected patients comes under the same heading but is discussed in Chapter 18.

Control of Insect Vectors
Destruction of insect vectors plays a large part in the control of many diseases—notably of rickettsial infections (Chapter 10), yellow fever (p. 174) and malaria (p. 207). While it may be difficult or impossible to eradicate an insect species from an area permanently, it is often possible to reduce its numbers to a very low level for a time, and during that time to treat any remaining human cases of the disease and so abolish the reservoir from which the insects might otherwise become infected on their return.

When the relevant insects cannot be destroyed, it may be possible to prevent them from acting as vectors. For example, mosquito nets, fly screens and insect repellants can keep biting insects from attacking prospective hosts, and flies which cannot reach human faeces or human food cannot transmit dysentery bacilli from one to the other.

Communal Hygiene

The spread of disease is made easier when human beings live closely packed together in homes into which little bactericidal sunlight penetrates; in which fleas, lice and bugs abound as vectors; in which accumulated refuse encourages the breeding of disease-carrying vermin; in which lack of water supply discourages personal and domestic cleanliness; and in which there is no adequate provision for sewage disposal. In other words, it is generally true that a well-housed community with a main water supply and proper provision for the disposal of refuse and sewage is also a community relatively free from microbial diseases, and the provision of such conditions must be the aim of those interested in the prevention of such diseases. But transmission of infection is not, of course, limited to the home. In schools, shops, meeting halls, places of amusement, public vehicles, swimming baths and wherever else human beings come together they exchange their microbial parasites. Some of the factors concerned in such transmission are mentioned below under 'Personal hygiene'; public responsibility is generally limited to preventing gross overcrowding and seeing that the individual has the necessary facilities for hygienic behaviour and is encouraged to use them. During serious epidemics, particularly of droplet-borne diseases, it may be wise to prevent people from congregating indoors.

The communal and personal aspects of the proper treatment of food and drink are discussed in Chapter 19.

Personal Hygiene

The individual has a double responsibility in relation to the transmission of disease—to do his best to avoid being either a recipient or a donor. Much of what he has to do about protecting himself relates to the maintenance of his general health and specific immunity, and so is not the concern of this section; but there are some ways in which he can reduce or eliminate his risks of acquiring certain infections—e.g. he can avoid promiscuous sexual intercourse (without which the serious problem of venereal diseases would cease to exist), and if he lives in an area where diseases are transmitted by biting insects he can protect himself from them as indicated above. In many everyday matters it is hard to decide how far hygienic precautions should be taken. Theoretical considerations suggest scrupulous care to keep all potentially infected objects away from the lips and mouth; but since this includes virtually everything except food which has just been cooked or has been kept in a sterile container since being cooked, some compromise with practical reality has to be reached which involves avoiding only those things that are most likely to be contaminated. From a purely microbiological standpoint kissing is a deplorable habit!

Precautions against transmitting pathogens to others are of course most important when one knows that one has an infection to transmit, and at such times it may be one's duty to stay at home or in some other way to reduce one's social contacts to a minimum. However, personal hygiene should also take into consideration the possibility of carrying and disseminating a pathogenic organism without knowing about it. Particular attention needs to be paid to the excretions of the respiratory and alimentary tracts. Airborne droplets, which are the means of transfer of many bacterial and virus infections, can be intercepted to some extent by following the advice of the slogan: 'Coughs and sneezes spread diseases; trap the germs in your handkerchief'. However, the handkerchief itself, replaced in a warm pocket for a period of incubation and then shaken out vigorously before its next use, can make a considerable contribution to the microbial population of the air. There is much to be said for using (and disposing of) disposable tissues. Spitting of sputum on to the ground, where it is allowed to dry, is a potentially dangerous practice at all times and a serious menace if the sputum contains tubercle bacilli. Faeces may contain pathogenic bacteria and viruses, and so good personal hygiene includes proper disposal of faeces and the washing of hands after defaecation. Food-handlers must be particularly careful to avoid transfer of their intestinal bacteria to food—which may prove a good culture medium for pathogens and so an excellent way of transmitting them to large numbers of people.

RAISING HOST RESISTANCE

General Considerations
It is certain that malnutrition (p. 68), and virtually certain that fatigue and lowering of the body temperature by exposure to a cold environment (chilling) decrease resistance to infection, though there is a surprisingly small amount of clear-cut experimental evidence to support long-established clinical impressions about the latter two factors. These probably operate more by allowing latent infections to develop into overt diseases than by increasing susceptibility to fresh infection. Potential hosts who are well fed, well rested, well housed and well clothed are therefore relatively resistant to microbial diseases—though excess of food, rest or warmth may be harmful. Treatment of non-microbial diseases—notably of diabetes—may be important in raising resistance to infection.

Prophylactic Medication
Indiscriminate use of antimicrobial drugs to prevent infection can be dangerous and costly (p. 305); but there are some clear indications for such prophylactic medication. Examples are the taking of suppressive drugs by those visiting or living in malarial areas (p. 206), and the use of metronidazole to prevent wound infection following bowel surgery (see pp. 307–8, where other examples of the correct prophylactic use of antibacterial drugs are given).

Immunization

This very important part of the raising of host resistance has a chapter to itself (Chapter 20). Here it is sufficient to stress (*a*) the duty of the individual, for his own sake and that of the community, to see that so far as possible he and his family are immunized against any disease which is a potential menace in his particular environment; (*b*) the responsibility of public health authorities to see that he has the necessary information and facilities to carry out that duty; and (*c*) the responsibility of the employing authorities to ensure that doctors, nurses, ambulance drivers, medical laboratory technicians and others who are specially at risk because of the nature of their work are adequately immunized against such infections as tuberculosis and poliomyelitis.

Suggestions for Further Reading

Detailed information about the control of a wide range of infectious diseases is to be found in *Control of Communicable Diseases of Man*, ed. A. S. Benenson 13th edn. (American Public Health Association, New York, 1981).

CHAPTER 17

STERILIZATION AND DISINFECTION

This chapter deals with sterilization and disinfection in relation to clinical and laboratory practice. As an introduction to it, the section of Chapter 5 entitled 'Survival and Death' should be looked at again (pp. 30–6).

STERILIZATION

Sterilization is an absolute term, meaning the removal or killing of *all* micro-organisms (p. 31). It can be achieved by using *heat, irradiation* or *filtration*, under carefully defined and observed conditions. The killing of a microbial population is a continuous process, not an instantaneous event. The time taken to complete it depends on the size of the population (among other things). Therefore if a sterilizing procedure kills 90 % of a particular bacterial population every minute, 5 minutes of such treatment would be virtually certain to eliminate a population of 100 organisms (failing only once in a thousand times) but would be unreliable against a population of 10 000 (failing once in ten times) and could not be expected to kill all of 1 million organisms. Several hours of such treatment could be expected to deal with astronomical numbers of organisms of that strain; but in fact prolonged exposure to heat selects increasingly resistant individuals from the bacterial population, and the sterilizing process has to be restricted to that which gives a reasonable degree of safety without doing excessive damage to the article or material that is being sterilized. 'A reasonable degree of safety' depends on the dimensions of the problem (in terms of bacterial populations and numbers of items to be sterilized) and upon the possible consequences of failure. For example, failure to sterilize 1 % of bottles of culture media is of little consequence, but such a failure rate would be potentially disastrous among bottles of fluids for intravenous administration to patients, or ampoules of vaccines meant to contain dead pathogenic organisms. Thorough cleaning of instruments and apparatus before submitting them to a sterilization process decreases the risk of sterilization failure, because it reduces the number of micro-organisms likely to be present and removes material that might protect them against the process.

When in the following paragraphs we say that items 'can be sterilized' by the temperature–time combinations named, we mean that these combinations are commonly used because they can be relied on to sterilize the types of item mentioned, yet are not excessively destructive to them.

Heat Sterilization

For all articles to which it is applicable, *heating is the recommended means of sterilization*. Dry heat kills micro-organisms by oxidation, moist heat by denaturing their proteins.

(a) Dry Heat

INCINERATION   Total destruction by burning in a furnace is a useful means of eliminating the microbial content and consequent infection hazard of such disposable items as dirty dressings, pathological specimens in destructible cartons, some forms of laboratory cultures and the bodies of small dead animals.

FLAMING   Bacteriological wire loops and various other metal instruments can be sterilized by heating them to redness in a flame, but such treatment blunts cutting instruments. A less destructive modification, which is not a fully reliable means of sterilization but is sometimes useful as a 'first-aid' measure when proper facilities are not available, is to dip the instruments in methylated spirit (or pour it on to them) and set fire to the spirit—taking care to keep one's fingers out of the resulting conflagration!

DRY HEAT IN AN OVEN   Glassware, surgical and laboratory apparatus and instruments of many kinds, some forms of dressing and many other solid heat-resistant items can be sterilized by heating them at 160°C for one hour in a hot-air oven. They are usually packed in containers or paper wrappings that are impenetrable to bacteria so that they remain sterile after removal from the oven. To ensure uniform heating of the contents of the oven, there must be room for free circulation of air between the items (overloading prevents this) and the circulation should be maintained by a fan. Time must be allowed for the entire load to reach 160°C before starting to measure the hour. The measures for ensuring proper use and for monitoring the performance of ovens are much the same as those for autoclaves (see below).

(b) Moist Heat

STEAM UNDER INCREASED PRESSURE   Many materials, instruments and pieces of apparatus which cannot tolerate being heated to 160°C can be sterilized by exposing them to pure steam at more than atmospheric pressure (and therefore at more than 100°C). The instrument used to achieve these conditions is the *autoclave*—essentially an enlarged and sophisticated version of the domestic pressure cooker (which itself can be used for the same purpose on a small scale). The efficacy of steam as a means of killing micro-organisms depends on the fact that on reaching the surface of an object that is cooler than itself the steam condenses, giving up latent heat and rapidly raising the temperature of the object. The sudden decrease in volume draws in more steam, and so penetration into porous structure is good. For steam to be effective, it must be free of air, since this reduces its partial pressure and therefore the temperature achieved. Upward displacement of the air by rising steam, as in the pressure cooker, is an inefficient process because air is heavier than steam. Downward displacement autoclaves, with steam entering at the top and displacing the air downwards and out at the bottom, are adequate for some purposes, provided that the load is not packed in such a way as to retain the air (e.g. in upward-facing bowls). In the most efficient autoclaves the air is evacuated by suction before the steam is allowed in. After the load has been exposed to pure steam for long enough to reach the appropriate temperature and has been at that temperature for the appropriate time, the steam is evacuated and the vacuum is maintained for long enough to dry the load, after which dry air is introduced and the load is allowed to cool. Adequate time/pressure combinations for sterilization of appropriate items are 15 minutes at 15 lb/sq. in. (temperature 121°C), or 3 minutes at 30 lb/sq. in. (134°C)—the latter being attainable in modern high-vacuum autoclaves.

Clearly an oven or an autoclave (or any other form of sterilizing apparatus) can sterilize its load only if it is correctly loaded and correctly controlled throughout the sterilizing process. Loading depends on human attendants, but subsequent control can be maintained by thermometers, thermostats, clocks and other devices. Automatic recorders can show whether these mechanisms are working or have worked correctly, but the human attendants must take due notice of the recordings in order to decide which loads have been properly processed. As a protection against mechanical and human errors, *indicators* should be incorporated in the load. (It may be thought necessary to do this for every load, or only from time to time.) Chemical indicators which change colour when adequately heated are in common use; some are designed for testing hot air ovens and some for testing autoclaves. The chemical indicator can be incorporated in adhesive tape as stripes that are the same colour as the tape until heated. The appearance of coloured stripes on such a tape that has been wrapped round or strapped across a package is an indication that the article has been heated to an appropriate temperature. In the Bowie – Dick test for autoclaves, a diagonal cross of indicator tape is placed in the middle of a standard pack of towels to be sterilized; by the end of the cycle the stripes on the tape should have changed colour uniformly to the centre of the cross, indicating adequate steam penetration. Such methods indicate indirectly whether bacteria should have been killed, but a more direct approach is to use bacterial indicators (which can also be used for checking other means of sterilization, such as irradiation or gas steriliz-ation). These consist of standard numbers of viable spores of suitable *Bacillus* species, commonly carried on filter-paper strips or threads, which are placed inside appropriate containers at selected points within the load, and which should fail to grow when placed in culture media after undergoing the sterilization process.

STEAM AT ATMOSPHERIC PRESSURE Many culture media and other aqueous liquids which would boil in an oven can be sterilized in an autoclave. However, some are damaged by temperatures more than a little above 100°C. Twenty minutes at this temperature kills all vegetative micro-organisms. Cotton wool-stoppered bottles or tubes of liquid can be heated in a *steamer*; free steam is generated by boiling water and is retained under a conical lid which has a small escape vent at the top. Such treatment does not kill spores; but if these are present and the liquid is suitable, they will germinate after it has been removed from the steamer and allowed to cool. The vegetative cells can then be caught and destroyed by similar heating on the next day. Further heating on the third day is usually added for extra security. This process of intermittent steaming is called *Tyndallization* after its originator.

LOW-PRESSURE STEAM WITH FORMALDEHYDE A combined physical-chemical method of sterilization applicable to many heat-sensitive materials is exposure to steam and formaldehyde in a special chamber at sub-atmospheric pressure (temperature about 80°C).

BOILING WATER Boiling-water-baths have been commonly used in hospital wards and operating theatres for the treatment of bowls, instruments, etc., and were often described as 'sterilizers'. They cannot sterilize consistently, since some sporing organisms can survive boiling. Such pieces of apparatus may have their uses, provided that their limitations are remembered and that they are not, for example, expected to sterilize instruments used in wounds with possible clostridial infections.

Radiation
This subject is briefly discussed on p. 32. Ionizing radiations kill micro-organisms by damaging chromosomal DNA. Gamma-rays are exten-sively used for sterilization of the many disposable items used in medical practice; but the need for a radiation source (cobalt 60) and strict safety precautions means that sterilization by ionizing radiations is carried out only in a few special centres. The use of ultraviolet radiation is discussed on p. 32.

Filtration
Air and liquids can be sterilized by passing them through filters that remove bacteria and larger particles. Free virus particles are small enough to pass through the majority of filters in common use, but for many

purposes this is of no importance. Many viruses are arrested by the filters because they are contained in droplets or in cells.

(a) Filtration of Air
If a glass tube is tightly plugged with cotton wool, bacteria and other particles contained in air which enters the tube become entangled in the fibres of the cotton wool. This must have been sterilized by heating before use as a filter, and must be non-absorbent because motile organisms can swim through it if it becomes wet. Such simple filters are used in microbiological laboratories to allow sterile air to enter tubes and flasks containing cultures. Larger and more elaborate filters are used to provide sterile air for operating theatres and other places where it is particularly important to avoid airborne contamination. These are 'absolute' filters; whereas those used to provide clean air for wards, etc. remove particles and most micro-organisms but do not sterilize.

(b) Filtration of Liquids
Liquids can be sterilized by passing them through cellulose membrane filters. The liquid to be sterilized is drawn through a funnel into a sterile bottle or flask which is connected via an air filter to a vacuum pump. For small volumes a small membrane filter in a plastic holder can be attached to a syringe. Filtration is more time-consuming than heat-sterilization, the filter assemblies have themselves to be heat-sterilized beforehand, and there is always a risk of accidental contamination of the material because of leakage of unsterile air into the apparatus. It is used only for materials such as serum and yeast extracts which would be adversely affected by heat. Cellulose membranes of known pore size can also be used to determine the sizes of microbial particles or to separate organisms of different sizes. *Seitz* filter pads (made of compressed asbestos) can be used to remove bacteria from liquids, but are not sterilizing filters, as viruses can pass through them.

DISINFECTION

For the meanings of the terms *disinfection* and *disinfectant* see pp. 31 and 32. Disinfectants are widely used in clinical and laboratory medicine to treat objects and materials which are potential sources of infection or contamination but for which sterilization by heating is impossible, inconvenient or unnecessary. The properties listed in Table I (p. 33) play a large part in determining the suitability of a disinfectant for a particular task. Examples of appropriate uses are:

1 Treatment of Excreta that may contain Pathogens, of Discarded Microbial Cultures and Preparations, etc.
Unusually dangerous items should always be sterilized in the autoclave or by some other effective form of heating before disposal, but for routine use the clear phenolics are appropriate because of their powerful and rapid action even in the presence of organic matter. However, they are

ineffective against most viruses. Formalin is often used for the treatment of faeces in chemical closets, but its usefulness for other purposes is restricted by its pungent smell.

2 Treatment of Surfaces of Dressing Trolleys, Bedside Lockers, Laboratory Benches, etc.

A detergent-hypochlorite mixture has the advantages of physically removing adherent and possibly contaminated matter from the surfaces and of being effective against viruses—including hepatitis viruses, which have to be constantly remembered when blood may have been spilled. However, hypochlorite may cause corrosion of metal and is inactivated by organic matter. Other disinfectants sometimes appropriate for such purposes include alcohols, alcoholic solution of chlorhexidine and cetavlon or (where the virus hazard can be ignored) clear phenolics.

3 Treatment of Instruments and Apparatus that would be damaged by Heat-sterilization

Such items must be thoroughly cleaned before any attempt at chemical sterilization. This reduces the number of organisms present and deprives them of protection by blood clot, pus and other extraneous material. Hollow tubular instruments such as cystoscopes and catheters, and more complex devices such as heart-lung machines, are difficult to clean, but prolonged flushing with running water immediately after use often decreases the problem. They can then be exposed to low-pressure steam with formaldehyde (p. 265) or, if that is not possible, to a 2% solution of glutaraldehyde. This is a powerful bactericidal agent given adequate time (20 minutes for vegetative bacteria and 3 hours for spores), but it is expensive and unstable in the alkaline pH range in which it is active; and instruments immersed in it need to be rinsed in distilled water to remove the disinfectant. The gas ethylene oxide is a sterilizing agent that penetrates into relatively inaccessible sites in complex pieces of apparatus, and is also used for sterilizing objects as different as bone grafts and disposable plastic syringes. It is used in a special chamber, and requires a high humidity to be effective. It is toxic, and when mixed with oxygen in a wide range of proportions it is highly explosive.

It was formerly a common practice in busy surgeries, clinics and wards to put frequently used instruments into a 'sterilizing solution' for a short while after each use and then to remove, rinse and re-use them; and to keep syringes and needles in alcohol between uses. Such procedures do not sterilize, and are an improper use of disinfectants. If instruments must be re-used, a sufficient supply should be held to permit resterilization by heat or some other adequate treatment between uses; but whenever sterile disposable items are available and appropriate, it is safer to use them. (Radiation is extensively used commercially for sterilising these—p. 265.)

4 Treatment of Skin

Although the term 'skin sterilization' is often used, there is no reliable way of rendering skin sterile without severely damaging it. There are, however, various sets of circumstances in which steps must be taken to reduce its bacterial population, and in particular to eliminate pathogens. (The term *antiseptic* has often been used for a substance that can achieve this purpose, but it has also been used in other meanings—for example, in early editions of this book, in the meaning that we now give to *disinfectant*.)

(*a*) When there has been known or possible contamination of the skin—usually of the hands—as a result of contact with patients or with laboratory cultures, the organisms in question are on the surface of the skin and can be relatively easily removed with soap and water. For additional safety, the hands can be first immersed for a few minutes in a disinfectant such as a 5 % aqueous or alcoholic solution of chlorhexidine. Alternatively, an alcoholic solution of a skin disinfectant can be rubbed over the skin *after washing* and allowed to evaporate; but this is not a means of decontaminating unwashed skin.

(*b*) A more difficult problem is the treatment of the hands of doctors and nurses in order to minimize the chances of their passing on their own resident flora, possibly including pathogens such as *Staph. aureus*, to their patients during surgical procedures. Vigorous 'scrubbing up' removes surface organisms but drives others up from the hair follicles and sweat glands; culture of the skin after this procedure may yield more bacteria than before. A satisfactory approach to the problem is to wash the hands, wrists and fore-arms carefully with a 'surgical scrub', consisting of a detergent and either chlorhexidine or povidone-iodine (iodine carried on an 'iodophor', which retains the efficacy of the long-established tincture of iodine but does not cause staining or sensitization of the patient's skin); and then to rub 70 % isopropyl alcohol or some other suitable alcoholic preparation over the washed skin.

(*c*) A patient's skin can be satisfactorily prepared for surgical incision by first cleaning it with soap or detergent and then painting it with povidone-iodine or chlorhexidine in 70 % alcohol. This is also appropriate preparation for needle-puncture for special purposes—notably for lumbar puncture or for setting up a blood culture (pp. 236 and 238)—but on most other occasions application of 70 % isopropyl alcohol to the skin is sufficient. For efficacy and also the patient's comfort, the alcohol should be given time to dry before the needle is inserted.

Note that antibiotics have not been mentioned in this chapter. Because of limited ranges of organisms against which they are active and their relative or total inefficiency against those which are not multiplying, they are not to be regarded as sterilizing agents or general disinfectants.

PRESERVATIVES

For many purposes the prevention of microbial growth is an adequate substitute for sterilization. For example, in the laboratory serum can be preserved by adding chloroform (1:400) or 'Merthiolate' (1:10 000), the former having the advantage that it can be driven off by warming when it is no longer required. In the kitchen, sugar, salt, vinegar, alcohol and certain ingredients of smoke have been used as preservatives from very early days. Sodium sulphite, calcium propionate and a small number of other non-toxic chemicals are used in commercially produced foodstuffs. Again, antibiotics are unsuitable for such purposes, for various reasons, including their instability.

Suggestions for Further Reading
See references at the end of the next Chapter.

CHAPTER 18

SOME SPECIAL PROBLEMS OF HOSPITALS

The population of a hospital necessarily includes many disseminators of pathogenic organisms and many people whose illnesses or injuries make them particularly susceptible to infection. In the past, before the nature and modes of spread of micro-organisms were understood, hospitals were fearful places into which patients were loathe to go. Highly infectious diseases such as cholera were liable to spread uncontrollably among the overcrowded patients and their attendants; childbirth was commonly followed by puerperal fever which might well be fatal; and wounds all too often became gangrenous and gave rise to fatal septicaemia. 'Let him bear in mind,' wrote the early nineteenth-century surgeon, John Bell, concerning hospital gangrene, 'that this is a hospital disease; that without the circle of the infected walls the men are safe; let him therefore hurry them out of this house of death . . . let him lay them in a schoolroom, a church, on a dunghill or in a stable . . . let him carry them anywhere but to their graves.' This terrible position was transformed by the introduction of Lister's antiseptic techniques (p. 8) and then of aseptic surgery, and by the development of other ways of controlling infection. Antimicrobial drugs have played a part in this control, though early hopes of their dramatic success in this field have been disappointed by the emergence of drug-resistant strains, especially of *Staph. aureus* and of enterobacteria. But the fact remains that hospitals are by their nature places in which infection is a grave menace that can be reduced to a minimum only by constant care on the part of all concerned.

The term *hospital infection* (or, in American literature, *nosocomial infection*) is used for any infection which a patient acquires in hospital, whether it becomes apparent during his stay there or only after his discharge and whether the organism came from another patient (*cross-infection*), or was one that he himself was formerly carrying in another site (*self-infection* or *auto-infection*). In cross-infection the organism may have been brought into the hospital by the other patient, but commonly it is resident in the hospital or in a particular ward, to be found on the floors, walls, bedding, etc., and maintained by infection of successive generations of patients. Self-infection is illustrated by infection of a wound with a *Staph. aureus* which the patient was carrying in his nose when he was admitted to hospital, or by urinary infection with an *Esch. coli* from his own intestine. While such infection is not due to hospital organisms, it may well have been made possible by operative or other procedures carried out in the hospital and hence be a direct consequence of hospital admission; and in practice it is often impossible to distinguish the two types of hospital infection because the sources of infecting organisms are not known.

Available evidence from this and other countries suggests an actual increase in recent years in the frequency and severity of hospital infections, particularly of those due to antibiotic-resistant enterobacteria, *Staph. aureus* or *Ps. aeruginosa*. The size of the problem is illustrated by a survey of 3354 operation wounds in 38 hospitals in Birmingham, England, during 1967–73. The overall infection rate was over 15 %, rising to nearly 50 % for wounds liable to faecal or other heavy contamination and with post-operative drains. Wound sepsis and other forms of hospital infection cause the death of some patients, and prolong the stay in hospital of many others. Such prolongation may be a serious matter for the patient and for his family; his maintenance in hospital and treatment are expensive; and meanwhile a bed is occupied which might otherwise be used for another patient.

Of course, problems similar to those encountered in hospital arise with patients nursed at home, and much of what is said in this chapter applies also to them. But they are less liable to cross-infection, and any bacteria that they do acquire are more likely to be sensitive to antibiotics. Multiple drug-resistance is a feature of 'sophisticated' organisms bred in the highly selective environment of a hospital (p. 317). However, antibiotic-resistant strains of *Staph. aureus* and other bacteria are increasing in frequency among the general population, presumably derived from patients who were discharged from hospital, carrying them.

PATIENTS REQUIRING ISOLATION

It is obvious that patients with easily transmissible and serious diseases such as Lassa fever, diphtheria, typhoid or even open tuberculosis should not be nursed in open wards among patients suffering from other diseases. In accordance with the circumstances prevailing, they should be isolated either in special hospitals, in special wards for patients with the same condition or in separate rooms or cubicles. Similarly, children with such conditions as measles or whooping cough should not be nursed in general children's wards, though in many cases there is no reason why they should not be nursed at home. The desirability of isolating patients with *Staph. aureus* infections is less widely recognized. In most hospitals these are so numerous and the number of suitable cubicles is so small that there would be no possibility of isolating them all, and in most cases this is not necessary. But some, such as those with staphylococcal pneumonia or with large infected areas of dermatitis or burns, liberate very large numbers of staphylococci into their environment and certainly require to be isolated if possible. This is particularly important if the *Staph. aureus* in question is resistant to a number of antibiotics and belongs to one of the phage-types known to be able to cause serious epidemics of hospital sepsis (p. 83). If such a patient is in a ward, the staphylococci become freely distributed throughout the ward, colonize and multiply in the noses of other patients, invade wounds and respiratory tracts, and may make it necessary for the ward to be closed; attempts, not always successful, must then be made to rid the ward of its staphylococci by extensive washing with disinfectants. *Staph. aureus* can be particularly troublesome in the nursery of an obstetric unit, and babies with even minor lesions should be isolated. Isolation is also desirable for babies with *Esch. coli* gastro-enteritis, and indeed for patients of all ages with diarrhoeal diseases; and for many patients with *Ps. aeruginosa* infections.

An isolation cubicle should be so designed, equipped and managed that so far as possible no micro-organisms can pass from it to a ward. Since for administrative reasons it is usually close to a ward and the patient is usually cared for by the ward staff, the success of isolation depends on the thoughtfulness and scrupulous carefulness of *everyone* concerned. The ventilation of the cubicle must be so designed that all air from it passes to the outside of the building, not into the ward or corridors. Washing facilities for the patient and attendants must be provided inside the cubicle. Attendants should put on gowns on entering the cubicle and remove them on leaving, remembering that this is not a mystic rite but an attempt to prevent contamination of themselves or their clothes and consequent carriage of pathogens out of the cubicle. Everything inside the cubicle should be regarded as contaminated; dressings should be discarded into paper bags in which they can be removed to an incinerator; bedding and clothes should be placed and sealed in distinctive bags before being sent to the laundry; excreta should be treated with appropriate disinfectants; and cutlery and crockery should be disposable and go into the incinerator bags, or (if that is not possible) should not be allowed to return to a kitchen without sterilization. When the patient finally leaves the cubicle, it should be thoroughly washed with a detergent–disinfectant preparation and all equipment should be sterilized so far as possible.

When isolation is necessary but no cubicle is available, *barrier nursing* of patients in open wards is commonly used. The patient's bed is surrounded by screens and a routine similar to that for true isolation is applied to the area inside the screens. While this procedure serves as a reminder to the patient's attendants to use special care, it is not a satisfactory alternative to the use of cubicles, particularly as air-borne micro-organisms are not impressed by the 'barrier'.

Protective isolation is used for patients whose resistance to infection is seriously impaired by extensive burns, severe bone-marrow disease, treatment with immunosuppressive or cytotoxic drugs, heavy radio-therapy or any other cause of marked immunodeficiency (p. 66). Such patients can be protected to some extent by nursing them in cubicles with sterile air constantly supplied under sufficient pressure to ensure that airflow at all doors and windows is outwards from the cubicles at all times (*positive pressure ventilation*); this prevents entry of airborne organisms. Far greater protection can be provided by enclosing patients and their beds in plastic isolator tents, again with sterile air supplied under pressure, and with access ports to allow feeding, nursing procedures, etc. If microbial contamination of all items entering the isolator is minimized, such immunodeficient patients are protected against virtually all micro-organisms except their own. Even these need to be reduced in number in some cases, to lower the risk of opportunist infections (p. 38). The bacterial population of the intestinal tract can be substantially reduced by oral administration of non-absorbable antibiotics; it seems to be best to aim these at the aerobic organisms and to leave the anaerobic flora intact as a protection against overgrowth by opportunist invaders of the intestine, and frequent monitoring of the faecal flora is advisable. Reduction of the normal skin flora by application of disinfectants may be helpful to some severely immunodeficient patients.

GENERAL WARD HYGIENE

Even the patients who do not require isolation must always be regarded as potential sources or recipients of infection with pathogenic organisms. Overcrowding increases the ease with which organisms can pass from one bed to another, and lack of ventilation allows a high concentration of micro-organisms to be built up in the ward air. Bedding, particularly blankets, can become heavily loaded with bacteria, which are thrown off into the air by vigorous bed-making. For this reason it is bacteriologically desirable, though not always administratively convenient, that dressings which have to be changed in the ward should be dealt with before beds are made, and indeed as early in the day as possible since any movement of a patient in bed adds to the bacterial content of the air. Blankets should be made of cotton, and laundered before being used for another patient. Ward dust is often rich in pathogenic organisms and should be removed by a vacuum cleaner rather than a brush; and the vacuum cleaner must be fitted with a suitable filter so that it does not fill the ward air with bacteria collected from the floor. Appropriate steps should be taken to prevent transmission of pathogens by bed-pans and other common utensils, and each patient should have his own thermometer, or disposable thermo-meters should be used.

HOSPITAL STAFF AS CARRIERS OF PATHOGENS

Nurses or medical staff or students can easily act as vectors of organisms from one patient to the next by allowing their clothes to be contaminated or by failing to wash their hands after attending to or examining a patient.

This, however, is probably of little importance by comparison with the possibility of their being true carriers—i.e. those in or on whose bodies pathogenic organisms are multiplying. There are many microbial species which can be carried and disseminated around a hospital in such a way— *Str. pyogenes*, salmonellae and shigellae and the viruses of respiratory infections, for example—but once again *Staph. aureus* is by far the most important species in this context in present-day Britain. There is little point in routine swabbing of hospital staff aimed purely at detecting carriage of this species, since it is very common (p. 80) and there is little that can be done about it or indeed needs to be done about it in most cases. There is some point in such routine swabbing of the staff of special units if the phage-types and antibiotic sensitivities of carried strains can be determined. In this way it may be possible to pick out an occasional member of the staff who is carrying an organism which could be really troublesome. Frequently, however, the search for carriers of such strains is carried out not as a routine but in an attempt to find the cause of an outbreak of staphylococcal sepsis. It may be that the number of cases of staphylococcal infection in a ward or unit has been abnormally high and that at least a proportion of them were due to strains of the same phage-type. Swabbing of the staff and of all other regular visitors to the ward may reveal one or more carriers of the appropriate phage-type. It does not follow that these were the source of infection for the patients—they may in fact have acquired their staphylococci from the patients or from a common source—but as carriers of organisms which have shown themselves capable of causing an outbreak of sepsis these people must be excluded from contact with patients, and may be allowed to return only when such carriage ceases. This may occur spontaneously after a few weeks, or may be assisted by application of antiseptic or antibiotic creams or sprays to the nose. The use of systemic antibiotics for such a purpose is seldom justified. Medical, nursing or other hospital staff who have staphylococcal lesions such as boils must be removed immediately from duties in which they may infect patients, since the nature of their lesions proves the pathogenicity of their staphylococci. Similarly, members of staff who develop diarrhoea must be removed from such duties until it can be established that they are not excreting pathogens, as should any who are found to have *Str. pyogenes* in their throats or noses or in skin lesions.

SOME VARIETIES OF HOSPITAL INFECTION AND THEIR PREVENTION

Wounds and Burns

Any breach of the skin surface, whether accidental or surgical, provides an open door for bacterial infection. Bacteria can establish themselves more easily in damaged than in healthy tissue, and it is therefore important to remove all tissue debris from accidental wounds and burns and to reduce to a minimum the amount of tissue crushed, bruised or otherwise harmed during operations. Aseptic surgical technique is aimed at preventing entry of bacteria from any source into wounds during operations, and dressings should be so designed and applied that they fulfil the protective function of the missing skin barrier. A drain in a wound makes it more difficult to exclude air-borne organisms and also is liable to predispose to infection by damaging the tissues. When dressings are changed, great care must be taken to protect the wound or burn from infection and to dispose of dressings from already infected wounds in such a way that organisms from them are not transferred to other patients. While there are considerable advantages in changing dressings in special side-rooms rather than in open wards, careless technique which allows contamination of the air and equipment of such dressing rooms can be the means of extensive cross-infection. Many wound and burn infections are endogenous and could have been prevented by good technique—assisted where relevant by antibacterial prophylaxis. Patients with extensive burns need particular care, as they provide large areas of potential culture medium for bacteria, and infection of their lesions may result in delayed healing, rejection or breakdown of skin grafts, or even death of the patients. They are best cared for in special burns units.

The Urinary Tract
The passage of a catheter or other instrument into the bladder is liable to cause infection of the urinary tract, usually with *Esch. coli* or other Gram-negative bacilli. Such instrumentation should therefore be carried out only when it is essential, and with full aseptic technique, using pre-sterilized disposable catheters whenever possible. When it is necessary to drain the bladder continuously through an indwelling catheter, a closed drainage system should be used, so as to prevent ascending infection by organisms from the air or environment. Such a system must provide some means of drawing off an uncontaminated specimen of urine, for bacteriological examination, at a point near to the end of the catheter; and it should end in a plastic collecting bag with a non-return valve, and preferably with some means of emptying it without allowing entry of organisms, as frequent changing of bags is a common means of introducing infection. Care must be taken to see that infection does not develop in the urethral orifice around the catheter.

The Respiratory Tract
Patients who lie still for long periods as a result of unconsciousness, major operations, paralysis or other causes, and some who have respiratory tract virus infections or other predisposing conditions, are liable to acquire pneumococcal, staphylococcal or other infections of their respiratory tracts. Endotracheal and tracheostomy tubes increase their risks of infection by by-passing the normal defences of the respiratory tract. Apart from general hygienic measures there is little that can be done to prevent these infections. Attempts at antibiotic prophylaxis often do

more harm than good (p. 309); antibiotic treatment of an established infection is a different matter.

The Alimentary Tract

Outbreaks of *Esch. coli* gastro-enteritis among babies and of *Sh. sonnei* dysentery occur from time to time in hospitals. They can be prevented or controlled by measures already outlined in this chapter—isolation, general hygienic precautions and exclusion of carriers. The scale of catering required in hospitals makes them potential sites for large outbreaks of food-poisoning, affecting patients and staff and usually found to be due to salmonellae or *Cl. perfringens* (but to campylobacters in some recent outbreaks). The high proportion of elderly, debilitated or otherwise vulnerable people in hospitals means that fatalities are relatively high in such outbreaks. It is important that all hospital food-handlers should be adequately trained, and that the precautions outlined on pp. 288–9 should be scrupulously observed.

Infection Due to Injection or Transfusion

Introduction of a needle and extraneous fluids into a patient's subcutaneous or muscular tissues or his blood stream may involve the introduction of pathogens. This can be avoided by adequate skin preparation (p. 268), aseptic technique including particular care not to contaminate the prepared skin with organisms from the operator's respiratory tract or hands, and use of properly sterilized syringes, needles, blood-giving sets and fluids. Since there is little that can be done about sterilization of blood, donors must be chosen with care to avoid any likelihood of their blood containing pathogens—in other words, they must be in good health and give no history or serological evidence of virus hepatitis or syphilis. When injections or transfusions are being given to patients with jaundice, known hepatitis B carriers, drug-addicts, homosexual males and those who have been extensively tattooed, there is an increased hazard to the attendant staff (p. 192); and blood taken *from* such patients must be transmitted as indicated on p. 219.

Baths as Means of Cross-Infection

To minimize the chances of cross-infection via baths, they should be cleaned and disinfected after each patient use. A scouring powder containing hypochlorite can be employed for porcelain or enamel-surfaced baths, but for plastic, fibre-glass or stainless steel baths a non-abrasive hypochlorite/detergent preparation should be used. Patients who are particularly likely sources of pathogens should not use communal baths. There is a strong case (slightly and perhaps only temporarily weakened in recent years by the problem of legionellosis—p. 129) for the more general use of showers rather than baths for ambulant patients. Bathing of a series of babies in the same bath or sink can result in dispersal of *Staph. aureus* and other pathogens through a nursery; if newborn babies need to be bathed at all, this should be done in stainless-steel bowls which can be autoclaved after each use.

INVESTIGATION OF OUTBREAKS OF HOSPITAL INFECTION

We can deal only very briefly with this large and complex subject. Investigation of such an outbreak is a detective operation, and begins with the accumulation of evidence—the number of patients involved; their distribution in the hospital or ward; the times of onset of their symptoms and the probable times at which they were infected; whether all or the majority of cases followed operation and, if so, whether they were operated on in the same theatre or by the same team; and any other clues as to the way in which they became infected. If their infections are all due to apparently identical bacteria, a human carrier or other source of the appropriate organism must be sought, whereas an outbreak of infection due to various organisms suggests a breakdown in theatre or ward ventilation, in aseptic technique or in the sterilization of dressings or instruments. In many hospitals today a member of the medical staff (a clinician or a bacteriologist) is appointed Control of Infection Officer, and is assisted by a Control of Infection Nurse in the task of keeping a record of all cases of sepsis and continually reviewing the cross-infection situation. Such work can be valuable provided that there is some mechanism for ensuring that appropriate administrative action is taken when there is evidence of trouble. A small committee—including, for example, a surgeon and a bacteriologist, the Control of Infection Officer (if he is not one of the first two), the Control of Infection Nurse (who must be of adequate seniority to speak for the nursing administration) and a hospital administrator, with other members co-opted as the occasion demands—can be a suitable body for dealing with such episodes, and can also be responsible for defining the hospital's policies for preventing cross-infection. (It is, of course, easier to define policies than to ensure that they are carried out by all concerned!)

Suggestions for Further Reading

Hospital Hygiene by Isobel Maurer, 2nd edn. (Edward Arnold, London, 1978)— an excellent small book, full of good practical advice.

Control of Hospital Infection: A Practical Handbook, ed. E. J. L. Lowbury and others, 2nd edn. (Chapman & Hall, London, 1981).

CHAPTER 19

THE BACTERIOLOGY OF WATER, MILK AND FOOD

WATER

Water, particularly drinking water, has enormous potential as a means of spreading microbial diseases; and provision of safe drinking water is thus of great importance to public health. Bacteriological monitoring of a water supply is an essential part of the procedure for ensuring its continuing safety.

Many factors influence the total bacterial content of a water supply, including the following:

(1) Rivers fed by surface drainage contain many bacteria, some collected from the air by the water as it fell in the form of rain or snow and many collected from the soil or other surfaces on to which it fell or over which it passed.

(2) Water from deep wells or springs usually has a low bacterial content because it has undergone filtration as it percolated through the soil to reach underground lakes or rivers.

(3) Bacterial multiplication may occur in running water if it contains suitable organic nutrients and if the temperature and other conditions are appropriate.

(4) When water comes to rest in large lakes and reservoirs, its bacterial content is as a rule greatly reduced as a result of sedimentation and other factors.

(5) Supplies to most developed human communities are usually first stored, then further purified by filtration through sand-beds (which owe their efficiency as filters to a surface layer of protozoa and algae), and finally chlorinated. Chlorine, in a concentration as low as 1 : 5 000 000, rapidly kills nearly all vegetative bacteria provided that there is very little organic matter present.

It is not merely the total bacterial content, however, which is important in assessing the suitability of a water supply for human consumption, though a high total count certainly suggests unsuitability. What matters is the possibility that it contains potential pathogens. Important among these are the bacilli of typhoid, paratyphoid, dysentery and cholera; some pathogenic viruses can also be water-borne—notably those of poliomyelitis and hepatitis A. Presence of such organisms results from contamination with human excreta, or in some cases with animal or bird droppings. There are a number of obvious precautions which can be taken to reduce the risk of such contamination—e.g. drawing supplies only from relatively uninhabited catchment areas; ensuring that one community is not discharging its untreated sewage into a river upstream from the point at which another is drawing off its supply; or, in places where there is no main water supply or main drainage, seeing that wells are so situated and protected that there cannot be any leakage into them from pit-latrines and the like. A dangerous level of contamination is highly improbable in the case of water taken from a fast-running stream in a hill or mountain area above the level of human habitation. With this exception it is virtually always unwise to drink unboiled water derived from a source that has not been subjected to thorough and repeated testing, as described below, or to filtration and chlorination with adequate bacteriological control.

Routine examination of water supplies aimed directly at detection of bacterial pathogens is impracticable. With very rare exceptions (e.g. when urine from a renal carrier of *S. typhi* has entered the water), any bacterial hazard in drinking water is due to faecal contamination. Where this has occurred, pathogens are likely to be heavily outnumbered in the water by other faecal bacteria, and the latter are therefore easier to detect. In any case, the presence of recognizably faecal organisms in water implies that, even if no pathogens are currently present, they may well appear on other occasions. Most non-chlorinated water supplies contain assorted bacteria, including enterobacteria of various species and from various sources; but water bacteriologists are particularly concerned with those enterobacteria that fulfill their special criteria for designation as *Esch. coli*—which include growth in the presence of bile salts at 44°C with production of acid and gas from lactose. Presence of such organisms indicates faecal contamination, and so the possible presence of pathogens. Such a water is not safe for human consumption, and its source should be checked. Other bacterial species that have a similar significance are faecal streptococci and *Cl. perfringens*; though, since the latter is a sporing organism and survives longer than faecal *Esch. coli* or streptococci, its presence without them suggests that the faecal contamination was not recent. The significance of enterobacteria that resemble *Esch. coli* when grown at 37°C but fail to grow at 44°C (known to water bacteriologists as 'other coliform organisms'—see p. 109) is less certain. They are suggestive, but not clearly indicative, of faecal contamination, and therefore their presence in more than trivial numbers must be a cause for concern. The precise criteria for declaring a sample from a non-chlorinated water supply to be bacteriologically acceptable are too complex for brief summary. Since contamination may be intermittent, a single satisfactory bacteriological examination does not guarantee the safety of the supply. Regular testing of any supply to be used for drinking is essential, and in the case of a non-chlorinated supply any deviation from the pattern of results obtained over the course of previous years must be taken as indicating that there has been a change in the source of the supply and that it must be regarded with suspicion.

Almost all piped drinking water in Britain is chlorinated. The presence of any coliform organisms in a 100 ml sample of chlorinated water collected at its point of entry into a public supply (i.e. before there is any chance of mixing with unchlorinated water) indicates that the chlorination procedure was defective.

BACTERIOLOGICAL EXAMINATION   If a suitable broth, containing bile salts and lactose, is inoculated with part of a water sample and incubated at 37°C for 48 hours, production of acid and gas indicates the presence of coliform organisms in the water. If several such cultures are made with different volumes of water—e.g. one with 50 ml, five with 10 ml and five with 1 ml—and acid and gas are produced in some but not in all, the 'most probable number' of coliform organisms per ml of the original water sample can be worked out statistically. Further cultures are set up at 44°C to determine whether the coliform organisms are faecal *Esch. coli*.

An alternative procedure for the bacteriological sampling of water is to pass a known volume of water under pressure through a special porous cellulose acetate membrane which holds back all bacteria. The membrane can then be placed in a Petri dish on top of a pad of filter paper or other suitable absorbent material which is saturated with a fluid culture medium. On incubation, colonies form on the surface of the membrane. By using appropriate media and incubation temperatures it is possible to carry out total counts, counts of lactose-fermenting organisms that will grow on bile-salt lactose medium and counts of those which will do so at 44°C.

SEWAGE   From what has been said above it is obvious that proper management and disposal of sewage is important for the safety of a water supply. Sewage collection and water distribution systems inevitably follow similar routes in residential areas, and it is therefore important to ensure that there can be no leakage from the one to the other, even in times of heavy rainfall or flooding; and the processing of sewage must be such as to minimize the number of potential intestinal pathogens contained in effluent that is discharged into rivers which provide the water supplies of communities downstream.

MILK

Human milk taken by the baby straight from the mother is seldom a vector of pathogens, though transmission of cytomegalovirus and other viruses to unprotected infants by this route is possible. In human milk banks the milk is pasteurized to prevent feeding of contaminant micro-organisms to the infants, but this process may deprive them of passive immunity by destroying maternal antibodies. Cow's milk, on the other hand, presents many important problems. It may contain pathogens derived from the cow; the circumstances of its collection, unless carefully controlled, permit it to become heavily contaminated with a wide variety of micro-organisms; it is a good culture medium for many of these; it may spend hours or days at temperatures suitable for bacterial multiplication before it is consumed; and, as the result of pooling, milk from a single cow may be distributed to a large number of human beings.

Organisms which may be present in cow's milk include the following:

(1) *Pathogens excreted in the milk or derived from the animal's udders.* The most important of these are *Myco. tuberculosis* and *Br. abortus* (*Br. melitensis* being transmitted similarly in goat's milk in some countries). Other pathogens which occasionally come under this heading are *Staph. aureus, Str. pyogenes* (including scarlet fever strains), salmonellae and *Coxiella burneti.*

(2) *Pathogens derived from the animal's faeces.* The risk of such faecal contamination, and of consequent transmission of salmonellae or campylobacters, is greatly increased during an outbreak of scours in the herd.

(3) *Pathogens derived from the hands or respiratory tracts of dairy workers during or after milking; from utensils or bottles washed inadequately or with water from a contaminated supply; or from airborne or other contamination.* These include *Staph. aureus, Str. pyogenes,* salmonellae and shigellae, campylobacters and possibly viruses such as those of poliomyelitis and hepatitis A.

(4) *Non-pathogens* of many varieties and from many sources, which may multiply in the milk and cause souring or other changes in it. Souring, which is due to the production of lactic acid from lactose by such organisms as *Str. lactis* and lactobacilli, is deliberately encouraged for such purposes as the production of butter and cheese, but is otherwise undesirable.

Regular tuberculin-testing of cattle and examination of milk for brucella antibodies (see p. 283) make possible the detection and slaughter of animals with these infections. Scrupulous attention to the general health of the cattle and to any local lesions of the udders are other important steps towards eliminating pathogens of the first category. Subsequent contamination of the milk can be reduced by a high standard of hygiene in cow-sheds and by efficient washing and sterilization of all utensils and containers. Multiplication of organisms can be kept to a minimum by cooling the milk as soon as it is collected, keeping it cool during transmission, and delivering it to the consumer early in the day while the atmospheric temperature is still low. But even a combination of all these measures does not guarantee that the milk will be safe to drink. This can be achieved only by heating it, as described below.

Pasteurization

A process which Louis Pasteur devised to deal with a problem of the wine industry has been generally adopted as the most satisfactory treatment for milk. If milk is heated to $63-66°C$ and kept at this temperature for 30 minutes (the *Holder process*) or is heated to $71°C$ for at least 15 seconds (the *High Temperature Short Time process*), all vegetative pathogens are killed; spore-forming pathogens are of no importance in this context. The milk must then be rapidly cooled to $10°C$ or less, so that surviving organisms do not multiply. The adequacy of the treatment which a specimen of milk has received can be tested by a simple procedure—the *phosphatase test*. This depends upon the fact that the enzyme phosphatase is constantly present in fresh milk and is destroyed by heat treatment that just conforms with the above standard. Inability of treated milk to liberate phenol from disodium phenylphosphate is therefore evidence that it has been effectively pasteurized.

Pasteurization does not impair the taste of milk, and there is no evidence that it appreciably lowers its nutritional value. It does make the milk entirely safe to drink, provided that it is delivered into sterile bottles immediately after treatment and is kept sealed until it is consumed.

Sterilization

More vigorous heat treatment is required in order to destroy all bacteria in milk and so prevent it from being soured or otherwise spoiled by bacterial multiplication. Such treatment inevitably causes a change in the taste of the milk, due to caramelization. True sterilization by steam under pressure is necessary for such products as condensed milk, which must be able to survive prolonged storage in tins at room temperature, but heating at or around boiling point, which destroys all but the most resistant spores, is adequate for less long-term purposes. Such treatment causes coagulation and precipitation of proteins and therefore the *turbidity test* can be used to check that it has been carried out efficiently. In this test ammonium sulphate is added to the milk, which is filtered five minutes later and then boiled for five minutes and cooled. 'Sterilized' milk should show no sign of turbidity at the end of this procedure.

'Ultra Heat' Treatment (UHT)

In Britain 'ultra heat treated' is the official designation of milk which has been treated to $132°C$ for 1 second under specified conditions, has been delivered aseptically into sterile containers which are then sealed so as to be air-tight, and has a very low bacterial count as determined by specified tests. Such milk has a shelf life of several months.

Bacteriological Examination

Milk can be examined for its content of coliforms and other bacteria by tests similar to those used for water. Its total bacterial content can also be assessed by microscopic examination of stained films (since the number of bacteria is likely to be very much higher than in samples from water supplies) or by the *methylene blue reduction test*. This is a non-specific test for the presence of organisms producing enzymes that reduce and thereby decolorize methylene blue. Milk collected with reasonable care to avoid contamination, and therefore suitable for distribution or pasteurization, should not have a bacterial population that is able under standard conditions to decolorize methylene blue in less than 30 minutes. Examination for individual pathogenic species such as *Myco. tuberculosis* or *Br. abortus* is carried out by culture on suitable media. Milk from cows with brucellosis may contain brucella agglutinins. Even when such milk has been mixed with a large volume of milk from healthy cows, these agglutinins can be detected by the sensitive *brucella ring test*. In this test, haematoxylin-stained dead brucellae are added to a sample of the milk; if they are agglutinated, they rise up in the fat globules and form a blue ring in the cream layer.

Milk products, such as butter and cheese, and milk-containing foods, such as ice-cream and custards, are of course liable to contain pathogens similar to those found in milk, and are exposed to greater risks of contamination by handlers. It is, however, very much more difficult to devise bacteriological standards and tests for these products, apart from cultures to exclude the presence of named pathogens.

FOOD

Many foods make good microbial culture media and 'go bad' unless protected from the deleterious effects of multiplying bacteria and fungi. This protection can take the form of cooking, refrigeration, drying or the addition of sugar, salt or other preservatives (see p. 269).

The role of food as a vector of pathogenic organisms is not closely associated with obvious deterioration. Food which has been made unpalatable by the activities of multiplying organisms is not necessarily harmful to eat, and on the other hand food may contain large numbers of pathogens and yet be normal in appearance and pleasant to eat; if this were not so, there would be few outbreaks of food-poisoning.

What we said above about the difficulties of devising bacteriological standards and tests for milk products applies even more strongly to other food substances, because of their great diversity.

Salmonella, staphylococcal, clostridial and *B. cereus* food-poisoning are discussed separately below, and *V. parahaemolyticus* and the campylobacters were mentioned on pp. 122–3. The organisms of bacillary or amoebic dysentery may be carried by food—including lettuce and other uncooked vegetables, especially in communities where human excreta are used as fertilizers. Meat and poultry are the foods incriminated in the majority of food-poisoning incidents in Britain.

Treatment of food-poisoning is mainly symptomatic. Antibiotics are liable to do more harm than good in cases of salmonella food-poisoning (p. 116) and are irrelevant to forms of food-poisoning due to preformed bacterial toxins. The use of *Cl. botulinum* antitoxin is discussed on p. 104.

Salmonella Food-Poisoning

AETIOLOGY   Contamination of food with salmonellae can arise in many different ways and can come from a wide range of natural sources.

Salmonella infections are common among chickens, ducks and turkeys, and the organisms may be found in their eggs. Occasional cases of food-poisoning result from eating lightly-cooked individual eggs, but far more serious trouble arises from the mixing and spray-drying or freezing of large batches of eggs for use in the catering trade. Eggs often travel from one country to another in these forms, and can carry large numbers of salmonellae with them. The danger of such egg preparations is increased by the fact that they are often used in preparing food items that undergo little cooking. The carcasses of the birds themselves, especially of those reared in the crowded conditions of modern intensive production, are often heavily contaminated with salmonellae by the time that they reach the kitchen. They can then contaminate kitchen utensils and surfaces, and if these are not properly cleaned they can later recontaminate food items that have been cooked.

Pigs and cattle may have salmonella infections, and some human infections are due to eating inadequately cooked meat. In connection with this and all forms of food-poisoning it is important to appreciate that heat penetrates very slowly to the centre of large joints of meat or other large volumes of solid or semi-solid food during cooking, so that even vegetative organisms. may still be alive at the centre long after the periphery is well cooked. Similarly, turkeys and other large birds may not be cooked right through if air circulation is prevented by stuffing; and the same is true of frozen poultry or joints of meat that are not adequately thawed before cooking.

Oysters grow particularly well near sewage outlets, and readily become contaminated with faecal bacteria and viruses. Since they are eaten raw, it is important that they should be kept for long periods in clean water before they are marketed.

Rats and mice are commonly carriers of salmonellae and must therefore be kept away from food stores.

Finally, human carriers may contaminate food with salmonellae, of the food-poisoning or the enteric varieties. Transmission can easily occur via a substance such as ice-cream, which is readily contaminated during manufacture, is a good culture medium and is not cooked before it is eaten. Sometimes the route from man to man is long and complex. For example, salmonellae have been known to travel from Ceylon to Britain in desiccated coconut.

Although typhoid is not strictly 'salmonella food-poisoning', international transmission of salmonellae is well illustrated by the 1964

Aberdeen typhoid outbreak, which was the largest of several that occurred in Britain within a few years in association with the distribution of corned beef imported in large cans from South America. These cans were in effect cultures of typhoid bacilli, which they had presumably acquired from river water, contaminated with human excreta, that had been used to cool the cans after sterilization and had been sucked into them through faulty joints, as described below in connection with an outbreak of staphylococcal food-poisoning. The large scale of the Aberdeen outbreak—507 cases—was a result of contamination of a slicing machine and other utensils in the shop in which the corned beef was sold, and consequent transfer of typhoid bacilli to various other foods sold in the same shop. A fortunate feature of this series of outbreaks was the very low frequency of secondary cases—i.e. of patients who had not themselves eaten the contaminated food but had acquired their infection from those who had.

Salmonellae usually produce gastro-enteritis only when ingested in large doses. Their multiplication, which is encouraged if infected foods of appropriate composition are allowed to stand for some hours in a warm room, is even further stimulated by 'warming up' the food for too short a time to kill the bacteria and then allowing it to cool slowly through the temperature range that suits their growth.

CLINICAL PICTURE   The presenting symptoms are headache, fever, abdominal pain and diarrhoea. They usually come on 12 to 36 hours after eating the offending food. Vomiting may occur but is not commonly a prominent feature. Recovery may take a week or two, and convalescents may remain carriers for long periods. In a small proportion of cases the infection is invasive, leading to an 'enteric fever' type of septicaemic illness (p. 112), which is sometimes fatal.

Staphylococcal Food-Poisoning

AETIOLOGY   In contrast to the 'infection' type of food-poisoning caused by salmonellae, this is a 'toxin' type—i.e. it is due to the ingestion of preformed toxin, not to any action of the organisms themselves upon the patient. Milk may be contaminated with *Staph. aureus* from cows (rarely in Britain today) or from human beings, so cream-filled cakes and other foods containing uncooked milk products are prominent in the literature of this disease. Cooks with staphylococcal finger infections may infect various other 'culture media' which are left to stand in a warm room or are 'warmed up'—notably cooked ham. Multiplication may also occur inside tins of food. For example, one outbreak was traced to the following sequence of events: In a certain factory tins of vegetables were placed in cold water immediately after they were sealed, in order to cool them down before labelling; the cooling process produced a partial vacuum in the tins, and one of them had a small leak, through which it sucked in some of the water; the worker responsible for lifting the tins out of the water had boils on her arms and had contaminated the water with *Staph. aureus*; labelling sealed the small leak, and the staphylococci were left to multiply in an apparently normal sealed tin. Once formed, the staphylococcal enterotoxin is more heat-resistant than the organism itself, and will even withstand 100 °C for 30 minutes. Many of the *Staph. aureus* strains that have been shown to cause food-poisoning belong to a small number of types in phage-group III (p. 83).

CLINICAL PICTURE   Vomiting, which may be violent, comes on within 2 to 6 hours of eating the food. Diarrhoea often follows. The patient may be prostrated and usually has abdominal pain. Complete recovery takes place by the next day.

Clostridium perfringens (*Cl. welchii*) Food-Poisoning

AETIOLOGY   As indicated on p. 107, many of the *Cl. perfringens* strains responsible for this condition differ from other members of type A in that their spores are able to survive prolonged boiling. They are also antigenically distinct. They are found in the intestines of man and animals, and meat is often contaminated with them either in the slaughter-house or at some other stage before it reaches the consumer. This type of food-poisoning is usually associated with mass catering. The story of a characteristic outbreak begins with a large quantity of meat or stew being simmered for some hours and then left to cool. The clostridia find themselves in an excellent anaerobic culture medium, similar to the cooked meat medium which is used for growing such organisms in the laboratory (p. 222). Cooling in the centre of a large mass of food is slow, especially if it is not immediately refrigerated. Multiplication of the clostridia begins when the temperature falls below 50° C, continues until it reaches 20° C or lower, and is resumed if the food is gently heated on the next or subsequent days before being served. The bacilli are commonly found in very large numbers in food which has caused outbreaks of this form of poisoning. They are there in the vegetative form, but on ingestion they sporulate in the intestine. The final stages of sporulation involve lysis of the remainder of the vegetative cell, with liberation of an enterotoxin that was formed during the earlier stages and is the cause of the clinical manifestations.

CLINICAL PICTURE   Abdominal pain and diarrhoea, which is often violent, come on within 8 hours (the minimum sporulation time) to 24 hours of eating the food. Prostration is common, but there is no fever and seldom any vomiting. In most cases recovery is complete by the next day, but occasional fatalities occur among the old and infirm.

Botulism

AETIOLOGY   *Cl. botulinum* is another organism that can survive prolonged boiling and can multiply in the anaerobic environment provided by food that has been treated in this way. Unlike *Cl. perfringens* it is not found in the intestines of animals but is a soil saprophyte in many parts of the world, notably in the USA, and may contaminate vegetable foods as well as fish and meat. Home-preserved vegetables, particularly beans, have figured in a number of incidents; careful supervision of commercial canning of such items ensures that they are raised to temperatures that are lethal to clostridia. Botulism, the very severe human illness that results from eating food in which this organism has multiplied is described on p. 103. It is due entirely to the exotoxin, the organisms themselves being harmless; and can be prevented by quite gentle cooking immediately before the food is eaten, as the toxin is destroyed in 10 minutes at 100°C. It is very rare in Britain; an outbreak consisting of four cases, two of them fatal, occurred in Birmingham, England, in 1978, and was found to have been due to eating tinned salmon imported from North America.

Bacillus cereus Food-Poisoning

AETIOLOGY   *B. cereus* is a common soil organism, found on many sorts of vegetable matter destined for human consumption (notably rice), and is a spore-former and consequently resistant to drying and heating. Episodes of food-poisoning associated with its presence in food have been reported from as far back as 1906, and have been more frequently recognized since 1950, but since 1971 a special association with Chinese fried rice has been noted in many countries. The typical story behind an outbreak of this kind is that the rice has been boiled (which does not destroy *B. cereus*) and then allowed to remain warm for many hours before being lightly fried. The organism multiplies briskly in the warm rice if it is in the range 30–37°C, and produces one or more enterotoxins, which are not destroyed by the final frying.

CLINICAL PICTURES   Two distinct pictures can be recognized, and are probably due to differences between strains of *B. cereus* in the number and proportions of toxins that they produce. Most of the rice-associated outbreaks are characterized by nausea and vomiting coming on 1 to 5 hours after eating the rice. In contrast, vomiting was uncommon in most of the outbreaks of the kind recognized in earlier years, which were characterized by abdominal pain and diarrhoea coming on 8 to 16 hours after eating the food responsible.

LABORATORY INVESTIGATION OF FOOD-POISONING

The nature of the organism responsible for a food-poisoning outbreak is often suggested by the pattern of the outbreak—whether it is confined to a household or involves large numbers of people, the time relationships, the nature and severity and duration of the symptoms, and so on. Except in salmonellosis the investigation of an outbreak has little bearing upon treatment and is principally concerned with finding out what went wrong and preventing further outbreaks. The laboratory's contribution is to try to isolate the responsible organism, by culture of faeces and vomit (if available) from a manageable proportion of the patients and by microscopy and culture of the offending food if it can be identified and if some of it is still available. Precise identification of the organism isolated—e.g. by phage typing (p. 83) or serotyping (p. 113)—may help to pinpoint the source of contamination of the food. Sometimes the history of the outbreak clearly incriminates a particular item or at least a meal, but in other cases detailed detective work is necessary. If the food is available and either a salmonella, a heat-resistant *Cl. perfringens* or a *B. cereus* is involved, there is not usually much difficulty in growing the organisms from the food and from at least some of the patients, and in showing that they are identical. *Cl. botulinum* is also likely to be recoverable from the food, and although it is unlikely to be recovered from the patients it produces a highly characteristic clinical picture. The case against a staphylococcus, however, may be difficult or impossible to prove. These organisms, being less heat-resistant than their enterotoxin, may have been killed during cooking, and there is no simple and satisfactory procedure for demonstrating the presence of the enterotoxin, though it can be detected by tests used in specialized food-hygiene laboratories.

PREVENTION OF FOOD-POISONING

The responsibility for preventing food-poisoning is shared by many people, including public health authorities, wholesale and retail food distributers, caterers and their staffs, and housewives. The following are among the more obvious precautions:

(1) All animals should be inspected before being slaughtered for human consumption, and their meat should be inspected afterwards, for evidence of relevant disease.

(2) All consignments of potentially dangerous food ingredients such as spray-dried or frozen eggs should be tested bacteriologically.

(3) All food should be protected from flies, rodents and other possible vectors of pathogens at all times—during distribution and storage and after being cooked.

(4) All food in or on which bacteria could multiply should be kept in a refrigerator, or at least cool, at all stages. This applies particularly to such excellent culture media as ice-cream mixtures and synthetic cream.

(5) Meat, poultry, etc. that have been stored uncooked in the frozen state must be allowed adequate time for complete thawing before being cooked, otherwise the heat may fail to penetrate them adequately.

(6) Cooking, especially of meat, should be thorough, and food which is not to be eaten immediately after cooking should be cooled rapidly. If reheating is necessary, temperatures of more than $60°C$ should be attained with a minimum of delay. These precautions are particularly important with large quantities, especially of meat.

Cooling of large joints is accelerated if they are cut into several pieces immediately after cooking.

(7) Cooked food must be protected from the risk of contamination by contact with uncooked food, or with instruments or surfaces that have been used for uncooked food and not subsequently cleaned. In large kitchens the work-flow should ensure that uncooked and cooked foods are dealt with in separate areas.

(8) If there is any ground for doubting the effective sterilization of home-preserved foods in a part of the world in which botulism occurs, they should be raised to 100°C for more than 10 minutes immediately before consumption. This destroys *Cl. botulinum* toxin, and even if the organism itself is still alive, it can be eaten with impunity if it is given no time to make more toxin. (But see p. 103—infant botulism)

(9) Known carriers of salmonellae, shigellae or *Ent. histolytica* and people with known staphylococcal lesions, especially of the hands, should be excluded from work involving the handling of foods. Appropriate laboratory tests for the intestinal pathogens should be carried out on all those about to be engaged in the kitchens of institutions, restaurants, etc., or in the food-distribution trade at points at which contamination of the food could have serious consequences.

(10) A high standard of personal hygiene, especially the careful washing of hands after defaecation, should be observed by all food handlers (and indeed by all!).

Suggestions for Further Reading

Food Poisoning and Food Hygiene by Betty C. Hobbs and Richard J. Gilbert, 4th edn. (Edward Arnold, London, 1978).

CHAPTER 20

IMMUNIZATION

Immunological theory has been considered in Chapter 8. Here we are concerned with the artificial enhancement of immunity—i.e. immunization.

ACTIVE IMMUNIZATION

This is the administration of an antigen which stimulates the recipient's own immunological mechanisms. The speed and vigour of his response depend on the dose of antigen, the route of administration, his age and whether he has met the antigen (or something closely similar) previously. The *primary response* to an antigen not previously encountered may take 1–3 weeks to manifest itself, and if antibodies are produced they are predominantly IgM (p. 246). The *secondary response* on meeting it again weeks, months or even in some cases many years later is more vigorous and much faster, and if it involves production of antibodies they are predominantly IgG; alternatively, or in addition, the T-lymphocyte responses are enhanced and accelerated. These differences between primary and secondary responses, which are of central importance in the design of immunization regimens, are the result of immunological memory, as described on p. 54. For adequate and lasting immunity it is necessary, with many antigens, to give an initial course of three doses and a *booster dose* a few years later; and even then immunity may wane unless further doses are given every few years. Other antigenic stimuli—e.g. measles or mumps virus—may stimulate life-long immunity. There are some antigens that provoke adequate primary responses, but with no accompanying immunological memory that enhances the response to a second encounter. For example, immunization with pneumococcal or *Haemophilus influenzae* capsular polysaccharide results in a good and sustained antibody response (except in infants—p. 65), but the response to a second injection is virtually indistinguishable from that to the first. The primary/secondary distinction is of course blurred if the antigen persists in the tissues, and particularly when it is a live organism that not only persists but proliferates. As in natural infections, there is then a period of continuous, and at least for a time increasing, stimulation; and the pattern of immunological response is modified accordingly. Substances such as alum are added to some injected immunizing agents, in order to delay their absorption and so prolong their effectiveness; the name *adjuvants* is given to such substances which, when administered with antigens, enhance their immunogenicity.

In general it is probably desirable that an immunization regimen should simulate as closely as possible the corresponding natural infection, and in particular the mode of entry of the pathogen into the host. Thus, while non-living antigens are most effective when injected, live attenuated vaccines are increasingly given orally or intranasally. For example, of the vaccines available for immunization against poliomyelitis (p. 298), the inactivated vaccine is given by injection and stimulates production of much antibody in the serum but virtually none in the intestinal secretions, whereas oral administration of live attenuated vaccine results in high levels of secretory antibody at the site at which natural infection would otherwise occur as well as some serum antibody. Secretory antibody responses appear to be accompanied by little or no immunological memory.

Antibodies already in circulation, especially IgG, can suppress the response to active immunization. This is of practical relevance to the immunization of infants who still have placentally transmitted maternal IgG antibodies in their blood (pp. 57–8 and 65). Such serum antibodies can impair the response to parenteral immunization, but do not affect the response to oral vaccines, whereas the latter can be impaired by maternal antibodies in breast milk (p. 59).

Another complication of active immunization is illustrated by responses to influenza virus vaccines. One might expect that immunization with a vaccine containing a range of currently prevalent influenza A virus strains might result in protection against them all; but in fact the response is far from uniform, and is dominated by production of antibodies to the first influenza A virus strain the recipient ever encountered—perhaps many years before. The term *original antigenic sin* has been applied to such behaviour. It is characteristic of human responses to any virus with numerous cross-reacting types; and it has important implications for natural as well as artificially induced immunity, as exposure to a new variant of a virus may lead to production of antibodies which are not of the right specificity and give poor protection against the new strain. (See p. 301 for an example of a somewhat similar phenomenon in connection with the use of combined vaccines.)

Since active immunization of a subject who has no previous experience of the antigen takes several weeks to produce effective protection, it is of prophylactic but not of therapeutic value. Boosting of existing immunity may be of immediate value—e.g. in prevention of tetanus (p. 297).

PASSIVE IMMUNIZATION

This is the giving of ready-made antibodies, formed by another person or an animal in response to artificial immunization or to natural infection. If formed in an animal, they are to their human recipients foreign proteins and potential allergens. The antitoxin used in treatment of diphtheria is produced in horses, and causes few problems because nobody is likely to need repeated courses of it. This is not true of tetanus antitoxin, which may have to be given to the same individual prophylactically after a series of relevant injuries (unless he has been actively immunized). Repeated injection of horse proteins has led to hypersensitivity reactions to these foreign proteins—Type I reactions such as anaphylactic shock, which may be fatal, if the host produces IgE antibodies, or Type III reactions such as serum sickness if he produces IgG (see pp. 63 and 65). Tetanus antitoxin is therefore now prepared by repeatedly immunizing human volunteers with toxoid (p. 298).

The γ-globulin fraction of pooled plasma from healthy blood donors, known as *human normal immunoglobulin*, contains antibodies that reflect the prevalence of infectious diseases in the community. Injections of this material are used for such purposes as giving travellers a few months' protection against hepatitis A; reducing the severity of reactions to measles vaccine; or giving general temporary protection to patients with hypogammaglobulinaemia. Similarly, *human specific immunoglobulin*, derived from convalescents or from immunized volunteers (as mentioned above in relation to tetanus), can be used to confer temporary protection against a particular infection on exposed immunodeficient patients or those for whom active immunization is contra-indicated—e.g. by severe skin disease. Such specific immunoglobulin is also an important means of conferring protection against rabies or hepatitis B on normal people, if it is given soon after exposure.

Passive immunization begins to be effective as soon as the antiserum enters the recipient's circulation, but its effect lasts at most for only a few

Table VIII

	Active	Passive
Immunizing agents	Live or dead organisms, toxoids	Sera from immunized animals or humans
Rapidity of protection	2 to 3 weeks' delay if no previous immunity	Immediate
Duration	Usually several years	At most a few months
Complications	Various (see later) but rarely serious	Anaphylaxis, serum sickness (animal sera)
Uses	Long-term prophylaxis Treatment only if previously immunized	Short-term prophylaxis Treatment

months. This is because the antibody molecules, like all protein molecules in the body, have only a short life, and they are not replaced as are those produced in response to active immunization. Consequently passive immunization is of use only for short-term prophylaxis or for treatment of existing infection.

The main differences between active and passive immunization can be summarized as in Table VIII.

VACCINES

The words *vaccine* and *vaccination*, derived originally from the use of material from the cow (Latin *vacca*) for immunization against smallpox, have gradually extended in meaning to include all immunizing preparations of living or dead organisms or of materials derived from organisms. Vaccines can be classified as follows:

(*a*) *Live organisms of limited virulence*—usually attenuated derivatives of pathogens, but sometimes naturally occurring organisms closely related to pathogens (e.g. cowpox virus, or the vole tubercle bacillus which has been used for immunizing humans against tuberculosis). Because live cultures are used, it is important to ensure that they do not contain contaminant pathogenic organisms (see p. 294—the Lübeck disaster). A particular hazard of virus vaccines that have to be grown in primary tissue cultures—i.e. in cell populations directly derived from animal embryos or organs—is that they may contain wild viruses that were already in the tissues. Provided that a live vaccine 'takes' and multiplies in the recipient's tissues, a single dose usually gives a satisfactory degree of immunity, since it provides a prolonged antigenic stimulus.

(*b*) *Dead (or inactivated) organisms.* Suspensions of dead bacteria have on the whole been disappointing as inducers of immunity, though some are misleadingly successful in stimulating the production of measurable antibodies. The position may be improved by research aimed at finding for each organism the culture conditions and method of killing which give the best yield, not just of organisms but of those antigenic components which stimulate protective responses. Inactivated virus vaccines have been somewhat more successful, but disasters have resulted from failures of the inactivation processes and consequent inadvertent administration of live virulent viruses. Because a dead or inactivated organism does not multiply in the recipient's tissues, several suitably spaced and relatively large doses have to be given, usually by injection.

(*c*) *Purified microbial products.* The classical examples of these are *toxoids*, which are bacterial toxins—e.g. of diphtheria or tetanus—that have been made harmless by heat or formalin treatment, but are still effective as antigens and stimulate the production of antibodies which neutralize the corresponding toxins. Also in this category of products are the *B. anthracis* protein antigen mentioned on p. 102 and the pneumococcal and meningococcal capsular polysaccharides. The ultimate aim in active immunization must be the maximum of protective response with the minimum risk of unpleasant or harmful reactions. Administration of whole organisms, alive or dead, is a somewhat crude approach to this aim as compared with administration of refined preparations of 'protective' antigens, from which virtually all irrelevant and potentially 'reactogenic' material has been removed.

IMMUNIZATION AGAINST PARTICULAR DISEASES DUE TO BACTERIA

Tuberculosis

Immunization against tuberculosis, using the living attenuated bovine-type tubercle bacillus of Calmette and Guerin (BCG), has been in use since 1922, but its widespread adoption was greatly delayed by the 1930 Lubeck disaster, in which 72 of 251 BCG-vaccinated infants died of tuberculosis soon afterwards. There is little doubt that this was due to contamination of one batch of vaccine with virulent tubercle bacilli. In recent years BCG has been given to many millions of people with few complications; a very small number of generalized and fatal infections have been attributable to unsuspected T-cell immunodeficiency.

The vaccine is given as a small intradermal injection of a suspension of the live bacilli—usually a reconstituted freeze-dried culture. For a variety of reasons the upper arm is the most satisfactory site for this and most other forms of vaccination. BCG vaccination in Britain (and in many other countries) is preceded by tuberculin testing, and is confined to those giving negative results. This is partly because a positive result is presumptive (though not conclusive) evidence that the subject is already protected against tuberculosis; but mainly because BCG vaccination in the presence of tuberculin hypersensitivity may result in a destructive Type IV reaction (p. 132). The omission of preliminary tuberculin testing in large-scale BCG immunization programmes in developing countries speeds up the programmes, and hypersensitivity reactions have not been found to be a serious problem. In the absence of pre-existing hypersensitivity, a small tuberculous ulcer develops a few weeks after vaccination and persists for several months before it heals, leaving a small scar. The recipient usually gives a positive tuberculin reaction from the sixth week after vaccination.

While BCG vaccination does not give complete protection against tuberculosis, there is clear evidence from trials in Britain and many other countries that it decreases the chance of contracting the disease and virtually eliminates the danger of developing it in its more virulent primary form (p. 132). How long this protection lasts is not so clear. Reversion to tuberculin negativity after 3 or 4 years or less is quite common, and may be regarded as an indication for revaccination, but there is in fact no certainty that protective immunity has also waned at the same time as the hypersensitivity. Some trials in other countries—notably the USA and India—have failed to show any protective effect following BCG vaccination. A possible explanation of this failure is that the populations concerned were already enjoying, as a result of natural infection with non-tuberculous mycobacteria, a degree of protection against tuberculosis comparable to that conferred in less fortunate communities by BCG vaccination. As with any form of immunization, the cost-effectiveness of BCG immunization is decreasing as the risk of tuberculous infection decreases.

Whooping Cough

This disease can be serious, even lethal, in the first year or so of life, and responds poorly to antibiotic treatment. Effective prophylaxis is therefore clearly desirable, and ideally would give protection even in the first months of life, since there is little transfer of maternal immunity to this disease. Vaccines consisting of killed suspensions of *B. pertussis* have been available since the 1930s, and are given by intramuscular or subcutaneous injection. Early trials showed that they were effective, and some (though by no means all) of those in use in Britain and elsewhere in the 1950s were shown (in excellent Medical Research Council trials) to give good levels of protection. However, since then there have been conflicting reports, especially in Britain, about the efficacy of available vaccines. Much of the confusion is attributable to variations in their composition and lack of any satisfactory method of testing their potency in the laboratory; but it has been suggested that antigenic variation of prevailing *B. pertussis* strains might have played a part. There has also been fierce controversy in Britain about the safety of pertussis immunization. There is no doubt that it does sometimes cause encephalopathy, but the true frequency of this complication is very difficult to assess, since comparable brain damage can occur in unvaccinated children, either from unrelated causes or following an attack of whooping cough. Unfortunately but under-standably, public discussion of all these doubts about whooping cough vaccination has caused many parents to doubt the wisdom of having their children vaccinated at all—against any disease, not merely against whooping cough. On the basis of recent appraisals of the available evidence it seems reasonable to recommend parents to have their children vaccinated against this disease, starting at 3 months old, in the absence of such specific contra-indications as a history of epilepsy in the family or of convulsions or cerebral irritability in the child during the neonatal period, or central nervous system abnormalities, or a current febrile illness (a contra-indication for any form of immunization).

Typhoid and Paratyphoid

Immunization against enteric fever by injecting killed suspensions of the causative bacilli was introduced at the end of the last century and has been very widely used, especially in war-time, ever since then; but for many years there was surprisingly little definite evidence that it gave any protection. This was in part because army units and other groups of people with high vaccination rates have usually also had high standards of general hygiene which could equally well have been responsible for their low incidence of enteric fever; and in part because the effectiveness of such a vaccine varies with its method of preparation. However, carefully controlled large-scale trials in Yugoslavia in 1954–55 established that recipients of a heat-killed phenol-preserved *S. typhi* vaccine developed typhoid significantly less often than did those who received either a *Sh. flexneri* vaccine (presumably irrelevant) or an alcohol-killed *S. typhi* vaccine (which, on the evidence of this trial, was of little or no value).

Subcutaneous injections of heat-killed suspensions of *S. typhi* and of *S. paratyphi* A and B or A, B and C (TAB or TABC) have been extensively used in the past. These commonly produce painful local swellings, often accompanied by fever, and they provoke vigorous antibody responses to all of the species used, as measured in the Widal test (p. 248); but since there is no evidence that the paratyphoid components evoke any useful level of protection, and since they undoubtedly increase the adverse reactions, a monovalent *S. typhi* vaccine is now used. It is given intradermally, since this further reduces the adverse reactions; and an acetone-killed suspension is recommended, since it has been shown to give better protection than those killed by heat.

Diphtheria and Tetanus

Both active and passive immunization against these diseases date from the pioneer work of Behring and Kitasato at the end of the last century (p. 9), and from the time of their discovery there has never been any room for doubt about the efficacy of these procedures. In both diseases the damage is done by toxins and immunization is aimed at neutralizing these.

ACTIVE IMMUNIZATION   In each case toxoid for active immunization is made by heat- and formalin-inactivation of toxin obtained from a culture of the relevant organism. Elaborate steps are taken to purify this *formol toxoid* so as to eliminate unnecessary ingredients which might act as antigens and give rise to hypersensitivity reactions, or else might be directly toxic.

Diphtheria formol toxoid is an inadequate antigen when given on its own, but whooping cough vaccine given with it acts as an adjuvant (p. 291). Of various other means used to enhance the efficacy of the formol toxoid, adsorption onto aluminium phosphate or hydroxide is the most successful. Two intramuscular or deep subcutaneous injections of such an adsorbed vaccine, given 4–6 weeks apart, constitute an adequate primary course, and adverse reactions are uncommon and virtually never serious in children up to 10 years old. Older children and adults are more likely to have trouble from it. It is therefore best to carry out Schick tests (p. 252) on such subjects, so as to discover those for whom diphtheria immunization would be unnecessary or unwise, and to immunize the rest with the preparation known as toxoid antitoxin floccules (TAF), to which they are much less likely to react adversely. However, this preparation consists of formol toxoid that has reacted with antitoxin from an immunized horse, and therefore must not be given to anyone who is allergic to horse protein; and it is a less potent antigen than the adsorbed vaccines, so that 3 doses are required.

'Provocation poliomyelitis' is a possible complication of diphtheria immunization in a community in which polioviruses are circulating—as in Britain in the 1950s, before vaccination against poliomyelitis had been carried out here on a large scale. At that time it was found that paralysis of the injected limb occurred with a frequency of about 1 per 37 000 injections of diphtheria toxoid, and that it could follow use of formol toxoid with whooping cough vaccine or of alum-precipitated or aluminium-phosphate-adsorbed toxoid without whooping cough vaccine. It apparently depended on local tissue damage converting a non-paralytic poliovirus infection into a localized paralytic form of the disease.

Tetanus formol toxoid is itself a potent antigen, but an adsorbed vaccine is also available. For either the recommended primary course consists of 3 intramuscular or subcutaneous injections, with 6 to 12 weeks between the first two and 6 to 12 months between the second and third.

As we shall see later, diphtheria and tetanus vaccines are commonly used in combination with one another and with other vaccines, and the timing of doses is therefore a matter of finding the best compromise between the optimal schedules for individual components of the mixture.

PASSIVE IMMUNIZATION The danger to life in *diphtheria* depends largely upon circulating toxin, and there is a good chance of neutralizing this by giving intravenous diphtheria antitoxin (usually horse serum) as soon as the diagnosis is made or suspected. Since this is the only effective treatment, it must be given with the minimum of delay, but it must be preceded by a small subcutaneous dose of the serum to ensure that the patient is not sensitive to horse protein. If the test does cause any systemic reaction, desensitization must be attempted. There is virtually never any call for the prophylactic use of diphtheria antiserum.

Lesions potentially infected with *tetanus* spores are common, and their treatment would be simpler and safer if everyone was actively immunized in infancy and received regular booster injections. An injured patient could then be safely and efficiently protected by giving him a further dose of toxoid. As it is, all too often the patient either does not know or is incapable of telling the doctor that he has been actively immunized. When the immunization status of a potentially infected patient is not known, or when he is known not to have been recently immunized, it is now widely agreed that anti-tetanus serum (ATS) prepared in horses should not be given (p. 292), and that it is better to rely on preventing multiplication of the bacilli by careful surgical toilet of wounds including removal of damaged and avascular tissue and by use of antibiotics, until active immunity has been established. Human ATS is much safer to use, but more expensive and less readily available, than horse ATS used to be.

Therapeutic use of ATS is of little value, because toxin already fixed in the nervous system cannot be neutralized even by a large amount of intravenous antitoxin. All that this might be expected to achieve is neutralization of further toxin released by the bacilli, and it is better to prevent this from happening by using antibiotics. It is important to remember that an attack of tetanus does not confer immunity (probably because of the small amount of toxin involved and its inappropriate localization), and that therefore the recovered patient needs to be actively immunized to prevent further attacks.

IMMUNIZATION AGAINST PARTICULAR DISEASES DUE TO VIRUSES

Smallpox
When nearly 200 years ago Jenner introduced a safe means of immuniz- ation against smallpox (p. 9), he began the first (by many years) and one of the greatest of medicine's success stories; but it was not until 1980 that the World Health Organization's campaign for the eradication of this disease culminated in the declaration that the world was now free of it (p. 256). For the first time, therefore, we are able in this edition to omit all reference to the technical details of the procedure that gave us the word 'vaccination' (p. 293).

Poliomyelitis
Immunization against this disease, as introduced by Salk in 1953, involved repeated injections of formalin-inactivated suspensions of all 3 poliovirus types. Salk-type vaccines made a great contribution to the control of poliomyelitis, but Sabin-type vaccines, consisting of live attenuated viruses, are now in general use in the UK, the USA and many other countries, with the inactivated vaccine used only when live vaccines are contra-indicated—e.g. in pregnant women and in those with im- munodeficiencies. Live vaccines are cheaper to prepare, are taken by mouth, and have other merits (p. 291). The live viruses establish themselves in the recipient's intestinal wall, and in addition to providing him with an antigenic stimulus they are for some weeks excreted in his faeces and may be transmitted to other people around him. Immunity develops sooner and lasts longer after live-virus than after inactivated-virus vaccination, and it includes resistance to propagation of wild polioviruses in the intestine, whereas after inactivated-virus vaccination wild viruses are prevented from reaching the nervous system but are permitted to propagate in the intestine and so can be disseminated through the community. If live-virus vaccination is attempted in a community in which certain other enteroviruses are prevalent, it may be unsuccessful in

some cases because of interference (p. 161). Similarly, when vaccine strains of all 3 poliovirus types are administered simultaneously, that of one type (commonly type 2) may establish itself in the intestine to the exclusion of the other two, and the resultant immunity is against only the one type. However, the strain that 'takes' on the first occasion is in consequence unable to do so if a further dose of the trivalent vaccine is given after a suitable interval, and immunization against all 3 types can be achieved by giving 3 doses of the trivalent vaccine at monthly intervals. It is important that the course should be completed, so as to achieve protection against polioviruses as a whole, not just some of them. The phenomenon of interference can be put to good use during an outbreak, since oral vaccine given to all contacts will protect them against the wild viruses long before they have developed protective levels of antibodies.

When, as in Britain at present, the circulation of polioviruses within the community is insufficient to maintain herd immunity (the importance of which is outlined on p. 51), it is essential that it should be maintained instead by a high level of vaccination—otherwise imported viruses can cause havoc. Furthermore, the community may need protection against the vaccine strains themselves. There has been no confirmation of early fears that the virulence of these might be rapidly enhanced by a few passages through human contacts of those who had been given the vaccine. However, a slower change is going on; some of the polioviruses circulating in Britain today, and capable of causing clinical illness with neurological symptoms, have genetic characters which indicate their derivation from vaccine strains that have been able to adapt to life in the community. A falling level of herd immunity might permit such strains to cause more serious trouble. Non-immune parents should be offered vaccine at the same time as their children, to avoid any danger of the vaccine strain being transmitted to them with enhanced virulence, though the risk of this is very small. Vaccination is clearly indicated for previously unvaccinated individuals going from a country with a low prevalence of polioviruses to one where they are common.

Measles
Measles may be a severe infection, complicated by otitis media, broncho-pneumonia and even in a few cases by encephalitis. Active immuniz-ation, by means of a single injection of a chick-embryo culture of a live attenuated virus, is commonly followed by fever and rash and sometimes by bacterial infection of the respiratory tract, but these complications are far less serious than those of the natural measles which virtually every unvaccinated child acquires. Vaccination in the early months of life commonly fails to prevent subsequent development of measles, probably because maternal antibodies neutralize the vaccine. The beginning of the second year of life seems to be the best time for routine vaccination. American experience indicates that vaccination is highly effective, and that protection is still good after 14 years; but

eradication of the virus from a community requires immunization of nearly 100 % of its members.

Rubella

Immunization against this disease is discussed on pp. 175–6.

IMMUNIZATION PROGRAMMES

Active immunization of a large proportion of a population can be used either to bring a disease under control or to prevent its return to a community from which it has been eradicated. Such use of any immunizing procedure must be governed by the answers to the following questions:

(1) *Is it effective?* Smallpox vaccination had been widely used for over a century, and often with the backing of legal compulsion, before there was any formal proof of its efficacy. Today any prophylactic procedure must be tested in carefully designed trials, to ensure that any apparent benefit is not in fact due to other factors such as improved nutrition or hygiene. Part of the problem of assessing the value of whooping cough immunization (p. 295) is that the marked fall in the incidence of this disease in Britain following the introduction of general immunization occurred at a time of rapidly improving living standards.

(2) *Is it safe?* No form of vaccination is entirely free from risk—there are very few things in life which are! Safety in vaccination has to be assessed by comparison with the risks of being unvaccinated. Again, this point is illustrated by the pertussis controversy (p. 295). Poliomyelitis, on the other hand, is a disease in which the benefits from vaccination outweigh (except in a community with negligible risk of infection) the small risk of complications.

(3) *How great is the need?* In general, the need for immunization against a disease depends on the risk of acquiring it, the likelihood that the illness will be serious, and the effectiveness of available means of treating it. Yet again, whooping cough provides a clear illustration: small children need protection against it, since it is potentially lethal to them; but there is no need to immunize adults, to whom the disease presents no serious hazard, though it may be an unpleasant experience.

(4) *Is it practicable?* This depends on many social and economic factors. Repeated small outbreaks of diphtheria, with quite high death rates, have occurred in some countries which could, in theory, have prevented them, but which could not in fact afford to divert their available medical, administrative and financial resources from larger and more urgent problems.

(5) *Can it be made acceptable?* No programme of mass-immunization can succeed without popular support. This depends largely upon successful propaganda, and is much easier to secure when

the disease is still prevalent and its dire effects are known. 'Diphtheria is deadly', an effective slogan in Britain of the early 1940s, is today liable to produce the reply, 'What is diphtheria? Surely it doesn't happen any more.' Popular support also depends upon absence of disfigurement (such as large vaccination scars) and absence of unpleasant (even if harmless) reactions. One reason for never immunizing anyone who is at all unwell is that any illness which he may be incubating will be attributed to the injection. A single death *following* (not caused by) immunization outweighs much expensive propaganda. Finally, immunization is made more acceptable by minimizing the number of visits to the clinic or surgery which are necessary. This means using potent and, where possible, combined vaccines.

Immunization of large numbers of people is made easier and safer by giving intradermal injections in the form of a high-pressure jet, from an instrument which does not touch the patient and therefore cannot transmit infections such as hepatitis B (p. 276).

Combined Vaccines
In Britain it is currently recommended that young children should be immunized against diphtheria, tetanus, whooping cough, poliomyelitis and measles. If immunization against each of these diseases was carried out separately, the primary courses alone would require at least 12 administrations of vaccine. However, three doses of *triple vaccine* (diphtheria and tetanus toxoids and a killed suspension of *Bord. pertussis*) constitutes an effective primary course for the first three diseases, the whooping-cough vaccine acting as an adjuvant to enhance the efficacy of the toxoids as well as fulfilling its primary function. Three doses of oral live poliovirus vaccine can be given at the same times as the injections, so that after three visits to the doctor the child needs only to be immunized against measles (one visit). The increasing use of combined vaccines makes it necessary to consider the theoretical possibility of *antigenic competition*—impairment of response to one or other of two vaccines when the two are given together or sequentially. In practice, studies with combined vaccines have failed to show that this does occur.

Timetable for Immunization of Children
Attempts at immunization of a new-born baby are generally unsuccessful both because of the immaturity of its immune mechanisms and because maternal antibodies in the baby's circulation may interfere with the induction of an active immune response (pp. 58 and 291). BCG is an exception to this, and is effective when given at birth. If advantage is to be taken of the triple vaccine, there is a problem about when to use it. Whooping cough immunization should start as early as possible, in order to protect the infant during the dangerous period; but diphtheria and tetanus immunization are more efficient if started when the child is at least

6 months old, so a compromise is necessary. The schedule of immuniz-
ations currently recommended for use in Britain is as follows:

At 3 months old	
Again 6–8 weeks later	Triple vaccine (see above)
Again 4–6 months later	and oral poliovirus vaccine
At 1–2 years	Measles vaccine
At 5 years (school entry)	Single booster doses of diphtheria/tet-anus toxoids and oral poliovirus vaccine
At 10–13 years	BCG for tuberculin-negative children
At 11–13 years	Rubella vaccine for all girls
At 15–19 years (school leaving)	Single booster doses of tetanus toxoid and oral poliovirus vaccine

In any community in which infants run a high risk of tuberculous
infection, BCG should be given at or soon after birth. In Britain this
applies to some immigrant groups, but for most people adolescence is the
period of greatest risk.

Vaccination for International Travel
To pass from one country to another a traveller may need to produce
certificates of recent vaccination against one or more diseases. The details
depend on his country of origin and his route, and vary from country to
country and from time to time in accordance with the distribution of foci
of active disease and the current anxieties of health authorities. The
prospective traveller should make sure of the prevailing regulations by
asking travel agents or official representatives of the countries to which he
is going. Vaccination against yellow fever (obtainable only at specially
designated centres) and an International Certificate of such vaccination
are required for entry into some of the Central African countries in which
this disease is endemic, and also for entry into many countries when
travelling from the endemic zones of Africa and South America. The
certificate becomes valid 10 days after primary vaccination or immediately after revaccination, and remains so for 10 years. Vaccination
against cholera, though of little efficacy, is required for entry into some
countries, and immunization against typhoid, poliomyelitis and various
other diseases may be recommended. Travellers to any of the numerous
countries where hepatitis A is common should be given human normal
immunoglobulin (p. 292), which protects against this disease for a few
months. Chemoprophylaxis against malaria (p. 206), though it does not
belong under the heading of vaccination, must be included in the
provisions made for travel to any country where there is a risk of
acquiring this disease.

Contra-indications to Vaccination
Live vaccines should not be given to patients with defective immunity,
whether primary or due to such causes as leukaemia, lymphoma, other

widespread malignant disease or treatment with immunosuppressive drugs; and oral poliovirus vaccine should not be given to family contacts of such patients. Live virus vaccines should not be given to pregnant women, because of the risk (theoretical at least) of damage to the foetus. Patients allergic to eggs may have serious hypersensitivity reactions to vaccines grown in eggs, which include yellow fever vaccine and some rabies vaccines.

Suggestions for Further Reading
Immunisation by George Dick (Update Books, London/New Jersey, 1978).

CHAPTER 21

ANTIBACTERIAL DRUGS*

PERSPECTIVE

Up until 1935 no drugs were available for the treatment of systemic bacterial infections other than syphilis. Doctors could do no more than treat symptoms and, with the invaluable help of nurses, look after the patient's general condition while he overcame the infection himself, or failed to do so. Then came the sulphonamides and other drugs for systemic treatment of bacterial infections, notably the antibiotics. The situation was rapidly transformed, and the morbidity and mortality of bacterial infections were dramatically reduced (p. 10). It is hardly possible to overestimate the importance of antibacterial drugs.

However, this is far from meaning that today the correct answer to a bacterial infection is simply to give the right antibacterial drug. In many cases, as we shall see, choosing the right drug is by no means simple. Furthermore, choosing the right drug is only part of the right management of the patient. The doctor who treats pneumonia merely by giving a suitable antibiotic, and forgets the principles of general medical and nursing care and the importance, for example, of giving oxygen for anoxia, may lose his patient even though he cures the infection. Similarly, the surgeon who ignores the rules of aseptic surgery and relies on antibiotics to prevent or cure wound sepsis is on the way to disaster. Antibacterial drugs must be seen in proper perspective. To use them is to intervene in the struggle between the host's defences and the invading organisms. If the weapons are rightly chosen and rightly used, such intervention is likely to be decisive; but at no time can we afford to neglect the defender's morale or supplies, or to allow the invaders to build up massive reinforcements.

---

* Information about drugs for use against viruses, fungi or protozoa is to be found in Chapters 11 to 13.

Hazards

Neither can we afford to forget that antibacterial drugs are foreign substances so far as the patient's body is concerned, and are potentially harmful to him. They vary in the frequency and severity of their adverse effects, but none of them is perfectly safe, and almost all of them have on occasions killed patients. Most of the troubles for which they are responsible fall into the following three categories:

(1) *Direct toxicity to host cells.* These drugs are necessarily toxic to living cells; but their clinical usefulness depends on *selective toxicity* (p. 35)—i.e. upon their being substantially more toxic to bacterial than to host cells. The β-lactams, which act on bacteria by interfering with a process not shared by mammalian cells (p. 35), are in general free from direct host toxicity, except at very high levels or by unrelated mechanisms (e.g. the nephrotoxicity of cephaloridine). In contrast, trimethoprim interferes with a process common to bacterial and mammalian cells (folate synthesis—p. 324), but its greater affinity for the relevant bacterial enzymes than for their mammalian counterpart ensures that only when given in prolonged high dosage does it interfere with the process in the host. Cephaloridine, mentioned above, is by no means the only antibacterial drug which is toxic to the host by a mechanism unrelated to its antibacterial action; the ototoxicity of aminoglycosides is one of very many other possible illustrations of such an effect. In the very early days of chemotherapy Ehrlich introduced the concept of the *therapeutic index*, which is (the maximum tolerated dose) ÷ (the minimum curative dose). As patients vary in tolerance and bacteria in drug-sensitivity, this index can never be given a precise numerical value, but the underlying concept is important; and for every antibacterial drug that has been developed for clinical use there are many that have been tested and rejected because this index was too close to or even below unity. (This problem is even more serious in relation to antiviral drugs—see p. 164—since the metabolic processes of virus replication are in fact host-cell processes.)

(2) *Hypersensitivity reactions.* Patients may become hypersensitive to almost any antibacterial (and indeed, almost any other) drug, but the antibacterial drugs with which this type of problem is most commonly encountered are the penicillins, otherwise the least harmful of antibiotics. Penicillin hypersensitivity may be of any of the four types described in Chapter 8—rashes (Type IV), serum-sickness-like reactions with urticaria, fever and arthralgia (Type III), haemolytic anaemia (Type II) or anaphylactic shock (Type I). Hypersensitivity is not merely unpleasant or dangerous in itself; it also means that the patient is in future deprived of the possibility of being treated with the drugs to which he has become hypersensitive—and in practice this all too often means that the use of an antibiotic for a condition for which it was unnecessary or inappropriate debars its subsequent use in a more

serious situation in which it might have been extremely valuable.

(3) *Alteration of the host's bacterial flora.* The doctor who prescribes an antibacterial drug is aiming it at a known or suspected pathogen, but the drug itself is by no means so selective! As we have indicated in earlier chapters, man's normal bacterial population is of great value to him, and any major interference with it can have unpleasant and sometimes serious consequences (pp. 19, 80 and 112). The availability of powerful antibiotics has made such interference possible, and indeed easy to achieve. Freed from the restraining influence of their more numerous but antibiotic-sensitive neighbours, more resistant organisms that are normally present only in small numbers—e.g. *C. albicans, Ps. aeruginosa* and some of the enterobacteria—may be able to proliferate vigorously and may become 'opportunist' pathogens, particularly if the patient is debilitated or immunologically deficient. Furthermore, antibiotic-resistant variants of the pathogen for which the patient is being treated, or of any other pathogen that he may be carrying, may be present as a result of mutation or plasmid-transfer (pp. 27 and 28); and if so, the selective advantage conferred on them by the antibiotic treatment may enable them to multiply and so both to cause serious trouble to the patient and to be transmitted to other patients or potential patients in his vicinity. We shall return later in the chapter to the problem of bacterial resistance to drugs; here we would simply point out that a large part of the problem has been created by their use (wise or unwise).

USE AND ABUSE OF ANTIBACTERIAL DRUGS

As far back as 1956 Professor Jawetz, one of America's leading authorities on this subject, hazarded a guess that not more than 5 to 10 % of the vast output of antibiotics was employed on proper clinical indications. He went on to give a vivid description of the various pressures, notably from the manufacturers and from patients and their relatives, which cause doctors to misuse such drugs. The number of new antibacterial drugs introduced since 1956 has increased our capacity both for effective treatment and for misunderstanding and mistakes, and it may well be that Jawetz's estimate is not far from the truth today. To provide his patients with optimal antibacterial therapy the doctor needs to answer a number of questions, which we can group under three headings: *Why?*, *Which?*, and *How?*.

WHY does this patient need antibacterial treatment?
This is the most important of the questions. Unless there is a valid reason—scientific, not just social or emotional—for giving an antibacterial drug, the patient would probably be better off without it. (For a placebo effect it is usually possible to choose something safer and cheaper.) Valid reasons include the following:

(1) *Treatment of a known or suspected bacterial infection* that is unlikely to undergo rapid and satisfactory spontaneous resolution, and that can be expected, on the available evidence, to respond to the drug given.

Patients in the early stages of acute upper respiratory tract infections are commonly given oral penicillin or some other antibiotic. This is often a clear example of the misuse of such drugs, since the infection is usually caused by a virus and is likely to be rapidly self-limiting; the antibiotics cannot therefore be expected to do good but may well do harm. However, if the patient has tonsillitis or pharyngitis and there are clinical, epidemiological or bacteriological reasons for suspecting that it is due to *Str. pyogenes*, penicillin treatment is indicated.

Sometimes a patient is known to have a bacterial infection due to an organism which is sensitive to antibiotics *in vitro*, but their clinical use is contra-indicated by existing knowledge. For example, attempted antibiotic treatment of enteritis due to the 'food-poisoning' salmonellae commonly results merely in prolonged carriage and excretion of the offending organism (p. 116).

On many occasions, however, use of antibacterial drugs is clearly indicated. Patients with lobar pneumonia, purulent meningitis, serious post-operative wound infections, or specific bacterial infections such as typhoid, tuberculosis, syphilis or gonorrhoea—to name but a few of many possible examples—must receive prompt and effective anti-bacterial treatment. In many other cases the indications are less clear, but one or more antibacterial drugs should be given because of the probability that the patient has a bacterial infection, or of the possibility that he has such an infection which could be serious unless treated promptly. However, as we shall see more clearly when we come to our next question, if there is any doubt about the presence or nature of a bacterial infection it is the doctor's duty to ensure that so far as possible all necessary specimens for precise bacteriological diagnosis are collected before antibacterial treatment is given.

(2) *Prevention of bacterial infection.* There are a few definite indications for prophylactic administration of antibacterial drugs, such as the following:

(*a*) Patients who have had rheumatic fever need to be protected, especially during childhood, from *Str. pyogenes* infections which might precipitate further attacks. Fortunately this species is always highly susceptible to penicillin and nearly always to the sulphonamides, and either of these can safely be given in prolonged low dosage for prophylaxis.

(*b*) Patients with congenitally abnormal, diseased or prosthetic heart valves run the risk of developing bacterial endocarditis. This risk is increased by procedures that result in bacteraemia, notably major dental treatment—especially extraction—and tonsillectomy.

In such cases the offending organism is usually an oropharyngeal streptococcus, often of the viridans group (p. 88). Similarly, enterococcal endocarditis may follow prostatectomy or other genito-urinary tract surgery or instrumentation in such patients. It is debatable whether they are at increased risk following gastro-intestinal tract instrumentation. Prophylaxis against such risks consists of ensuring that on entering the blood the bacteria encounter antibiotic concentrations that will kill them before they reach and establish themselves on the heart valves. Such antibiotic cover should begin only just before the relevant procedure, so as to allow no time for proliferation of resistant bacteria; and probably does not need to be continued for more than 12 hours. Work with animal models has suggested that the most effective cover might be penicillin or ampicillin + streptomycin or gentamicin, by injection; but there is evidence from studies in man that a single large oral dose of amoxycillin (a very well absorbed oral penicillin) may be all that is needed.

(c) Operations involving the intestine, particularly the appendix, colon and rectum, almost inevitably result in some contamination of the peritoneal cavity and incised tissues with mixed intestinal flora. Various procedures for pre-operative 'gut sterilization' have been tried, without convincing evidence of success; but 'peri-operative prophylaxis', starting just before or during operation and continued for a few days, can reduce the frequency of wound infections. Its aim is not to alter the intestinal flora but to prevent intestinal organisms from colonizing and invading the incised tissues. Metronidazole (p. 325) is highly effective in such prophylaxis, because of the special importance of *Bacteroides* and other anaerobes in the establishment of these wound infections (p. 130), because of its selective activity against such organisms, and because it is well absorbed from the intestine and has little effect on anaerobes there but does achieve effective levels in the tissues.

(d) *Cl. perfringens* and other clostridia are predictably sensitive to penicillin (and to metronidazole, but the value of this drug in the situations that we are about to describe has not yet been assessed). Patients at special risk of developing gas-gangrene (clostridial myositis) include: those who have suffered major trauma with soil contamination; those who have lower limb amputations for vascular disease; and those who have operations on their hip-joints or femoral heads. These 3 classes of patient have in common the presence of devitalized muscle or bone fragments and the likelihood of clostridial contamination of these—due, in the last two classes, to the frequency with which the patient's intestinal clostridia are to be found on the skin of the thigh and the difficulty of eradicating these sporing organisms by pre-operative skin preparation. For all such patients penicillin prophylaxis is indicated.

Antibacterial prophylaxis can be justified in a few more conditions—e.g. extensive burns, open heart surgery, leukaemic patients with severe marrow depression, and some patients with recurrent urinary tract infections—but in most others it is likely to do more harm than good. Antibiotics are frequently given to patients with virus infections, in order to prevent superinfection by bacteria. This is nearly always unwise; its most likely result is to ensure that the superinfection is by antibiotic-resistant bacteria and therefore more difficult to treat. Attempted prophylaxis against pneumonia in paralysed, unconscious or debilitated patients has much the same effect. In general it is better to wait until bacterial infection occurs and then treat it with an appropriate drug.

WHICH drug or drugs should this patient receive?
This question breaks down into a number of subsidiary questions:

(1) *What is the pathogen, and to which drugs is it sensitive?*
Proper use of antibacterial drugs requires that the problem be defined as closely as possible, so that the best tool or tools for dealing with it can be selected. Sometimes the patient's clinical condition is characteristic of the activities of a particular pathogen—e.g. a typical staphylococcal abscess, typhoid or syphilis—and the drug sensitivities of that organism are predictable enough for a suitable drug to be chosen without waiting for laboratory help. Sometimes an illness could be due to any of a number of organisms but stained smears of pathological material give all the information that is needed; pneumococci may be recognized microscopically, for example, in pus from otitis media or in cerebro-spinal fluid from meningitis, and can be relied upon to be sensitive to penicillin (in most countries). But in many cases in which immediate drug treatment is necessary, it has at first to be based on informed guesses as to the organism and its sensitivities. Except in an emergency or when no laboratory facilities are available, *all specimens necessary for the isolation of the causative organism should be collected before treatment is started.* If this is not done, treatment may obscure the diagnosis without being adequate to effect a cure. For example, a patient may have a streptococcal endocarditis which has not yet been diagnosed. If he is given bacteriostatic tetracycline treatment before blood cultures have been set up, it may then be impossible to isolate the organism. His clinical picture may be temporarily improved, but it is highly unlikely that cure will result (p. 310). When tetracycline treatment stops, he is likely to relapse, and his proper investigation and treatment will have been delayed by some weeks. Whenever initial treatment has been based on guesses, it needs to be reviewed in the light of subsequent laboratory reports about the nature and sensitivities of the organism isolated. However, the ultimate test of a drug's suitablity is its therapeutic effect; laboratory sensitivity reports are at best only an indication of probabilities, and if the patient is responding well to the initial treatment, it is usually unwise to act upon

a report which suggests that he ought not to be doing so! In many cases there is no urgent need to start treatment until the laboratory report is available.

(2) *Narrow or broad spectrum?*

The ultimate in precision tools for dealing with identified pathogens—a dream in Ehrlich's time and still no more than a dream—would be an array of drugs, each one of which would with antibody-like precision attack one pathogenic species, leaving other micro-organisms and the host intact. At the other extreme would be a drug which would deal with all bacterial (and preferably other) pathogens. This might be a pharmaceutical manufacturer's dream, as he might hope that all doctors would give it to most of their patients; but to a bacteriologist it is more like a nightmare, because of its inevitable complex side-effects. Real-life antibacterial drugs come between these hypothetical extremes. Cloxacillin, benzyl penicillin, the macrolides and the polymyxins have useful levels of activity against only some parts of the 'spectrum' of bacterial genera, whereas some of the other penicillins, the aminoglycosides, chloramphenicol, the tetracyclines and others are effective against at least some members of most genera, and are often referred to as 'broad spectrum' antibiotics (particularly by manufacturers, who are naturally concerned to promote their wide-spread use). In practice, when the identity of the infecting organism is known or virtually certain the doctor's primary question about any particular antibiotic is not about the width of its spectrum but about its suitability for dealing with this pathogen; though when there is a choice between drugs that are equally appropriate in other respects, narrowness of spectrum is an asset, at least in theory. On the other hand, when the pathogen has not been identified or when there is more than one pathogen to be treated, it may be best to use a drug with a spectrum wide enough to cover all the probable or known organisms. The alternative approach is to use more than one drug—see below.

(3) *Cidal or static?*

It appears to be true of the treatment of most bacterial infections that there is no need to use drugs that can kill the invading organisms; if they are prevented from multiplying, the patient's own defence mechanisms can eliminate them. However, there are exceptions to this general statement. It is essential to use bactericidal therapy when the patient's immunological defences are seriously impaired, or when the infection is overwhelming. Chronic bronchitics may have longer spells free of bronchial suppuration if the offending organisms, in the bronchial lumen and so apparently beyond the reach of the host's defences, are eradicated by treatment rather than merely suppressed (p. 337). But the classic, and in some ways the most surprising, example of a disease in which bactericidal treatment is required is bacterial endocarditis. It might seem that organisms in fibrinous vegetations in the heart and major blood vessels were well within the reach of blood cells and antibodies, but in fact all available evidence indicates that in such a site they are unusually well protected against both of these. Bacteriostatic treatment, so long as it is continued, may bring about apparent cure; but the organisms persist inside the vegetations, ready to resume activity when the treatment stops. They require treatment with drugs that can kill them (p. 335).

(4) One drug or drugs?

It is possible to demonstrate *in vitro* four types of results when antimicrobial drugs are mixed: *indifference*, the combined effect being indistinguishable from that of the more powerful drug used alone; *addition*, the combined effect being the sum of the individual effects; *synergy*, the combined effect being greater than can be explained by simple addition; and *antagonism*, the combined effect being less than that of the more powerful drug used alone. The type of result depends upon drug concentrations, the microbial strain used and many other factors, and it is therefore meaningless to describe a drug combination as synergic or antagonistic without specifying the circumstances of such interaction. In general, synergy is likely to be observed only in a mixture of two bactericidal drugs (e.g. a β-lactam + an aminoglycoside) and antagonism only in a mixture of one bactericidal and one bacteriostatic drug (e.g. a β-lactam + tetracycline). In at least some instances the mechanism of antagonism appears to be that the bacteriostatic drug prevents the organisms from multiplying and so from entering the phase of growth in which they are susceptible to the bactericidal drug.

These various types of result also occur *in vivo*. Antagonism was clearly illustrated as far back as 1951 in one series of cases of pneumococcal meningitis, in which the mortality of patients treated with penicillin + tetracycline considerably exceeded that of comparable patients treated with penicillin alone. The possibility of such an interaction is a strong warning against the use of drug-combinations without definite reasons. Furthermore, use of more than one drug increases the likelihood of adverse reactions; and when these occur in such circumstances it may be difficult or impossible to decide which of the drugs should be discontinued and might be dangerous if given to this patient on future occasions. Drug incompatibilities are also possible (see below), and the expense is of course increased—a factor which we have not mentioned so far in this chapter, but which needs to be considered in many decisions about antibacterial therapy. However, there are situations in which it is justifiable and may even be essential to use combinations of antibacterial drugs, including the following:

(a) When the patient is suffering from infection with two or more organisms and no single drug is likely to be effective against both or all.

(b) As a temporary measure in a severe acute illness which might be due to any of several organisms and when again no single drug is likely to be effective against them all—see p. 336 (meningitis).

(c) To prevent the emergence of resistant strains—see p. 317 (drug resistance), p. 335 (*Staph. aureus* infections) and p. 338 (tuberculosis).

(d) When synergy can be expected—see p. 324 (cotrimoxazole), p. 335 (bacterial endocarditis).

(e) When there is empirical evidence that a particular combination gives the best results—see p. 128 (treatment of brucellosis).

(5) *Is it compatible with other medication?*
Even when an antibacterial drug is appropriate in all other respects for treating an infection, it may be contra-indicated or may have to be given with special precautions because of its possible interactions with other drugs that the patient is receiving. Some combinations of drugs are physically or chemically incompatible when mixed in high concentrations. Thus when a doctor prescribes two or more antibiotics which are to be mixed before injection or are to be given together in an intravenous infusion, he needs to be sure that they do not precipitate or inactivate one another. Similarly, when giving any antibiotic by slow intravenous infusion he must be sure that it is not adversely affected by other components of the infusion fluid (e.g. the aminoglycosides are incompatible with heparin, and ampicillin is fairly rapidly inactivated in the presence of 5% dextrose). This is clearly of great practical importance, since incompatibility may result in a patient never having an effective blood level of an antibiotic which is being given in apparently adequate doses. Also very important, and in general even more serious in their consequences, are the pharmacological incompatibilities of some drug combinations at the levels achieved in the patient. Renal damage may follow the giving of gentamicin with cephaloridine, for example, or of one of these with either of the diuretics frusemide or ethacrynic acid; and either nalidixic acid or cotrimoxazole may enhance the effects of anticoagulant drugs and lead to severe bleeding. As more new drugs are introduced, and more undesirable interactions between older ones are recognized, this subject becomes increasingly complex and worrying. Information about known incompatibilities involving antibacterial drugs is to be found in tables in the two books *Antibiotic and Chemotherapy* and *Antibiotics in Clinical Practice* mentioned at the end of this chapter.

HOW should the drug or drugs be given?
This question overlaps with the previous one at many points. For example, however appropriate a drug may be for dealing with a particular pathogen, it is not the right one for the patient if it can be given only in a form inappropriate to his situation—e.g. orally to a patient who is vomiting, intramuscularly to one with a severe bleeding tendency, or

intravenously to an out-patient. Nor is it sufficient to be able to give the drug to the patient; having been given, it must be capable of arriving at the site of the infection in adequate concentration. We therefore have to think about the route by which a drug can be delivered, not merely into the patient but to the place where it is needed; and also about dosage.

(1) *Route*

For a superficial infection of the skin or an accessible mucous surface it may be possible to apply the drug in high concentration directly to the lesion; but unfortunately such topical application, notably of the penicillins, is particularly liable to provoke a hypersensitivity reaction and so to deprive the patient of subsequent systemic use of the group of antibiotics in question. A different form of local application that gives less trouble and is sometimes indicated is direct injection into a body cavity—intrapleural, intraperitoneal, intrathecal or intra-ocular, for example.

Oral administration is possible only if the drug can be produced in a palatable form; if it survives the action of the gastric secretions (or can be protected from it in capsules that dissolve in the small intestine); if it does not provoke significant gastro-intestinal upset; and above all if it is reliably absorbed into the blood (unless its site of action is to be the bowel lumen) and passes through the liver without being inactivated. Sometimes an ester or other derivative, itself not an effective antibacterial drug but a 'pro-drug', meets all of these requirements and is converted into the active form after absorption. Oral preparations have, in addition to their unsuitability for patients who are vomiting or cannot swallow, the disadvantage that their absorption may be unreliable in very ill patients, in whom it is particularly important to achieve good levels rapidly and consistently. Some antibacterials, notably metronidazole, are well absorbed when given as rectal suppositories, provided that the patient does not have diarrhoea.

Parenteral (i.e. non-alimentary) administration is usually intramuscular or intravenous. For intramuscular injection it is necessary to produce a strong solution (so that the volume is tolerable) which is of physiological pH and which does not cause excessive pain, or damage the injected muscle; this is not possible for some antibiotics. Also, having been injected, the drug must be rapidly and reliably absorbed into the blood (unless it is deliberately given as a slow-release depot preparation, as is sometimes done with penicillin). Intravenous injection or infusion is in some ways the ideal way of getting a drug into the blood, but it is seldom the most practicable or convenient. Furthermore, some drugs are difficult to give repeatedly by this route because they cause local phlebitis and thrombosis and a consequent shortage of accessible veins.

Once in the blood stream, drugs vary in their distribution to tissues and body fluids and in their renal handling, and therefore a high blood level is no guarantee of good tissue levels. Indeed, a high and sustained blood level could well be due to the drug's inability to get out of the blood! Part of this variability in tissue penetration is related to differences in binding to plasma proteins. Virtually all antibacterials are bound to some degree, but some very much more than others—even others in the same group. There is a reversible equilibrium between bound and unbound drug, but it may be only the unbound portion that is free to diffuse out of the circulation—and even then its troubles are by no means over, as it may bind to tissue proteins. Bound drug may be inactive against bacteria, so two drugs may give comparable total levels but with one mostly bound and inactive and the other mostly free and active.

Rapid excretion of an antibacterial drug by the kidneys may make it highly suitable for dealing with urinary tract infections (p. 337), provided that it is not, like chloramphenicol, excreted mainly in an inactive form (p. 331). Such rapid excretion also necessarily means that blood and tissue levels are not well sustained—which may be an advantage, as we shall see below, under (2) (*a*). Conversely, persistent high levels will be achieved if a drug that is not excreted in bile or metabolized in the liver or elsewhere is only slowly excreted by the kidneys—either because of its nature or because of renal failure.

Antibacterial drugs also vary widely in their ability to pass into body fluids other than urine. For example, sulphadiazine or chloramphenicol levels in the cerebrospinal fluid are usually $40-80\%$ of the prevailing blood levels. On the other hand, only traces of the penicillins or of streptomycin reach the cerebrospinal fluid from the blood if the meninges are healthy; though much larger amounts go through and much higher cerebrospinal fluid levels are achieved when the meninges are inflamed, and high concentrations can be achieved by direct intrathecal or intraventicular injection (but see pp. 336—7). Similarly, when ampicillin is used in treatment of suppurative chronic bronchitis it may pass fairly readily into the sputum at first, but as the infection is brought under control and the sputum ceases to be purulent its ampicillin content falls sharply. Antibiotics vary greatly in their ability to cross the placenta and reach the liquor. Penicillins do it particularly well, and liquor concentrations may exceed those in blood. These examples indicate something of the complexity of a subject which is of great clinical importance but is far from being thoroughly understood.

(2) *Dosage*

Nowhere in this chapter do we go into details about dosage schedules for individual drugs; these are to be found in the books mentioned at the end of the chapter, as well as in the manufacturers' literature and in many other places. However, we do need to consider some general principles.

'Give enough, for long enough, and then stop'. This facile generalization embodies three important points:

(*a*) *'Enough'* The aim of antibacterial treatment must be to ensure a drug level at the site or sites of infection which is sufficient to kill or inhibit the pathogen. The patient must therefore be given his drug in doses adequate to achieve this, with due allowance for his size and other factors that may affect the distribution of the drug. To give him less than this is to deny him the help of the antibiotic without necessarily sparing him the hazards; it may well encourage development of drug-resistance by the pathogen or by other potential pathogens; and it is a waste of the drug and of money. When bacteriostasis is the aim, theoretical considerations suggest that an effective concentration should be maintained all the time. The same is not necessarily true for a bactericidal effect. For example, since the action of penicillins is on cell wall formation, they can do nothing to a bacterium which is inhibited and not trying to make cell wall; and it is still debatable, after all the years for which we have had penicillins to use, whether the best mode of attack is by a sustained high level or by a transitory high level ('peak'), followed by a period ('trough') during which the level is low enough to allow any survivors to resume multiplication and so to be susceptible to the next peak. Sometimes toxicity also has to be considered. For example, with gentamicin it is possible to produce toxic effects (mainly on the 8th nerve) by maintaining a blood level that is never high enough to be cidal to any but the most susceptible pathogens; it is therefore essential to achieve bactericidal peak levels but to ensure that for most of the time between doses there is a trough that is below the toxic level. With this and related drugs, laboratory monitoring of both peak and trough levels can be an important aid to treatment. This is particularly so when impaired renal function makes it difficult to predict the rate at which the drug will be excreted, and therefore the interval between peaks which is necessary to ensure adequate troughs.

(*b*) *'For long enough'*. The length of treatment necessary to eradicate a bacterial infection depends, obviously enough, on the nature and location of the pathogen. The tubercle bacillus, with its very long generation time by comparison with most bacteria, needs months or even years of treatment. A pathogen that is well 'dug in' in a fibrotic chronic lesion may call for considerably longer treatment than one that has just arrived and is causing an acute infection. The need for prolonged treatment in brucellosis is probably due to the relatively protected situation of the brucellae inside host cells. But so far as any generalization is permissible, it seems to be true that for many acute bacterial infections it is appropriate to give an antibacterial drug for 5–7 days. By then it will probably have done its job—or failed to do it, in which case a change of treatment is indicated and may well have taken place already. Unfortunately patients who are not closely supervised, including doctors themselves, commonly give up or forget their drugs as soon as symptoms are abating; relapse of infection following inadequate treatment is therefore all too common. Perhaps we need to learn more from the veterinary profession about the value of a single very large dose of an antibacterial. Venereologists, with their special problems,of patient supervision, have made some progress in this direction (pp. 95 and 141); and there is now evidence that acute urinary tract infections can often be treated effectively in one day, or even by a single dose.

(c) *'And then stop'*. No good purpose is likely to be served, and harm can be done, by continuing to give an antibacterial drug after it has had a proper chance to do its job. 'Tailing off'—i.e. continuing for a while with reduced doses—is even more deplorable.

DRUG RESISTANCE

Resistance of a given organism to an antibacterial drug is seldom absolute; it can usually be overcome by increasing the drug concentration. However, in the clinical context an organism is said to be resistant if it is not killed or inhibited by drug concentrations readily attainable in the patient. (This usually means blood and tissue concentrations; an organism resistant to these may of course be sensitive to the higher concentrations attainable in urine or by topical application.)

Even the broadest of broad-spectrum antibacterial drugs is ineffective against some bacterial genera, against some species of other genera, and usually against some strains of species that are in general sensitive to it. Bacterial resistance may be due to one or more of the following:

(1) Relative impermeability of the bacterial cell wall or cell membrane to the drug in question, so that it has difficulty in reaching its target site. For example, Gram-negative bacteria in general are resistant to penicillin and some related drugs, to some extent at least, because these cannot readily penetrate the lipopolysaccharide/lipoprotein outer membranes of their cell walls and reach the target enzymes at the mucopeptide-synthesis sites within the cell walls.

(2) Lack of a suitable intracellular target. Examples are sulphonamide-resistance due to possession of a dihydrofolic acid reductase that does not 'confuse' sulphonamides with PABA (p. 33); and streptomycin-resistance due to lack of a ribosomal protein to which streptomycin can bind.

(3) Ability of the bacteria to switch to alternative metabolic pathways unaffected by the drug.

(4) Ability of the bacteria (whatever their intrinsic sensitivity to the drug in question) to produce enzymes that destroy or inactivate it. Such enzymes may be cell-bound or may be released into the environment of

the bacteria; and their production may be constitutive or inducible (p. 21). Examples of such enzymes are the β-lactamases, which open up the β-lactam rings of penicillins and cephalosporins (p. 329); and the acetyltransferases that acetylate chloramphenicol, and in so doing inactivate it as an antibacterial agent.

Despite the limited range of effectiveness of any one antibacterial drug even when it is first introduced, a small selection from our present vast armoury of such drugs would have been sufficient, had they become available simultaneously in the 1930s, to deal with the great majority of pathogenic bacteria then in circulation. In fact, however, new drugs have appeared on the scene gradually; and in most cases the arrival of a newcomer and its widespread use have been followed by proliferation of bacterial strains, including pathogens, resistant to it. *Staph. aureus* has been notably successful in keeping pace with new discoveries. In relation to penicillin evolution of new strains has played a relatively small part, the increase in frequency of penicillin-resistant *Staph. aureus* being largely due to a 'take-over' by existing resistant strains as their more sensitive colleagues were eliminated. But with most other drugs a more important mechanism is that sensitive strains give rise to occasional resistant mutants; these normally have no particular survival value and indeed may be at a disadvantage when in a non-selective environment, but in the presence of an appropriate concentration of the drug in question they alone are able to multiply, giving rise to a new strain with increased drug resistance (p. 27). In most cases each mutation involves only a small increase in resistance, and therefore such selection depends upon the drug concentration being not much above the minimum to which the original strain is sensitive; but with streptomycin in particular a marked increase in resistance may develop by a single mutational jump rather than by a series of short steps.

Prevention of the emergence of resistant mutants is one of the main indications for the clinical use of combinations of drugs (p. 312). As a result of spontaneous mutation, one cell in every thousand million (10^9) might be resistant to drug A and one in 10^{12} might be resistant to drug B. 10^9 and 10^{12} are not very large populations by bacteriological standards. But provided that the mechanisms of action of the two drugs are unrelated, the incidence of cells resistant to both should be one in $10^9 \times 10^{12}$, which is a very large population. Therefore if both drugs are given in adequate dosage, the risk of the emergence of a resistant strain is very much less than if either is used alone.

Resistance to one or more antibiotics can be transmitted from one bacterial strain to a related but previously sensitive strain by bacteriophage transduction (p. 28). This is the main mechanism for transmission of antibiotic resistance between Gram-positive cocci, and occurs in other bacterial groups, but it is not yet clear whether it is an important source of therapeutic problems. *Transferable* or *infective resistance* among Gram-negative bacteria, on the other hand, is undoubtedly a major threat to the antibiotic control of bacterial diseases. As explained on p. 28, it depends on bacterial conjugation and transfer of plasmids. It is important for the following reasons:

(1) The transferable plasmids commonly determine resistance to several unrelated drugs, and organisms possessing them have a selective advantage in the presence of any one of these drugs. Thus, for example, the reduction in numbers of streptomycin-sensitive organisms in the intestines of a streptomycin-treated patient or animal may favour the growth of an enterobacterial strain resistant to streptomycin and also (incidentally) to other aminoglycosides, tetracyclines, chloramphenicol and sulphonamides, substances which the patient or animal has never received.

(2) Such plasmids are transferable not merely to related strains of the same species but to strains of other species and genera. Thus a patient under treatment with streptomycin for tuberculosis might have a large population of multiple-resistant but harmless *Esch. coli* in his intestine as a result of the mechanism described in the last paragraph; he might then ingest some shigellae or salmonellae to which the plasmids determining the multiple resistance could be transferred in his intestine; and these pathogens might then be unresponsive to treatment with any of the drugs concerned. Strains of *Sh. flexneri* resistant to chloramphenicol and various other antibiotics were current in Mexico before 1972, and in that year *S. typhi* strains with the same resistance pattern appeared there and were isolated in Britain and other countries from patients who had acquired them in Mexico. These *S. typhi* strains were resistant by virtue of plasmids which they had presumably acquired from the *Sh. flexneri* strains, either directly or via intestinal commensals, probably other enterobacteria. Furthermore, it is not only to one another that enterobacteria can transfer plasmids coding for resistance; *N. gonorrhoeae* and *H. influenzae* strains that produce β-lactamases by virtue of plasmids acquired from enterobacteria have become world-wide problems.

(3) It is possible for multiple-resistant enterobacteria to develop in farm animals and be transmitted to man. Some antibiotics are widely used as food supplements for young animals, since partial suppression of intestinal flora can accelerate their weight gain. Prophylactic and therapeutic administration of antibiotics to sick farm animals is also widespread, and often economically important, but it is uncoordinated. Resistant organisms that have proliferated as a result of such antibiotic usage have excellent opportunities for dissemination because of the prevailing conditions for maintenance and marketing of stock and because of the transfer of young animals from farm to farm. Multiresistant strains of *S. typhimurium* have arisen in recent years among cattle in Britain as a result of sequential acquisition of resistance

factors, and are now widespread among calves. There have been cases of infection with such strains among farm-workers and families who drank unpasteurized milk, and there have been several deaths—in part because of the difficulty of finding of suitable antibiotic for treatment of an invasive infection by such an organism.

(4) There is no reason to suppose that what happens among farm animals following widespread use of antibiotics does not also happen, in some measure at least, in human populations similarly treated. For some years development of resistance by man's bacterial flora was mainly a problem of hospitals, where antibacterial drugs are most heavily used and where they can be detected in the dust and even in the air! However, it now seems that widespread use of antibacterials in general practice encourages the spread through the community of multiple-resistant strains brought home by patients returning from hospital, and may even be responsible for adding others that are 'home-grown'.

Although the progressive sophistication of man's bacterial flora, including his pathogens, appears to be an inevitable consequence of the use of antibacterial drugs, we cannot afford to have a complacent or defeatist attitude to this growing problem of drug resistance. There are ways in which we can slow down or arrest its growth. As we have indicated repeatedly, antibacterial drugs should not be prescribed—to men or to animals—without valid indications for doing so. We have also indicated other precautions that should be observed so as to minimize the proliferation of resistant strains—such as isolating patients who are distributing these strains into their environments; always giving antibacterial drugs in adequate doses; and using drug combinations when appropriate. Another approach to the problem that has had some successes is to introduce an *antibiotic policy* for a hospital or area. This usually involves designating certain antibiotics as available for general use but withdrawing others from circulation or permitting their use only on rare and special occasions. If all goes well (and in particular, if all relevant clinicians abide by the policy), the incidence of strains resistant to the reserved antibiotics falls considerably in the months following institution of the policy, and in due course it may be judged right to reintroduce these drugs for general use and to withdraw others.

LABORATORY PROCEDURES

Sensitivity tests

We said on p. 309 that the proper use of antibacterial drugs requires that the problem be defined as closely as possible. Frequently an important part of that definition is to determine the antibacterial sensitivities of the pathogen. We described on p. 3 one of the rapid methods for doing this which may before long be in routine use, but at present most routine diagnostic laboratories use some form of disk-plate method. In essence, this involves inoculating the whole surface of a plate of suitable culture medium with the organism under test, and then placing at appropriate intervals on the surface of the plate a number of filter-paper disks impregnated with different antibacterials. The plate is then incubated, usually overnight. The antibacterials diffuse out of their disks into the medium, and bacterial growth is inhibited in a circular zone around any disk that contains a drug to which the organism is sensitive. 'Sensitive' is of course not an absolute term. The object of this type of test is to distinguish between strains susceptible to drug concentrations that are attainable in patients (and therefore designated *sensitive*) and significantly less susceptible strains (designated *resistant*)—with the option, thought by some authorities to be a useful one, of dividing the latter into those which might be treatable by achieving unusually high concentrations (designated *moderately resistant, moderately sensitive* or *intermediate*) and those that appear unquestionably resistant. For each drug the disk content should be such that a sensitive strain (as just defined) will give an inhibition zone large enough for any significant decrease to be readily detectable but not so large as to interfere with the zones around neighbouring disks. The amount that achieves this depends on the diffusibility of the drug through the culture medium and also on the levels of it that can be attained in the patient. (For most purposes this means attainable blood levels, but for tests on urinary tract pathogens it usually means the higher levels attainable in urine.) Zone sizes are at the mercy of many factors besides the amount of drug; these include the heaviness of the bacterial inoculum, the medium composition and pH, and the temperature and atmospheric conditions of incubation. Reproducibility of results depends on careful control of all of these factors. One method of standardization depends on faithful reproduction of precisely the right conditions and then the comparison of the inhibition-zone measurements with a table of the results to be expected from sensitive, moderately resistant and fully resistant strains of the species in question. The other approach is to compare the zone sizes given by the test organism with those given by a control sensitive strain tested at the same time and under the same conditions (indeed, on the same plate in the widely used Stokes procedure).

Like any *in vitro* method, the disk-plate method can at best only give an indication of what might happen in the very different circumstances prevailing inside the patient's body. In its basic form it does not distinguish between bactericidal and bacteriostatic action. This distinction can be made by the further procedure of transferring to fresh culture plates the bacteria that were originally inoculated on to the zones in which growth was inhibited, and so giving them a chance to show whether they are still alive. One anomaly of the disk-plate method is that resistance dependent on inducible enzyme (notably that of *Staph. aureus* to penicillin) is manifested not so much by a reduction in size of the zone of inhibition as by vigorous growth around the edge of the zone; bacteria near to the disk were overcome before they could produce enzyme, but those further out had time to defend themselves against the advancing drug, and then had the benefit of the additional nutrients diffusing from the nearby depopulated zone.

It is possible to use the disk-plate technique for *direct sensitivity determinations*—i.e. disks can be applied to plates inoculated with pus, sputum or other pathological material and inhibition can be observed in this primary culture. In such circumstances there is virtually no control of inoculum size, and difficulties of interpretation may arise if the specimen contains a mixture of bacteria; for example, it is impossible to assess the penicillin sensitivity of other strains in the presence of one which produces penicillinase. However, this method has the compensatory advantage of speed, since it may be able to provide a rough guide to appropriate therapy as soon as any visible growth is present—sometimes in as little as 6 hours from the time of the collection of the specimen, well before it would be possible to pick single colonies from the primary culture and set up a properly standardized test.

Sometimes it is desirable not just to classify an organism as sensitive or resistant but to determine more precisely the smallest drug concentration that will inhibit it—the *minimal inhibitory concentration (MIC)*. This is done by testing its ability to grow in the presence of the drug in a series of concentrations, either in tubes of broth or incorporated in solid media in plates. By appropriate subculture from such a series of tubes or plates it is possible to determine also the *minimal bactericidal concentration (MBC)*. Since MIC and MBC values are expressed in numbers (e.g. $0.5 \mu g/ml$ or mg/l) they appear more accurate than they are; with some organisms and some antibiotics in particular, they are markedly dependent on inoculum size and the precise techniques used.

The 'break-point' method, used by some as an alternative to the disk-plate method for routine sensitivity testing, is a simpler form of the incorporation MIC method. It is usually carried out on plates, using for each drug either one plate containing a concentration regarded as the most relevant break-point between sensitivity and resistance, or two plates with a 4-fold difference in concentration. 20–30 different strains can be tested on each plate by replicate spot-inoculation (which can be mechanized). Use of two plates allows strains to be called fully sensitive (i.e. to both concentrations), moderately sensitive (to the higher concentration only) or resistant (to both).

Assays of Drug Levels in Body Fluids

Chemical methods are available for the assay of some antibacterial drugs, but may give misleading results through failure to distinguish between biologically active drug and inactive derivatives. Immunological methods (e.g. RIA, p. 244) also fail to make this distinction, but they are highly sensitive and give rapid, accurate assays which are unaffected by the presence of other antibiotics. Biological methods (bio-assays) are more commonly used. A·simple bio-assay method is similar in general design to the disk-plate sensitivity test method. A plate is inoculated with an appropriate standard bacterial strain sensitive to the drug to be assayed. In place of the disks of the sensitivity test method, small cylindrical wells are cut in the medium; some of these are filled with various dilutions of the fluid under test, and others with fluid containing known concentrations of the drug in question. By comparison of the diameters of the zones of inhibition around the standard solutions after incubation and those around the dilutions of the fluid under test, the drug concentration in the latter can be calculated (provided that any other antibacterial that might be present in the specimen has been inactivated or is without effect on the test organism). More rapid results can be obtained by means of sensitive systems for early detection of either metabolic inhibition or enzyme production; these are used to compare the effects of dilutions of the test fluid and of standard solutions of the drug on a test organism.

Most antibacterial treatment can be carried out satisfactorily without any monitoring of the levels achieved in blood and other body fluids. This is because, by the time that an antibacterial drug is on the market, the ranges of levels to be expected following recommended dosage schedules have been reliably established. Monitoring may be required, however, when there is wide individual variation in the levels resulting from a standard dose, so that some patients need unusually high dosage in order to have levels within the therapeutic range. This is true, for example, of gentamicin and related drugs, and for them there is the additional complication of a narrow margin between dosage which is adequate and that which may give toxic levels (pp. 315 and 330). For these and many other antibacterial drugs, impaired renal function is one of the most important factors that may invalidate deductions based on results obtained in healthy volunteers, so that it is necessary to check the levels actually achieved in the patient (p. 339). Other reasons for monitoring include attempts to deal with a moderately resistant organism, for which unusually high concentrations of the drug are required; determining whether oral administration, the least reliable means of administration for most drugs but in some cases the most convenient or most acceptable, is giving adequate levels in a particular patient; and the need to discover whether a drug is penetrating in adequate amounts into some body fluid other than blood. In general, assays as part of patient management are aimed at determining either that the patient is having enough of the drug for a therapeutic effect to be likely, or that he is not having too much and therefore exposed to unnecessary hazard.

As an alternative to assay of a drug by use of a standard bacterial strain, it is sometimes more satisfactory to carry out a direct test of the effectiveness of the patient's serum or other body fluid against a culture of his own pathogen, isolated before he started the treatment. This approach is particularly useful when the patient is receiving more than one drug, since assay of one in the presence of others may be difficult. It is common practice in the management of bacterial endocarditis (p. 335) to expose a culture of the offending streptococcus (or other bacterium) to serial dilutions of the patient's serum in nutrient broth, and to test for cidal action by subculturing these serum dilutions after overnight incubation. Treatment may well fail unless for at least part of each day the concentration of drugs in the serum is such that a 1 : 8 dilution of the serum is cidal to the streptococcus (under defined test conditions).

THE DRUGS THEMSELVES

The contents of this section are subject to the following limitations:

(1) *Dosages* are not given. They are not necessary for a discussion of the principles of antibacterial therapy, and for its practice they would have to be considered in far greater detail than our present space permits.

(2) *Trade names* are also omitted. It is understandable that each manufacturer should want to promote the sales of his own product rather than those of identical or similar materials produced by other firms, but much confusion results from the consequent multiplicity of names. The marketing of mixtures of antibacterial drugs under names which suggest that they are single new compounds is another source of bewilderment. The wisest policy is to ignore trade names and to think entirely in terms of official names.

(3) *Antibacterial ranges* of drugs are impossible to define briefly in other than general terms. Strains of the same species may differ widely in their sensitivities, and strains resistant to a particular drug are likely to become far more common in any community in which that drug is widely used, as we have already noted. In this section we have merely indicated the important groups of organisms commonly sensitive to each drug or class of drugs.

(4) The drugs described here as bactericidal are those of which it is possible to achieve in the body concentrations that are lethal to susceptible organisms. They may have only a bacteriostatic action when used in lower concentrations or against less susceptible organisms. Some of the drugs described as bacteriostatic are in fact bactericidal *in vitro* but not in concentrations that have any relevance to their therapeutic use.

The meanings of the terms *chemotherapeutic agents* and *antibiotics* are given on pp. 34–5.

(a) CHEMOTHERAPEUTIC AGENTS

Sulphonamides (see also p. 34)
Sulphonamides are effective against a wide range of bacteria (though only bacteriostatic), cheap to produce, usually harmless to the patient (though

with occasional serious toxicity), and of such diverse pharmacological properties that there is likely to be at least one appropriate to any particular situation. Yet this once invaluable group of drugs is now of limited and decreasing medical importance—partly because of more widespread bacterial resistance but mainly because on almost all occasions when they might be used antibiotics are available that can be expected to do a better job. Sulphonamides that are rapidly absorbed when given by mouth and rapidly excreted into the urine, achieving high concentrations there without the problem of insolubility described below in connection with sulphadiazine, are still commonly used for treating acute urinary tract infections, because they have roughly the same high success rate as more expensive drugs; but even here it is arguable that trimethoprim should be given as well (see below). *Sulphadiazine* is also rapidly absorbed when given by mouth, or can be injected, but renal excretion is slow enough to give good blood levels and there is little protein binding; consequently it diffuses well into tissues, and also into the cerebrospinal fluid. This makes it the best sulphonamide for treating meningitis due to sensitive meningococci (p. 94). However, like many of the early sulphonamides it is poorly soluble in acid or neutral urine, and the patient must be given alkalis and plentiful fluids to prevent renal tubular obstruction by sulphonamide crystals. *Sulphacetamide*, one of the earliest sulphonamides, is not used systemically, but it is highly soluble and penetrates exceptionally well into the eye, so it is still widely used in the form of eye drops and eye ointment. Sulphonamides that are virtually non-absorbable when given by mouth have been extensively used, together with antibiotics, for pre-operative suppression of bowel flora, but with little benefit. Some other sulphonamides with special uses are mentioned on p. 325.

The occasional serious toxic effects of sulphonamides mentioned above include (in addition to renal tubular obstruction) the rare but often fatal form of erythema multiforme known as the Stevens–Johnson syndrome; other allergies, including an illness resembling serum sickness; and bone marrow depression, which has on a few occasions developed into a fatal agranulocytosis.

Trimethoprim, Cotrimoxazole

Sulphonamides block conversion of PABA to dihydrofolic acid—for many bacteria a necessary step in the production of tetrahydrofolic acid (p. 33). Conversion of dihydrofolic acid to tetrahydrofolic acid is blocked by trimethoprim in bacterial cells, but not to anything like the same degree in mammalian cells, in which it is also an essential process (p. 305). Sulphonamides and trimethoprim show marked synergy *in vitro* against many bacterial strains, including some that are resistant to one or other of them acting alone. Because of this, and because of fears that use of trimethoprim on its own would result in widespread resistance to it, from the time of its first release for clinical use it was available only as a 1 : 5

mixture with *sulphamethoxazole*; the mixture was given the name *co-trimoxazole*. Sulphamethoxazole was chosen from the many available sulphonamides because its rapid absorption after oral administration and rather slow excretion matched the behaviour of trimethoprim. The wide range of infections in which the combination has proved useful includes gonorrhoea, typhoid, brucellosis and nocardiosis. The 1 : 5 ratio was chosen because it becomes a 1 : 20 ratio in the blood, and *in vitro* studies had shown that this was the optimum ratio of the drugs for effectiveness against many (but by no means all) sensitive bacteria. The two components do not, however, penetrate comparably to all sites—for example, in sputum the trimethoprim is in effect left to work on its own—and it remains to be determined whether for some purposes other initial ratios should be used. Meanwhile, by 1979 fears about resistance developing after use of trimethoprim on its own had been largely dispelled, and it became generally available without an accompanying sulphonamide. This is an advantage when the patient is known to be hypersensitive to sulphonamides, or when sensitivity tests have indicated that the sulphonamide component of the mixture has nothing to contribute except the risk of toxicity—from which trimethoprim is relatively free (though folate depletion may follow its prolonged use without supplying the host with additional folate that cannot be used by bacteria). Also it is now possible to give the two drugs together in a ratio other than 1 : 5 when this seems appropriate.

Pyrimethamine, a compound related to trimethoprim but with more effect on human folate metabolism, is not a useful antibacterial agent. However, it is used in weekly doses for malaria prophylaxis—either alone, with dapsone (as for leprosy) or with *sulfadoxine*, a long-acting sulphonamide—and also for treatment of toxoplasmosis, again with a long-acting sulphonamide.

Metronidazole

This substance has been in use since 1959, in the form of oral tablets, for the treatment of trichomonas infections (p. 209). Later it was discovered also to be effective in giardiasis and in amoebiasis (pp. 210 and 213). Some years passed, however, before clinical use was made of its inhibitory action on anaerobic bacteria. Metronidazole itself is inactive against micro-organisms, but on entering the cell of an anaerobic organism—protozoal or bacterial—it is reduced to a form that interacts with DNA. All strictly anaerobic bacteria are affected in this way. Its widespread use has not yet been followed by the emergence of resistant strains in significant numbers. It is of particular value against strains of *Bacteroides fragilis*, which are highly susceptible to it and are often resistant to most of the commonly used antibiotics. Patients who cannot take it by mouth can have it in the form of rectal suppositories or intravenously. It has rapidly acquired an important place in prophylaxis for intestinal surgery (p. 308), and in treatment of wound infections, septicaemia and other conditions for which anaerobes might be responsible. Apart from an unpleasant metallic taste it rarely produces side-effects.

Nitrofurantoin and Nalidixic Acid

These two unrelated substances have in common that when given by mouth they are rapidly absorbed and are excreted in high concentration in the urine. They are of use only in treatment of urinary tract infections. Nitrofurantoin achieves urinary concentrations that are bactericidal to some members of most bacterial groups, especially if the urine is acid—a condition not likely to be fulfilled if the infecting organism is a *Proteus* or other urease-positive strain, converting urea into ammonia. Nalidixic acid is bacteriostatic. Its range does not include Gram-positive organisms or *Ps. aeruginosa*, and therefore its usefulness is restricted to enterobacterial infections. Thus although both of these drugs have been widely used in treatment of urinary tract infections they are not reliable for this purpose without laboratory evidence of a suitably sensitive pathogen, and even then resistance may develop during treatment.

Chemotherapeutic Agents for Treatment of Mycobacterial Infections

Information about these is to be found on pp. 136 and 338–9.

(b) ANTIBIOTICS (For modes of action see pp. 35–6)

β-lactams: (a) Penicillins (see also p. 35)

The name 'penicillin', used on its own, refers to the first-discovered member of the group, *benzyl penicillin* (penicillin G). This remains one of our most valuable antibacterial drugs. It is bactericidal to a range of bacteria that includes many streptococci, the neisseriae (though some *N. gonorrhoeae* strains produce penicillinase), most Gram-positive bacilli, some Gram-negative bacilli (especially when it is in high concentration), spirochaetes and actinomycetes. Most *Staph. aureus* were sensitive to it when it was first introduced, but penicillinase-producing and therefore resistant strains now predominate in many areas, especially in hospitals. It is a remarkable drug in that it is tolerated by the body in almost unlimited quantities; such adverse reactions as do occur are due to hypersensitivity and are virtually independent of dosage (apart from the toxic encephalopathy occasionally produced by giving very large doses to patients with poor renal function, in whom exceptionally high blood levels can be achieved, or by giving a large excess intrathecally). Two of its unsatisfactory features are that it has to be given parenterally because it is acid-labile and destroyed to an unpredictable degree in the stomach, and that high blood levels are hard to maintain because it is rapidly excreted in the urine. The latter feature is occasionally beneficial, since high urinary concentrations can be achieved; more often it is merely wasteful of a relatively inexpensive compound; but sometimes, when persistent high blood levels are required, it is necessary to give *probenecid* which blocks renal tubular excretion of penicillin.

It is still an open question whether the most effective way of using penicillin is to maintain continuous high blood levels. It is possible that as good or better results can be obtained in most cases by intermittent high levels (p. 315). These can be achieved by suitably spaced intramuscular or intravenous injections. A steady blood level can be maintained by continuous intravenous administration, provided that incompatibilities are avoided (p. 312). However, it is often sufficient and more convenient to give a daily intramuscular injection of a slowly absorbed compound which will maintain an adequate blood level throughout the day, and in some cases there is a considerable advantage in being able to give a single dose which will maintain a moderate blood level for many days (see for example p. 141, treatment of syphilis). *Procaine penicillin, benethamide penicillin* and *benzathine penicillin* are slowly absorbed compounds of benzyl penicillin which respectively give useful blood levels for many hours, several days and several weeks after a single injection.

By varying the substrate for growth of the moulds that make benzyl penicillin, the acid-resistant *phenoxymethyl penicillin* (penicillin V) can be produced. When given by mouth, salts of this compound are sufficiently well absorbed to give reliably useful blood levels.

In 1959 it was discovered that the 'nucleus' of all penicillin molecules, 6-aminopenicillanic acid, could be made by substrate variation or by enzymic removal of side-chains from benzyl penicillin or other existing penicillins. By attaching various side-chains to this nucleus it has been possible to make a vast range of new semi-synthetic penicillins, some of which have special properties that make them useful therapeutic agents. These include:

(a) *phenethicillin* and *propicillin*, acid-resistant and absorbed more efficiently than phenoxymethyl penicillin, but, correspondingly less potent and therefore comparable with it in effectiveness.

(b) *methicillin, cloxacillin* and *flucloxacillin*, penicillinase-resistant and therefore active against penicillinase-producing staphylococci. The cloxacillins are both acid-resistant, but the much more complete absorption of flucloxacillin makes it the obvious choice for oral administration.

(c) *ampicillin*, and for oral administration, its much better absorbed esters *talampicillin, pivampicillin* and *bacampicillin* ('pro-drugs' which are converted to ampicillin after absorption); somewhat less potent than benzyl penicillin against many Gram-positive bacteria, but markedly more effective against some of the enterobacteria (including salmonellae and shigellae) and against *H. influenzae*; liable to provoke rashes (distinct from those due to hypersensitivity to all penicillins), especially in patients with infectious mononucleosis.

(d) *amoxycillin*, structurally related and similar in range to ampicillin; better absorbed than ampicillin when given orally (comparable to the esters); more effective in eradicating some infections (see p. 115, treatment of typhoid, and p. 337, chronic bronchitis).

(*e*) *mecillinam* and its ester *pivmecillinam*, highly active against some enterobacteria by a mode of action on cell-wall formation different from that of other penicillins; synergy with ampicillin in treatment of resistant enterobacteria.

(*f*) *ticarcillin* (which has replaced the related but less potent carbenicillin), active against *Ps. aeruginosa*, *Proteus* species and some of the enterobacteria, but relatively ineffective against Gram-positive organisms. It has to be given by injection.

(*g*) the ureidopenicillins *mezlocillin* (more active than ticarcillin against various enterobacteria and comparable to it against *Ps. aeruginosa*), *azlocillin* (highly active against *Ps. aeruginosa*) and *piperacillin* (possibly the most active of the three against many enterobacteria and against *Ps. aeruginosa*). All have to be given by injection.

Apart from the adverse effects mentioned under (*c*) above, the penicillins all share the lack of toxicity of benzyl penicillin, but also share its liability to provoke hypersensitivity reactions (p. 305). When hyper-sensitivity occurs, it applies to all members of the group, so that none of them can be given to a patient who has become sensitive to one of them.

β-lactams: (b) Cephalosporins
Nearly 20 years after the mould *Cephalosporium acremonium* was found to be a source of antibiotics, the first semi-synthetic derivatives of one of these were released for clinical use in 1964. Others followed, with increasing frequency, and the array of cephalosporins now available or due for general release in the near future is bewildering—especially to those who have to grapple with their trade names as well as their official names!

Cephalosporins resemble penicillins structurally (notably in having a β-lactam ring) and have a similar mode of antibacterial action (p. 35). Their clinical relevance is most easily explained by considering them in historical sequence:

(*a*) Those which were in general use before about 1975 ('first generation') are similar to ampicillin in their antibacterial range, with the additional advantage of being in varying degree more resistant to the β-lactamases of *Staph. aureus* and of some enterobacteria. *Cephaloridine* is the most active against Gram-positive cocci, but is liable to be nephrotoxic, especially in patients with existing renal impairment or when given with an aminoglycoside or with certain diuretics (p. 312). *Cephradine* and *cephalexin* can be given orally, and have been widely used—largely for this reason. There are seldom any clear reasons for preferring any of these drugs to either ampicillin or ampicillin + cloxacillin; patient hypersensitivity to penicillins was once thought to be such a reason, but it now appears that cross-hypersensitivity to cephalosporins occurs in nearly 10 % of such cases.

(b) Following the widespread use of penicillins and the early cephalosporins, bacteria (notably enterobacteria) resistant to them became increasingly frequent in clinical specimens and as pathogens. Much of this resistance is due to production of β-lactamases. These enzymes differ from one another in the range of substrates that they hydrolyse and the rates at which they do so; some are penicillinases only and others attack cephalosporins. Ability to resist most enterobacterial β-lactamases is the distinctive feature of the 'second generation' cephalosporins such as *cefuroxime, cefamandole* and *cefoxitin* (which is structurally a cephalosporin, but also called a cephamycin because it was derived from cephamycin C, a streptomyces product). These drugs are active against a wide range of Gram-negative bacteria, including *N. gonorrhoeae, H. influenzae* and some anaerobes.

(c) *Cefotaxime, moxalactam* and *ceftazidime* are among the advance guard of a large new 'third generation' of cephalosporins. They are far more active (up to 100-fold) against many of the species that were sensitive to their predecessors; and have useful activity against some *Ps. aeruginosa* strains and against certain enterobacteria that, while not common pathogens, are important because they have been virtually untreatable with earlier antibiotics. The specific values of all these new drugs will take a considerable time to assess—and it is to be hoped that during that time they will be used with restraint and intelligence.

No cephalosporins are effective against enterococci.

β-lactams: (c) Clavulanic acid

This β-lactam has negligible antibacterial activity on its own, but it is a powerful inhibitor of β-lactamases. It is now commercially available in Britain in a mixture with amoxycillin. Protecting the older susceptible β-lactams against β-lactamases at the site of an infection was an interesting new approach, and has been shown by laboratory and clinical trials to be practicable; but it remains to be seen whether it has any advantages over using newer β-lactam antibiotics that are themselves resistant to the enzymes.

Fucidin

This sodium salt of fusidic acid derived from the fungus *Fusidium coccineum* is unusual among antibiotics in having a steroid molecular structure. It is well absorbed when given by mouth, is apparently free from serious toxic effects, and is highly effective against most strains of *Staph. aureus*, including penicillinase-producers. Claims have been made that it is particularly good at eradicating staphylococcal infections of bones and joints. Resistance to it develops readily among staphylococci in culture, and sometimes occurs during treatment also. In order to preserve its value, it seems best to use it against staphylococci only, and always in conjunction with another antibiotic so as to reduce the risk of developing resistance (p. 312)—e.g. with cloxacillin or flucloxacillin.

Aminoglycosides
Most antibiotics of this group (and indeed of other groups yet to be discussed) are derived from *Streptomyces* species. Aminoglycosides of such derivation have names ending in 'mycin', whereas those derived from *Micromonospora* species have names ending in 'micin'.

Like the β-lactamases, aminoglycosides are bactericidal. They are effective against many strains of *Staph. aureus* and of enterobacteria, though resistance among the latter is an increasingly common problem because they can produce an assortment of drug-degrading enzymes (cf. β-lactamases). Some are effective against *Ps. aeruginosa* (see below). They are not effective against anaerobes, or against streptococci (except when acting synergically with a penicillin—see pp. 311 and 335). They are not absorbed to a useful extent when given by mouth. Dosages have to be carefully controlled to avoid damage to the 8th nerve, and these drugs may also be nephrotoxic (see below).

When introduced in 1944 *streptomycin* was the first effective anti-tuberculous drug, and it remains important in this field (p. 339). For the various other purposes for which it was once used it has been almost entirely replaced—at first by *kanamycin*, which has a somewhat wider range of activity and perhaps less toxicity; and then by *gentamicin*. This drug is more active than other aminoglycosides against a wide range of bacteria, and was the first member of this group to be effective against *Ps. aeruginosa*. It is a most useful drug for treatment of proven or suspected septicaemia due to organisms presumably originating from the alimentary or urinary tracts—after surgery or as a complication of a malignant growth, for example; but for such purposes it needs the assistance of metronidazole or some other drug capable of dealing with *Clostridium* and *Bacteroides* species, and possibly also of a penicillin to deal with streptococci. We have mentioned the importance of monitoring levels of gentamicin (pp. 315 and 322). Its nephrotoxicity is enhanced if it is given with cephaloridine (and possibly with some other cephalosporins) or with certain diuretics (see p. 312). *Tobramycin* is less active than gentamicin against many species but rather more active against many *Pseudomonas* strains. However, there has been a marked increase in the frequency of *Ps. aeruginosa* strains that are resistant to gentamicin by means of enzymes that also destroy tobramycin. Such enzymes are not usually effective against *amikacin*, a derivative of kanamycin. *Netilmicin* is said to be useful against some gentamicin-resistant Gram-negative bacilli, and to be less toxic than gentamicin in animal experiments, but needs further clinical assessment.

Neomycin and *framycetin* are kanamycin-like drugs too toxic for systemic use. Neomycin is sometimes given by mouth as a means of attack on intestinal pathogens, but may do more harm than good (p. 116). Either can be applied topically in the form of powder, cream, ointment, eye or ear drops, etc., though prolonged and heavy topical application can lead to absorption of toxic amounts. Gentamicin has also been extensively used in such topical forms, but this practice seems to have been responsible for the increasing frequency of gentamicin-resistant strains of *Ps. aeruginosa* and other species.

Spectinomycin (an aminocyclitol, not an aminoglycoside but closely related to that group) has been widely and successfully used for treatment of penicillin-resistant gonococci. For this purpose it is given in a single large intramuscular dose. There are no established indications for its use in other ways or for other purposes.

Chloramphenicol

Originally derived from *Streptomyces venezuelae* in 1947, chloramphenicol is now made synthetically. It is well absorbed when given by mouth, and passes from the blood stream into the cerebrospinal fluid more readily than any other antibiotic. It can also be given parenterally, but the intravenous route should be used, as absorption after intramuscular injection is slow and gives relatively poor blood levels. It is effective against a wide range of bacteria, and also against rickettsiae and chlamydiae. It is bactericidal to *H. influenzae*, and a valuable drug for treatment of the life-threatening infections of children caused by type b strains of this species (p. 124). Against other genera it is bacteriostatic only. This may explain its failure to eradicate *S. typhi* infections (p. 115), even though it is highly effective in controlling the acute illness of typhoid (except when this is due to a chloramphenicol-resistant strain). In the years following its introduction it was widely used for infections of many kinds, but then came numerous reports of fatal bone marrow depression following its use. Since then there has been a general tendency in N. America, Britain and some other countries to regard it as highly dangerous and to use it almost exclusively for treatment of typhoid and paratyphoid (for which amoxycillin and cotrimoxazole are now valid alternatives—p. 115) and of severe infections due to *H. influenzae* or to bacteria resistant to all reputedly safer antibiotics. In other countries it has continued to be frequently prescribed or to be available without prescription. On the available evidence it is impossible to be sure how dangerous chloramphenicol is, or indeed whether all batches are equally dangerous. Possibly because it has been 'in disgrace', it can be of great value in treatment of life-threatening infections because most strains of staphylococci and of other troublesome bacteria are still sensitive to it. Caution is necessary when giving it to new-born infants, since they inactivate and excrete it very slowly and therefore high dosage may lead to excessive blood levels, collapse and death ('the grey syndrome'). Blood levels can be determined in a few hours by bio-assay. It is of little value in urinary tract infection because the kidneys excrete it mainly in a form that is not active against bacteria. Chloramphenicol drops or ointment are extensively and effectively used for treating eye infections; but there is evidence that this practice is leading to the emergence of *H. influenzae* strains with transferable multiresistance.

Tetracyclines

Chlortetracycline (first isolated in 1948) and its now numerous relations are all derived, directly or with subsequent chemical manipulations, from *Streptomyces* species. Like chloramphenicol, they are effective when given by mouth. They are purely bacteriostatic. They have much the same antimicrobial range as chloramphenicol, including the rickettsiae and chlamydiae. Bacterial resistance develops rather readily, and has become increasingly common even in species such as *Str. pyogenes* and *Str. pneumoniae* which do not readily become resistant to drugs of most other groups.

Chlortetracycline, oxytetracycline and *tetracycline* itself, the original members of this group, are all still in use. Their rather inefficient and irregular absorption when given by mouth necessitates high dosage, with frequent gastro-intestinal side-effects: nausea and vomiting are probably due to chemical irritation of the stomach, and diarrhoea results from derangement of the normal bowel flora by unabsorbed drug. In its extreme form this derangement may lead to intestinal moniliasis, or on rare occasions to staphylococcal enteritis (p. 80). The chief advantage of more recently introduced tetracyclines is that better absorption and slower excretion permits lower oral dosage. *Demeclocycline* is comparatively well absorbed and rather slowly excreted. Excretion of *doxycycline* is so slow that a daily dose is sufficient, as against 6-hourly doses for the older tetracyclines. *Minocycline* is very well absorbed and slowly excreted, so that it too can be given as a daily dose, and it has the additional interesting property of being effective against many staphylococcal and other strains that are resistant to other tetracyclines; but unfortunately it makes many patients giddy. Permanent yellow staining of teeth may follow administration of tetracyclines to children during the early years of life or to their mothers during the later months of pregnancy. Other reasons for avoiding these drugs during pregnancy are reports of severe liver damage in pregnant women following high dosage and unconfirmed allegations of teratogenic effects on foetuses. Because of these various forms of toxicity, tetracyclines are less widely used than formerly. In Britain their main use is in chronic bronchitis (p. 337). They are also the most effective drugs for treatment of *Myco. pneumoniae* infection and Q fever.

Erythromycin

This macrolide, produced by *Streptomyces erythreus*, has an antibacterial range similar to that of benzyl penicillin. In high concentrations *in vitro* it is bactericidal to susceptible organisms, but this probably has only limited relevance to its action in the body. It can be given orally as base, which is poorly absorbed; as estolate, which is better absorbed but may cause acute (reversible) liver damage; or as stearate, new formulations of which are said to be well absorbed without toxicity. Injectable preparations are available, but intramuscular injection is painful. Staphylococci in particular readily become resistant to erythromycin but this can be discouraged by giving another antibiotic at the same time (p. 312). Erythromycin is sometimes a valuable alternative to penicillin in patients hypersensitive to the latter; it has been widely used in paediatrics, largely because of its lack of toxicity and its availability in the form of an acceptable oral suspension; and it has recently acquired a new level of importance as the drug of choice for *Campylobacter* and *Legionella* infections. It is also used in prophylaxis against whooping cough.

Clindamycin
This is a synthetic derivative of another streptomyces antibiotic, *lincomycin*. It closely resembles the macrolide antibiotics in most of its properties, in spite of having a markedly different molecular structure. It is well absorbed when taken orally, and penetrates into bone better than most antibiotics; it is therefore a useful weapon for dealing with osteomyelitis. It is an effective alternative to penicillin for use against *Str. pyogenes*, and is also valuable for dealing with *Bacteroides* infections. Being better absorbed from the alimentary tract than lincomycin, it does not cause the immediate gastro-intestinal upsets commonly associated with use of that drug. Pseudomembranous colitis (p. 108) is perhaps more often induced by one of these two drugs than by any other.

Vancomycin
This is another streptomyces antibiotic. It has an assortment of toxic effects, has to be given intravenously for systemic action, and is difficult to give repeatedly by that route because it causes thrombophlebitis. Nevertheless, its high activity against staphylococci and streptococci means that it is sometimes useful—in treatment of severe infections due to organisms of these genera resistant to less toxic drugs; in peri-operative protection of heart valves (p. 307) when the patients have already been on penicillin, with modification of their resident bacterial populations; or in patients hypersensitive to β-lactams. Given by mouth, it is the treatment of choice for pseudomembranous colitis (see above and p. 108) and for staphylococcal enteritis (p. 80).

Rifamycins
Although the members of this group of antibiotics derived from *Streptomyces mediterranei* have promising antibacterial activities *in vitro*, their clinical usefulness is impaired by their rapid excretion in the bile and the consequent impossibility of maintaining adequate blood levels. *Rifampicin*, a synthetic derivative of one of them, is less rapidly excreted, is well absorbed when given by mouth, and is bactericidal to staphylococci and non-faecal streptococci (at remarkably low concentrations), to *Myco. tuberculosis* and to many other bacteria. However, its most serious limitation is the speed with which resistant mutants emerge, and because of this it should probably never be used alone. Its considerable value in treatment of tuberculosis (p. 338) and leprosy (p. 136) is likely to be best

preserved by using it only in exceptional circumstances for non-mycobacterial infections (e.g. in treatment of endocarditis due to a staphylococcus resistant to most other drugs). It has been used with some success to prevent spread and eliminate carriage of meningococci and of *H. influenzae* type b; but rifampicin-resistant meningococci have appeared following such use, the haemophili can be expected to follow suit, and there is at least a theoretical risk of a selective action on tubercle bacilli in populations so treated. When given in low dosage rifampicin is mostly excreted in the bile, but higher dosage saturates this excretory mechanism and it then appears in useful concentrations in the urine, which it colours red (as it may also do to the tears).

Polymyxins

These are polypeptides derived from bacteria of the genus *Bacillus* and first reported in 1947. *Colistin*, discovered in 1950 and at first thought to be a new antibiotic, is identical with polymyxin E. All are nephrotoxic but the toxicity of polymyxins B and E is not sufficient to preclude their systemic use when necessary. For this purpose they are administered intramuscularly. They are also used in the form of powders and ointments for the treatment of wounds and burns, and given by mouth for treatment of alimentary infections. They are not absorbed from the intestine. They are administered either as sulphates or as sulphomethyl derivatives (methane sulphonates), and the latter are preferred by some for parenteral use because they give less pain when injected and are less toxic. However, they are also less potent and more rapidly excreted by the kidneys—an advantage, perhaps, when treating urinary tract infections but not when sustained blood levels are needed. The polymyxins are bactericidal and are effective against *Ps. aeruginosa* and against Gram-negative bacilli of most other genera except *Proteus*, but unfortunately their efficacy against *Ps. aeruginosa* is markedly reduced in the presence of calcium ions in concentrations found in blood and other body fluids.

SOME SPECIAL PROBLEMS

Staphylococcus aureus Infections

This most adaptable species has continued to be a special problem throughout the antibiotic era. Apart from the strains mentioned in the next paragraph, *Staph. aureus* strains are all *intrinsically* penicillin sensitive, and benzyl penicillin remains the best antibiotic for dealing with those that cannot destroy it. However, most hospital strains and many of those from other sources can protect themselves against benzyl penicillin, ampicillin and related compounds by producing penicillinase that destroys them rapidly—but is much less effective against the cloxacillin group and the cephalosporins. Cloxacillins are the first choice for dealing with penicillinase-producers (usually reported as 'penicillin resistant'), or with strains that are inaccessible for testing (e.g. because they are in deeply placed lesions) or that require urgent treatment before results of tests are available. Other antibiotics that can be used against *Staph. aureus* (in combination with one another or with some other effective drugs, to prevent rapid emergence of resistant variants) are erythromycin, fucidin, clindamycin and the aminoglycosides, with the more toxic vancomycin in reserve for special problems.

There are some *Staph. aureus* strains, once very rare but encountered with increasing frequency in hospitals as penicillin usage increased, which show genuine penicillin resistance—as distinct from the ability to destroy penicillins. Their resistance includes all penicillins, and usually the cephalosporins as well. It depends on unusual cell-wall composition, and is as a rule shown by only a very small proportion of any given population of such a *Staph. aureus* strain when incubated at 37°C, but this proportion is greatly increased at lower incubation temperatures (e.g. 30°C). Perhaps because of this, such strains (in our experience at least) occur mainly in surface wounds and ulcers and seldom cause serious systemic disease. There are reports that when they do cause major infections they respond poorly to treatment with any of the penicillins.

Subacute Bacterial Endocarditis

The paradox of antibacterial treatment for this condition, and the need for it to be bactericidal, have been discussed on pp. 310–11. It seems probable that in order to attain bactericidal drug levels inside the vegetations it is best to have persistent high blood levels. High penicillin dosage, accompanied if necessary by use of probenecid to block renal excretion of the penicillin, is usually effective against highly or even moderately penicillin-sensitive organisms, such as the viridans streptococci that are the commonest cause of this disease. However, there is evidence that even these are eliminated more rapidly and more surely if in addition to the penicillin the patient receives an aminoglycoside (even in quite low dosage, which minimizes the risk of toxicity). When the causative organism is an enterococcus (p. 91) or other streptococcus which on routine bacteriostatic sensitivity testing is resistant both to penicillin and to the aminoglycosides, bactericidal penicillin-aminoglycoside synergy can often still be demonstrated in the laboratory. In such circumstances combined use of (for example) ampicillin and gentamicin is likely to be successful. For other organisms, however, it is necessary to test various antibiotic combinations for *in vitro* synergy in an attempt to find a form of treatment that might succeed.

A special form of heart-valve infection is that which follows open-heart surgery and installation of a prosthetic heart valve. The organisms are commonly 'non-pathogenic' bacteria, such as coagulase-negative staphylococci, but *Candida* species or other fungi are sometimes involved. Even when backed by laboratory tests to find synergic antibiotic combinations, treatment seldom eradicates the infection and the valve usually has to be replaced. (A closely similar problem often arises with Spitz–Holter valves and other prostheses used in treatment of hydrocephalus.)

Meningitis

This disease illustrates clearly the point, made on p. 314 and elsewhere, that a drug with *in vitro* activity against a pathogen cannot be useful in treatment unless it can reach the appropriate site. Presumably in meningitis one such site is in the meninges themselves, but drug levels in the cerebrospinal fluid are much easier to determine and are also important—probably because of the massive bacterial 'reinforcements' that can accumulate there. Some information about drug penetration into the cerebrospinal fluid is given on p. 314.

The common causes of bacterial meningitis—the meningococcus, *H. influenzae* type b and the pneumococcus—can often be detected and firmly identified very soon after the cerebrospinal fluid specimen reaches the laboratory (p. 237). Such rapid identification of the pathogen simplifies the choice of treatment. For meningococcal meningitis the first choice was for many years a sulphonamide that penetrates rapidly into cerebrospinal fluid, usually sulphadiazine; but in many parts of the world the frequency of sulphonamide-resistant meningococcal strains now makes such treatment unreliable, and penicillin has to be given as well (or instead). Penicillin itself, which is also the first choice for pneumococcal meningitis, can be made to achieve adequate cerebrospinal levels via inflamed meninges by ensuring a high blood level, and there is probably nothing to be gained by giving it also intrathecally—apart from the small gain in time that is made by giving it by that route at the time of the diagnostic lumbar puncture if turbid fluid is withdrawn. Unfortunately penicillin is never a suitable antibiotic for treatment of haemophilus meningitis, and ampicillin—which was for some years regarded by some authorities as a suitable first choice for dealing with any of these 3 organisms—is ineffective against the increasingly common penicillinase-producing strains of *H. influenzae*. Chloramphenicol is, for this and other reasons, the best drug for treating haemophilus meningitis, but haemophilus strains resistant to it are not unknown and may increase in frequency. To treat a case of acute meningitis with a drug that might not be effective against the pathogen is to take a serious risk, as the infection can rapidly cause irreversible damage. Therefore if there is doubt as to the pathogenic species, or as to the reliability of the sensitivity of local strains of that species to a particular drug, a combination of drugs is indicated. The example of penicillin–tetracycline antagonism quoted on p. 311 is a warning about the risks of such a bactericidal + bacteriostatic mixture, but there has as yet been no evidence of significant penicillin–chloramphenicol or ampicillin–chloramphenicol antagonism in connection with meningitis, or that sulphadiazine should not be given with any of these. However, the drug combination to be used on any occasion has to be chosen in the light of local circumstances and experience—there is at present no simple and generally applicable answer to the problem. (It remains to be seen whether such an answer will be provided by either cefotaxime or moxalactam, two of the 'third generation' cephalosporins that combine good penetration in cerebrospinal fluid with very high activity against meningococci, *H. influenzae* and pneumococci.) Neonatal meningitis may be enterobacterial, and gentamicin is then usually a good choice of drug, though in view of its very poor penetration from blood into cerebrospinal fluid there is a case for giving it intrathecally or directly into a cerebral ventricle as well as intramuscularly or intravenously. Treatment of tuberculous meningitis is mentioned below.

Chronic Bronchitis

A large proportion of Britain's drug bill is spent on antibiotics for patients with chronic bronchitis. This disease is not caused by bacteria, but bronchi affected by it lose their ability to keep themselves sterile, and are liable to recurrent or persistent bacterial infection. The commonest offending bacteria are *H. influenzae* and pneumococci. Some patients harbour these in their bronchi without any significant trouble. Others have episodes of increased respiratory difficulty and purulent sputum, with these organisms in profusion in the sputum. Such exacerbations are often precipitated by colds or other virus infections, and indeed can in many cases be aborted by a few days of treatment, from the onset of such a virus infection, with one of the drugs to be mentioned below. This is in fact probably prophylaxis on some occasions and early treatment on others. Some patients get over their exacerbations quite rapidly with the help of bacteriostatic treatment with a tetracycline or trimethoprim. In others the trouble is more persistent, but it may be possible to give them quite long remissions by means of bactericidal treatment to eradicate the pathogens from their bronchi. Amoxycillin is preferable to ampicillin for this purpose, since penetration of ampicillin into sputum falls off rapidly as bronchial suppuration subsides. Advanced bronchitics, with such poor bronchial defences that they have trouble with bacterial infections throughout each winter or even throughout the year, may be helped by long-term bacteriostatic treatment, but may then have trouble from antibiotic-resistant species that are encouraged to proliferate in their respiratory tracts.

Urinary Tract Infections

Acute urinary tract infection is another condition that is responsible, in all parts of the world, for a vast consumption of antibacterials—sulphonamides (alone or with trimethoprim), ampicillin, amoxycillin, cephalosporins, tetracyclines, nitrofurantoin, nalidixic acid and others. These drugs are used because they are excreted in high concentrations in the urine, and it is these urinary levels, rather than those in the blood, that are generally used as the basis for laboratory sensitivity tests—some organisms therefore being reported as sensitive which would be resistant to the levels attainable in the blood. This is reasonable if the object of treatment is to deal with organisms that are in the urine itself, which appears to be all that is necessary for the majority of acute urinary tract infections. However, for treatment of more chronic infections involving the renal parenchyma blood levels are probably more relevant.

Most isolated episodes of acute urinary tract infections in otherwise healthy people are due to strains of *Esch. coli* or other bacteria that are sensitive to most or all of the commonly used drugs. Furthermore such episodes are likely to resolve spontaneously within a few days, and the main function of antibacterial treatment is merely to shorten the period of discomfort. In such circumstances it is sufficient to choose a drug which is cheap, relatively harmless and known to be effective against the great majority of prevailing strains. Only a short course of treatment is needed; a single dose, e.g. of amoxycillin, is adequate in many cases, especially if given at bed-time with the bladder as empty as possible, so as to ensure a high drug concentration throughout the night when bacterial multiplication would otherwise be uninterrupted. It is a good idea to send to the laboratory a pre-treatment urine specimen in case all does not go well and a follow-up specimen to ensure that the infection has been eradicated. Relapses, recurrent infections and infections acquired in hospital following catheterization or operation are likely to be due to more sophisticated strains, which need to have their sensitivities determined as a basis for treatment. Recurrent infections also require thorough investigation of possible anatomical or pathological causes; when no treatable underlying condition is found, such patients can be protected from further recurrences by long-term antibacterial treatment, continued over months or years, and they may not need more than a single nightly dose. Patients with indwelling catheters because of neurological or other long-standing problems are liable to repeated bouts of infection of their urinary tracts, and the organisms involved show an increasing range of resistance to drugs that have been used. Such patients commonly reach the stage of permanent colonization of their urinary tracts by highly resistant enterobacteria or pseudomonads, but may be able to co-exist with these for long periods without any serious inconvenience or damage.

Tuberculosis

Antibacterial treatment of tuberculosis has three unusual features: the need for combinations of drugs at all times, to avoid the emergence of resistance; the need for prolonged treatment, related to the very slow metabolism and multiplication rate of the tubercle bacillus; and the nature of the drugs used.

To prevent emergence of resistance, it is necessary to use two effective drugs; and since the drug-sensitivity of the organism is not known until several weeks after starting treatment, it is standard practice to use three drugs initially, in case one of them is not effective. The 'first line' triad in Britain and many other countries today, all of which can be given by mouth, are:

(1) *rifampicin* (p. 333), undoubtedly the most potent antituberculous agent available; costly; liable to cause hepatitis.

(2) *isoniazid*, also highly effective, except that resistant strains are

relatively common; cheap; liable to cause hepatitis or peripheral neuritis.

(3) *ethambutol*, in low dosage a useful supporting drug and virtually non-toxic, but liable to cause optic neuritis when used in the higher dosage necessary if one of the others is contra-indicated.

Streptomycin (p. 330), the first drug to make an effective impact on the problem of tuberculosis, has the disadvantage that it has to be injected. It is the principal reserve drug after the first line triad, but it is also still widely used for initial treatment in countries where the high cost of rifampicin makes it unsuitable for this purpose. Other reserve drugs include *pyrazinamide* (particularly useful in tuberculous meningitis because of its good penetration into cerebrospinal fluid), *thiacetazone* and *cycloserine*.

The efficacy of modern antituberculous drugs—including the synergic bactericidal action of rifampicin and isoniazid against tubercle bacilli— means that it is no longer necessary to continue treatment for up to 2 years, as was the case not long ago. Three drugs for 2–3 months, with two of them continued up to a total of 9 months, give good results in terms of clinical cure and low relapse rates—provided that the patients continue to take their drugs consistently. Failure of compliance with regimens is a major problem, especially where patients have little understanding of their disease, and is a strong reason for continuing attempts to evaluate shorter courses with different dose combinations. Weekly or twice weekly supervised administration of high doses of drugs is more effective for some types of patient than unreliable self-administration of standard doses.

Patients with Impaired Renal Function

If a patient who needs antimicrobial therapy also has impaired renal function, additional factors must be borne in mind when selecting appropriate drugs and dosage schedules. The renal excretion rate is a major factor in determining the blood and tissue levels of many antimicrobial drugs. The aminoglycosides and the polymyxins are examples of drugs which are normally excreted mainly by the kidneys and which have serious toxic effects at blood levels not far above those required for therapy; impairment of their renal excretion calls for carefully calculated dose-reduction and close attention to the levels actually achieved. On the other hand, the penicillins and clindamycin are also mainly excreted by the kidneys, but their lack of toxicity at much higher levels than those usually required means that they can safely be given to patients with impaired renal function, though it is usually wise to keep down to modest dosage. Drugs that are themselves potentially nephrotoxic clearly need special care—e.g. cephaloridine (p. 328). Blood levels of chloramphenicol, as determined by bio-assay, are little affected by renal failure, as the main mechanism of removal of this drug from the blood is conjugation by the liver to an inactive form. Therefore if the drug is to be used in the presence of renal failure it should be given in normal dosage, but it is best to avoid it if possible, as in the absence of renal excretion the conjugates accumulate in the blood and they are not free from suspicion of toxicity. The tetracyclines too should be avoided in such circumstances, as they are liable to precipitate severe and sometimes fatal uraemia—by direct action on the kidneys and also by an anti-anabolic effect which increases the amount of urea needing to be cleared from the blood. Fucidin and the rifamycins are among the few antimicrobial drugs that are excreted almost entirely by non-renal mechanisms.

Suggestions for Further Reading

Antibiotic and Chemotherapy by L. P. Garrod, H. P. Lambert and F. O'Grady, 5th edn. (Churchill Livingstone, Edinburgh and London, 1981).

Antibiotics in Clinical Practice by Hillas Smith, 3rd edn. (Pitman Medical, Tunbridge Wells, 1977).

A Clinician's Guide to Antibiotic Therapy by Paul Noone, 2nd edn. (Blackwell, Oxford, 1979).

APPENDICES

A

GLOSSARY OF TECHNICAL TERMS

For the reader's convenience definitions of some terms in common use in medical microbiology are brought together here. Definitions, or at least indications of the meanings, of many of them are also given in the main text on the pages cited. The meanings of many other terms not quoted here can be found by reference to the Index.

Acid-fast (acid-alcohol-fast): Resistant to decolorization by acid (or by acid and by alcohol) after staining with hot carbol fuchsin, and so retaining a red colour when stained by the Ziehl–Neelsen method—*page* 132.

Active (immunity, immunization): Dependent upon stimulation of the subject's own immunological mechanisms—*page* 49. (Cf. *passive*.)

Adjuvant: A substance which, by delaying absorption of an antigen or by other means, enhances its antigenic efficiency—*page* 291.

Aerobe: An organism which can live and multiply in the presence of atmospheric oxygen—*page* 22.

Agglutination: Clumping together, e.g. of red blood cells or micro-organisms, on exposure to an appropriate antiserum—*page* 242.

Anaerobe: An organism which cannot multiply or survive for long in the presence of more than a trace of free oxygen—*page* 22.

Anamnestic reaction: A rise of an existing antibody level in response to an irrelevant stimulus, such as an infection with an organism unrelated to that against which the antibody was originally formed—*page* 247.

Antagonism (between antimicrobial drugs): Impairment of the efficacy of one of each drug in the presence of the other—*page* 311. (Cf. *synergy*.)

Antibiotic: A product of micro-organisms which, even when much diluted, is lethal or inhibitory to other micro-organisms—*page* 33.

Antibody: A globulin which is formed by the human or animal body in response to contact with some foreign substance and which reacts specifically with that substance—*page* 55. Synonym *immunoglobulin*.

Antigen: A substance which provokes formation of antibodies—*page* 52.

Antiseptic: Roughly synonymous with *disinfectant* (q.v.)—*page* 268.

Antiserum: A serum containing antibodies for a given organism or toxin—*page* 292.

Antitoxin: An antibody for a given toxin—*page* 292.

Asepsis: Avoidance of infection—*page* 270.

Attack rate: The proportion of people, within a group or population exposed to the risk of infection with a particular organism, who develop clinical illness as a result of that exposure.

Attenuated (organism): Reduced in virulence for a given host (but often retaining useful antigenicity for that host)—*page* 42.

Bacillus: A 'little stick', a rod-shaped bacterium—*page* 13.

Bacteraemia: Presence of bacteria in the blood-stream with or without resulting illness—*page* 47. (Cf. *septicaemia*.)

Bactericidal: Lethal to bacteria—*page* 32.

Bacteriostatic (bacteristatic): Preventing multiplication of bacteria—*page* 32.

Bacteriuria (bacilluria): Presence of bacteria (bacilli) in significant numbers in freshly voided uncontaminated urine—*page* 233.

Brownian movement: Passive to-and-fro movement of small particles such as bacteria when suspended in a fluid medium, due to irregular bombardment by molecules of the fluid or its solutes—*page* 15.

Capsid: The protein coat surrounding the genome (q.v.) of a virus—*page* 14.

Capsomere: One of the units of which a virus capsid is composed—*page* 155.

Capsule: A coating, commonly of polysaccharide, outside the cell walls of some bacteria and fungi—*pages* 13, 73.

Carboxyphilic (organism): Needing for growth a higher concentration of carbon dioxide in the atmosphere than is found in air—*page* 22. Synonym CO_2-*dependent*.

Carrier: One who is harbouring but not currently suffering any ill-effects from a pathogenic organism—*page* 38.

Cell line: An *in vitro* culture of mammalian cells of known origin, suitable for propagation of viruses—*page* 159. (The word 'mammalian' in this definition is of course appropriate only in connection with the study of viruses that are parasites of mammals.)

Chemotherapeutic agent: A synthetic chemical suitable for systemic administration and effective in the treatment of microbial infections—*pages* 33 and 324–6.

Clone: A 'race' of cells derived from a single ancestral cell and sharing a single function, e.g. of producing a particular antibody—*page* 54.

Coccus: A spherical or ovoid bacterium—*page* 13.

Coliform bacillus: Not, as the name ought to mean, one that is shaped like a colon but one that resembles *Esch. coli.*—*page* 109. Authorities differ, however, on the closeness of the resemblance which is required for use of this term.

Colony: A visible pile or mass of micro-organisms on the surface of a solid culture medium, resulting in most cases from the multiplication of a single organism or a very small number—*page* 75. (A clump or chain of bacteria that together give rise to a single colony are called a *colony-forming unit*, and bacterial counts based on the numbers of colonies on plates are in fact counts of such units, not of total bacterial numbers.)

Commensal: Deriving nourishment from a host without being either beneficial or harmful to him—*page* 18. (Cf. *pathogenic, symbiotic.*)

Complement: A heat-labile system with many components, present in the serum of man and of animals and playing a number of important parts in the mechanisms of immunity—*page* 60.

Conjugation (bacterial): Exchange of genetic material between bacteria, a primitive form of sexuality—*page* 28.

Constitutive (enzyme): Produced under nearly all circumstances, not dependent upon the presence of appropriate substrate—*page* 21. (Cf. *inducible.*)

Cytopathic effect: Degenerative changes occurring in tissue-culture cells as a result of virus infection, the nature of the changes sometimes indicating the identity of the virus—*page* 159.

Disinfectant: A substance, not an antibiotic, which has useful anti-microbial activity but is too toxic for systemic administration—*page* 32.

Elementary bodies: Single virus particles of some of the larger viruses, visible by ordinary light microscopy after appropriate staining—*page* 166.

Endemic (disease): Persistently present in a given community—*page* 38.

Endogenous (infection or disease): Originated by organisms or factors already present in the patient's body before onset of the condition—*page* 44. (Cf. *exogenous.*)

Endotoxin: A toxic component of a micro-organism , largely dependent for its release on the death and disruption of the organism. In particular, lipopolysaccharide derived from the cell walls of Gram-negative bacteria—*page* 24. (Cf. *exotoxin.*)

Enrichment medium: A medium used to encourage preliminary growth of an organism so as to enhance the chances of growing it on subsequent plate cultures. (Cf. *selective medium.*)

Epidemic (noun or adjective): A disease that temporarily has a high frequency in a given community—*page* 38.

Exogenous (infection or disease): Originated by organisms or factors from outside the patient's body. (Cf. *endogenous.*)

Exotoxin: A toxin released by living micro-organisms into the surrounding medium or tissues—*page* 24.

Facultative (organism): Able to multiply in the presence or absence of oxygen—*page* 22; *or* (in other contexts) adaptable in behaviour.

Fimbria (plural *fimbriae*): Hair-like protrusions from bacterial cells, shorter than a *flagellum* (q.v.). Synonym *pilus*—*page* 13.

Flagellum (plural *flagella*): Whip-like organ of motion possessed by some bacteria and protozoa—*pages* 14, 73, 209.

Fomites (Latin, 3 syllables): Literally 'kindling wood', hence personal properties liable to convey agents that initiate diseases—*page* 5.

Genome: The total genetic material of an organism; the nucleic acid core of a virus—*page* 14.

Genotype: Genetic composition, whether manifest or not—*page* 27. (Cf. *phenotype*.)

Gram-negative: Staining red by Gram's method, through losing the primary stain during decolorization and taking up the counter-stain—*page* 77.

Gram-positive: Staining violet or blue by Gram's method, through retention of the primary stain—*page* 77.

Growth factor: An ingredient of which at least a small amount must be present in a culture medium in order that it may support the growth of a given organism or group of organisms—*page* 23.

Haemolysis: Disruption of red blood cells. In connection with growth of streptococci on blood agar, destruction of all red cells around a colony and decolorization of the medium is called β-haemolysis, whereas destruction of most of the red cells and production of a green pigment is called α-haemolysis—*page* 85.

Hapten: A substance which acts as an antigenic stimulus only when combined with a protein or other carrier, but which, even in the uncombined state, can react with the resultant antibody in the manner of a true antigen—*page* 53.

Heterologous: Related to a different kind of organism, a different disease, etc.—e.g. an *anamnestic reaction* (q.v.) is due to a heterologous stimulus.

Homologous: Related to the same kind of organism, the same disease, etc.—e.g. diphtheria requires treatment with homologous serum, serum containing diphtheria antitoxin.

Hypogammaglobulinaemia: Deficiency of circulating γ-globulins, resulting from inadequate production by B-lymphocytes—*page* 66.

Immunoglobulin: See *antibody*.

In vitro: 'In glass', hence in laboratory apparatus.

In vivo: In a living animal or human being.

Inclusion bodies: Aggregates of virus particles, visible by light microscopy after appropriate staining, within the nuclei or the cytoplasm of infected cells—*pages* 162, 166.

Inducible (enzyme): Produced only in the presence of an appropriate substrate—*page* 21. (Cf. *constitutive*.)

Infection: The arrival or presence of potentially pathogenic organisms on the surface or in the tissues of an appropriate host—*page* 37.

Inoculation: (1) of man or animals: Introduction of material containing micro-organisms or their products into the tissues—usually for prophylactic purposes in the case of man.

(2) of culture media: Introduction into a fluid medium, or applications to the surface of solid medium, of material known or suspected of containing living organisms—e.g. Fig. 4—*page* 76.

Inoculum: The particular portion of material used for a single inoculation.

Interference (by viruses): Modification of host cells infected with one type of virus so that other viruses are unable to multiply in them—*page* 161.

L-form: Cell-wall deficient mutant bacterium—*page* 74. (Cf. *protoplast, spheroplast.*)

Lyophilization: Combined freezing and desiccation (freeze-drying), a means of long-term preservation of micro-organisms—*page* 31.

Lysis: Disruption (literally 'dissolving') of a microbial or other cell—*page* 57.

Lysogenic conversion: Alteration of the properties of a bacterium as a result of *lysogeny* (q.v.)—*page* 194.

Lysogeny: A temporary stable relationship between a bacteriophage and its bacterial host, in which the phage is reproduced in step with the bacterium and thus handed on to succeeding generations of bacteria—*page* 194.

Micro-aerophile: An organism which grows best in sub-atmospheric concentrations of oxygen—*page* 22.

Monolayer: A sheet of tissue-culture cells one cell thick—*page* 159.

Mutation: An alteration in genetic material—*page* 27.

Nucleocapsid: The *genome* and *capsid* (q.v.) of a virus—*page* 156.

Nucleoid (virus): Former synonym of *genome* (q.v.).

Opportunist (pathogen): Not normally pathogenic but able to become so because of some deficiency the host's defence mechanisms—*page* 38.

Pandemic (noun or adjective): World-wide *epidemic* (q.v.)—*page* 38.

Passage (French): Administration of a micro-organism to a host and its subsequent recovery from the host, usually carried out with a view to modifying the pathogenicity of the organism—*page* 164.

Passive (immunity, immunization): Dependent upon injection of ready-made antibodies and not upon the subject's own immunological mechanisms—*page* 49. (Cf. *active.*)

Pathogenic: Actually producing or capable of producing disease—*page* 18. (Cf. *commensal, symbiotic.*)

Petri dish: A shallow circular flat-bottomed glass or plastic dish used as a container for solid media—*page* 75.

Phage-type: The identity of a bacterial strain as indicated by its sensitivity or resistance to the lytic action of the members of a standard panel of bacteriophages (its 'phage-pattern'); *or* a group of strains having identical or closely similar phage-patterns—*pages* 83, 194.

Phenotype: That part of the *genotype* (q.v.) of an organism which is expressed in a given situation—*page* 29.

Pilus (plural *pili*): Synonym of *fimbria* (q.v.).

Plaque: A small roughly circular deficiency in the growth of a bacterial culture on a solid medium, resulting from local destruction of bacteria by bacteriophages—*page* 194.

Plasmid: An extrachromosomal portion of genetic material (DNA)—*page* 28.

Prophage: Bacteriophage in a lysogenic relationship with its host—*page* 194. (See *lysogeny*.)

Protoplast: A bacterium deprived of its cell wall and thus highly susceptible to osmotic distension and rupture—*page* 74. (Cf. *L-form, spheroplast*.)

Reagin(s): *Either* the serum component responsible for the Wassermann and related reactions—*page* 250; *or* the IgE antibodies associated with certain types of hypersensitivity reactions—*pages* 55, 63.

Replication: Virus reproduction, so called to emphasize that a virus does not reproduce *itself* but causes the host cell to make replicas of it— *pages* 14, 157.

Saprophytic: Living on dead organic matter—*page* 18.

Satellitism: Enhancement of bacterial growth on a solid medium around a source of a growth factor—*page* 123.

Selective medium: A solid culture medium on which all but the desired microbial species are wholly or largely inhibited—*page* 114. A *selective enrichment medium* is a fluid medium in which the desired species can multiply more rapidly than others likely to be present, so that a sample subsequently taken from it for inoculation of plate cultures is 'richer' than the original material in organisms of the desired species—*page* 114. (Cf. *enrichment medium*.)

Septicaemia: A serious clinical condition (including shock) associated with the presence of pathogenic organisms in the blood—*page* 47. (Cf. *bacteraemia*.)

Serology: Study of the antibody content of sera—*page* 245—and also use of antisera in the antigenic analysis of micro-organisms and their products.

Serotype: The identity of a bacterial strain as indicated by antigenic analysis: *or* a group of strains shown by serological tests to be antigenically identical or closely similar—*page* 113. (Synonyms: antigenic type, serological type.)

Specific: (1) relating to a species.

(2) relating particularly to some other unit—e.g. type-specific. Hence commonly used in much the same sense as *homologous* (q.v.).

Spheroplast: A bacterium similar to a *protoplast* (q.v.) except that the cell-wall damage is partial and reversible—*page* 74. (Cf. *L-form*.)

Spirochaete: A member of one of several genera of spiral bacteria—*page* 139.

Sterilization: The process of killing or removing all micro-organisms— *page* 31.

Strain (of an organism): A culture all members of which are believed to be the progeny of a single organism—*page* 71. (This is not an entirely satisfactory definition, and indeed the variations which inevitably accompany bacterial reproduction make the whole concept of a 'pure' strain fallacious.)

Symbiotic: Living in a mutually beneficial relationship with the host—*page* 18. (Cf. *commensal, pathogenic.*)

Synergy (between antimicrobial drugs): Action of a combination of drugs which exceeds the sum of the actions of the drugs used singly—*page* 311.

Temperate phage: A phage capable of a lysogenic relationship with its bacterial host—*page* 194. (See *lysogeny, prophage.*)

Titre: The highest dilution of a serum or an antigen preparation which gives a positive reaction under defined conditions—*page* 246.

Toxoid: Toxin rendered harmless but still effective as an antigen—*page* 293.

Transduction: Conveyance of genetic characters from one bacterial strain to another by means of a transfer of bacteriophage—*page* 28.

Transformation: Acquisition of genetic characters of one bacterial strain by a related strain grown in the presence of DNA from the first strain—*page* 28.

Transport medium: A medium which increases the chances of survival of a micro-organism during transit from the patient to the laboratory—*page* 221.

Vaccination: Originally, the use of cowpox material or of vaccinia virus in active immunization against smallpox; then all forms of active immunization using live organisms; now all forms of active immunization—*page* 293.

Vaccine: Material used in vaccination; therefore this term also has an expanding meaning—*page* 293.

Viraemia: Presence of viruses in the blood-stream—*page* 162.

Virion: A virus particle, the virus unit corresponding to a single cell of a larger organism—*page* 14.

Zoonosis (four syllables): A disease that man acquires from animals—*page* 38.

B

MEANINGS OF SOME ABBREVIATIONS

Convenient though abbreviations may be, they are liable to cause confusion by meaning different things to specialists in different fields. The meanings given below are those which the appropriate abbreviations customarily have when they are encountered in the field of medical microbiology.

AAFB	acid-alcohol-fast bacilli—*page* 132 and Appendix A.
AFB	acid-fast bacilli—*page* 132 and Appendix A.
AHG	anti-human globulin (antibodies, serum)—*page* 243.
APT	alum precipitated toxoid—*page* 296.
ASO	antistreptolysin O—*page* 87.
ATS	anti-tetanus serum—*page* 297.
BCG	Bacille Calmette Guerin—*page* 294.
CFT	complement-fixation test—*page* 242.
CFU	colony-forming unit—Appendix A.
CIE	countercurrent immunoelectrophoresis—*page* 241.
CPE	cytopathic effect—*page* 159 and Appendix A.
CSF	cerebrospinal fluid—*page* 236.
CSU	catheter specimen of urine—*page* 233.
DCA	deoxycholate citrate agar—*page* 114.
DNA	deoxyribonucleic acid—*page* 13.
EB	Epstein–Barr (virus)—*page* 187.
ECHO	enteric cytopathic human orphan (viruses)—*page* 171.
ELISA	enzyme-linked immunosorbent assay—*page* 245.
EMU (EMSU)	early morning (specimen of) urine—*page* 233.
FT	formol toxoid—*page* 296.
FTA	fluorescent treponemal antibody (test)—*page* 251.
GC	gonococcus—*page* 94.
GCFT	gonococcal complement-fixation test—*page* 95.
GLC	gas-liquid chromatography—*page* 3.

H	flagellar (antigens, antibodies)—from German *Hauch*, see *page* 110.
HBcAg etc.	antigenic components of hepatitis B virus—*page* 191.
HVS	high vaginal swab—*page* 235.
IDU	idoxuridine—*page* 164.
IgA, IgE, etc.	immunoglobulins of classes A, E, etc.—*page* 55.
INAH	isonicotinic acid hydrazide = isoniazid—*page* 339.
K	capsular or envelope (antigens, antibodies)—*page* 110.
LD 50	dose lethal to 50% of a group of experimental animals—*page* 42.
LF	lactose-fermenter—*page* 77.
LGV	lymphogranuloma venereum—*page* 153.
MBC	minimal bactericidal concentration—*page* 321.
MIC	minimal inhibitory concentration—*page* 321.
MLD	minimum lethal dose (of a drug or microbial preparation).
MSU (MSSU)	mid-stream (specimen of) urine—*page* 232.
NGU	non-gonococcal urethritis—*page* 154.
NLF	non-lactose-fermenter—*page* 114.
NSU	non-specific urethritis—*page* 154.
O	somatic (antigens, antibodies)—from German *ohne Hauch*, see *page* 110.
OT	old tuberculin—*page* 253.
PABA	*p*-aminobenzoic acid—*page* 33.
PGU	postgonococcal urethritis—*page* 154.
PPD	purified protein derivative (of old tuberculin)—*page* 253.
PTAH	purified toxoid, aluminium hydroxide—*page* 296.
PTAP	purified toxoid, aluminium phosphate—*page* 296.
PUO	pyrexia of unknown origin—*page* 249.
REO	respiratory enteric orphan (viruses)—*page* 172.
RNA	ribonucleic acid—*page* 13.
RPR	rapid plasma reagin (test)—*page* 250.
RS (RSV)	respiratory syncytial (virus)—*page* 180.
RTD	routine test dilution (of bacteriophage)—*page* 83.
TAB (TABC)	typhoid + paratyphoids A and B (and C) vaccine—*page* 296.
TAF	toxoid-antitoxin floccules—*page* 297.
TB	tubercle bacilli—*page* 131—and hence loosely used to denote tuberculosis.
TCBS	thiosulphate citrate bile salts sucrose (agar)—*page* 122.
TPHA	*Treponema pallidum* haemagglutination (test)—*page* 251.
TPI	*Treponema pallidum* immobilization (test)—*page* 250.

TRIC	trachoma and inclusion conjunctivitis agents—*page* 153.
TT	(1) tetanus toxoid—*page* 297.
	(2) tuberculin tested (cattle)—*page* 281.
UHT	Ultra heat treated (milk)—*page* 282.
UV	ultraviolet (light)—*page* 16.
Vi	virulence (antigen of *S. typhi*, etc.)—*page* 115.
VDRL	Venereal Disease Research Laboratory (test)—*page* 250.
VZ	varicella-zoster (virus)—*page* 186.
WR	Wassermann reaction—*page* 249.
ZN	Ziehl–Neelsen (staining method)—*page* 132.

INDEX

Folate synthesis, 34, 305, 324–5
Fomites, 5, 39
Food and transmission of pathogens, 39, 112–13, 116, 121, 122, 190, 212, 276, 283–9
Food, preservation of, 269, 287
-poisoning, 276, 283–9
Foot and mouth disease, 11, 170
Formaldehyde, 33, 165, 265
Formol toxoids, 293, 296, 297
Fracastorius, 5
Framboesia, 141
Framycetin, 330
Francisella tularensis, 128–9
Freeze-drying, 31, 165
Freezing, effect on organisms, 31, 165
Frei test, 153
Friedländer's bacillus, 111
Frosch, 10
Fucidin, 329
Fungi, 14–15, 27, 196–203
Furuncles, 80
Fusobacterium genus, 129

Gangrene, 92, 106–7, 130, 270
Gas-liquid chromatography (GLC), 3, 26, 225
Gastric secretions, 45
washings, 220, 230–1
Gastro-enteritis, 110, 112, 122, 231, 276, 284–7
Genetics, bacterial, 26–9, 317
Genital tract, microbiology of, 234–6
Genome, virus, 14, 155
Genotype, 21, 27
Gentamicin, 330
German measles (rubella), 156, 175–6
'Germ-free' animals, 20
Ghon focus, 132
Giant-cell pneumonia, 68, 180
Giardia intestinalis, 209–10, 215
Giemsa's stain, 147
Glandular fever (infectious mononucleosis), 187, 188, 208
Glomerulonephritis, 86, 87
Glossina (tsetse flies), 210
Glucose-phosphate broth, 110
Glutaraldehyde, 33, 267
Glycerol, 126, 134, 165
Gnotobiotic animals, 20
Goats as sources of pathogens, 126–7, 151
Gonococcus, 94–6
Gonorrhoea, 94, 234–6
Gordon, 6
Gram's stain, 16, 74, 77–9, 221
Granules, volutin, 97
Griffith types of streptococci, 86, 87
Griseofulvin, 201
Growth phases of bacteria, 29–30
Gruber, 9
Guarnieri bodies, 163

Guinea-pigs, 42, 106, 127, 129, 137, 143, 148, 151, 235
Gummata, 140

H agglutination, 248–9
H antigens, 110, 112–13, 115, 248–9
Haemadsorption viruses, 159, 179
Haemagglutination, virus, 160–1, 176–7
-inhibition tests, 169
Haemagogus mosquitoes, 174
Haemolysins, 24, 86, 243
Haemolysis, streptococcal, 85, 86
Haemophilus genus, 123–5
Hamsters, 143, 184, 212
Hand, foot and mouth disease, 171
Hansen's bacillus, 134
Haptens, 53
Hartmannella genus, 213
Hay fever, 63
Heaf test, 253
Heat, effect on micro-organisms, 32, 147, 165, 263–5, 282, 286, 287, 289
sterilization by 103, 263–5
Hedgehog and leprosy, 188
Henle, 6
Hens' eggs for culture of micro-organisms, 158–9 *and see* Chick embryos
Hepatitis A, 156, 171–2, 190–1, 281
amoebic, 212
B, 156, 191–2, 219, 276, 292, 301
non-A, non-B, 192
Herd immunity, 51, 300
Herelle, d', 193
Herpangina, 171
Herpesviruses, 156, 185–8
Heterophil antibodies, 188
Hexachlorophane, 33
High Temperature Short Time process, 282
Histoplasma capsulatum, 203
Holder process, 282
Hormones and immunity, 67
Horse serum in immunization, 63, 64, 292, 297
Horses as sources of pathogens, 149, 173
Hospital infection, 38, 40, 270–7
Host defences, 45–51
Hot-air oven, 263
Human immunoglobulin for immunization, 292
Humoral defences, 49, 53, 55–62
Hyaluronidase, 25, 50, 87
Hydrogen ion acceptors, 22
concentration, 23–4, 122
sulphide, 110
Hydrophobia, 181
Hydroxystilbamidine, 203
Hygiene, communal, 259
personal, 259–60
ward, 273
Hypersensitivity, 63–5, 303, 305
skin tests for, 65, 128, 134, 153, 204, 215, 252–4

Neutralizing antibodies, 57, 168–9, 244
Niacin production, 134
Nitrofurantoin, 326, 337
Nocardia genus, 137, 139
Nomenclature of bacteria, 70–2
   of viruses, 155–7, 169
Non-gonococcal urethritis (NGU), 154
Non-specific urethritis (NSU), 154
Normal bacterial flora, 19–20, 45–6, 223–236, 306, 319
Nosocomial infection, 270
Nuclear bodies, bacterial, 13
Nucleic acids (DNA, RNA), 13, 14, 27–8, 36, 147, 155–6
Nucleocapsid, virus, 156
Nutrient agar, 76
Nutrition, microbial, 22–3
Nystatin, 199

O agglutination, 248–9
O antigens, 110, 112, 115, 116, 121, 248–9
Old tuberculin (OT), 253
Ophthalmia, neonatal, 94
Opportunist pathogens, 38, 273
Opsonins, 48, 56
Optimal proportion, antigen–antibody, 241
Optochin, 90
Original antigenic sin, 178, 291
Orf, 189
Organ culture, 160, 172
Oriental sore, 211
Ornithosis, 152–3
Orthomyxoviruses, 156, 177–8
Osteomyelitis (osteitis), 80, 113
Otitis, 85, 89, 111, 119, 226
Otomycosis, 201
Oxidase test, 93, 119, 120, 122, 128
Oxidation, bacterial, 22
Oxygen requirements of micro-organisms, 22
Oysters, 122, 284

Pandemic diseases, 38
Papilloma viruses, 156, 183–4
Papovaviruses, 156, 183–4
Para-aminobenzoic acid (PABA), 34, 147, 222
Paracoccidioides brasiliensis, 203
Parainfluenza viruses, 156, 178–9
Paramyxoviruses, 156, 178–80
Parasitism, types of, 18–19
Paratyphoid, 115, 231–2, 248–9, 295–6
Paronychia, 198, 224
Parvobacteria, 123–9
Pasteur, 5, 7, 9, 10, 18, 102, 181, 282
Pasteurella genus, 128
Pasteurization, 128, 131, 282
Pathogenicity, 19, 37–40, 41–5, *and under many species*
Paul-Bunnell test, 188

Pebrine, 8
Penicillinases, *see* Beta-lactamases
Penicillins, 35, 326–8
Pentamidine isethionate, 208, 211
Peptidoglycan, 13
Peptococcus genus, 92
Peptostreptococcus genus, 92
Peptone water, 109
Pernasal swabs, 126, 227
Peroxides, 22
Pertussis (whooping cough), 125–6, 228–9, 295, 300–2
Petri dishes, 75
Pfeiffer, 124
Phages, 28, 193–5
Phage-typing of *Ps. aeruginosa*, 120
   of *S. paratyphi*, 115
   of *S. typhi*, 115
   of *Staph. aureus*, 83, 274, 288
   technique, 194
Phagocytes, 9, 47–50
Phagosomes, 48
Phase variation, flagellar, 113
Phenethicillin, 327
Phenotypic variation, 29
Phenoxymethyl penicillin (penicillin V), 327
Phlebotomus (sandflies), 176, 211
Phosphatase test, 282
Phospholipase C, 24, 107
Photochromogens, 136
Phototrophs, 22, 25
Physical agents, effects on micro-organisms, 31–2, 147, 165
Picornaviruses, 156, 170–2
Pigments, 25, 120, 131, 200
Pig-bel, 107
Pigs as sources of pathogens, 126, 142, 173, 214, 281
Pili, 13, 43
Pinta, 141, 252
Piperacillin, 328
Pityriasis versicolor, 201
Pivampicillin, 327
Pivmecillinam, 328
Plague, 117–18
Plaques, phage, 195
Plasma cells and antibodies, 55
Plasmids, 13, 28, 95, 318
Plasmodium genus, 205–7, 214
Plate cultures, inoculation of, 75–6
Pneumococcus, 89–91
Pneumocystis carini, 67, 208
Pneumonia, 68, 80, 88, 89, 103, 111, 118, 119, 124, 129, 144, 150, 153, 154, 180, 208, 229
Pneumonic plague, 118
Poliomyelitis, 51, 170, 236, 281, 297, 298–9
Polioviruses, 156, 170–1, 298–9
Polymyxins, 36, 334
Polyoma virus, 183–4
Polysaccharides, capsular, 13, 43, 53, 73, 87, 90, 94, 110, 111, 125
Post-gonococcal urethritis (PGU), 154